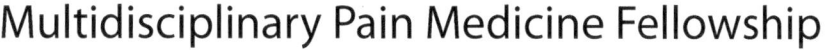

Multidisciplinary Pain Medicine Fellowship

Magdalena Anitescu

Editor

Multidisciplinary Pain Medicine Fellowship

Educational Guidelines by Program Directors

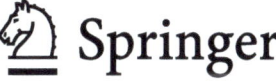 Springer

Editor
Magdalena Anitescu
Department of Anesthesia & Critical Care
University of Chicago Medicine
Chicago, IL, USA

ISBN 978-3-031-88356-9   ISBN 978-3-031-88357-6   (eBook)
https://doi.org/10.1007/978-3-031-88357-6

This Springer imprint is published by the registered company Springer Nature Switzerland AG
The registered company address is: Gewerbestrasse 11, 6330 Cham, Switzerland

If disposing of this product, please recycle the paper.

To my beloved husband, best friend, life coach, and my number one fan

To my parents who encouraged me to always be curious and ask questions

To my daughters with whom I became complete as a person by learning to be a mother.

Preface

Treating various pain conditions is one of the oldest activities of medicine. However, it was not until recently that the discipline of chronic pain medicine was introduced in clinical practice. As chronic pain is described as a very personal experience, pain fellowships around the globe experimented with assorted curricula with various degrees of a mix of procedures and medical management. In the United States alone, in the more than 100 fellowship programs, topics taught vary widely as detailed instructions on what is considered essential learning for pain fellows is lacking.

As such, the Association of Pain Program Directors (APPD), its executive board in collaboration with American Society of Regional Anesthesia and Pain Medicine (ASRA PM), decided that it is the time to standardize the requirements, at least their theoretical component, that are needed for pain fellows to graduate.

From this initiative came this book, *Multidisciplinary Pain Medicine Fellowship: Educational Guidelines by Program Directors*. Its editor, Magdalena Anitescu, in collaboration with the APPD contributors, designed the curriculum in 11 parts, each with an essential topic that is explored in detail and supported with extensive references for up-to-date information on the subject explored. Part I explores the diagnosis and non-interventional treatment of chronic pain conditions while Part II addresses approaches to various interventions, procedures, and surgeries that can be used in treating chronic pain conditions. Additionally, it describes in detail common challenges and their potential resolution that fellows face upon graduation from a pain fellowship; those include, among others, contract negotiation, enhancing practice through research, and how to start a solo practice.

We believe that this book offers a comprehensive view of what the pain fellows will need to know upon graduation, and we strongly advise using this comprehensive review to enhance local curriculum in pain fellowships across the nation and to be used for practitioners and trainees worldwide. In the time where pain medicine is such a dynamic and innovation incubator, we need to ensure that next generations of pain practitioners speak the basic common language of our specialty.

This book is intended as a massive reference for pain fellows preparing for the pain boards, for pain Program Directors who need to ensure pain fellows are learning the latest developments in pain management, for junior practitioners in need of quick review of conditions that they have not seen often, as well as for more established practitioners that need to update their practice in a quick review.

As such we believe this book will be useful for all physicians that practice pain management as it includes all topics essential to function as a competent pain physician. We hope this book will establish the basic common chronic pain guidelines that every pain physician will be required to know upon graduation. Furthermore, we hope that it will serve as a go-to reference for fellows as they make the transition from trainee to independently practicing physician.

Chicago, IL, USA   Magdalena Anitescu
December 15, 2024

Acknowledgments

The Editor and the contributors would like to recognize the American Society of Regional Anesthesia and Pain Medicine (ASRA PM) leadership, in particular Dr. Samer Narouze, past-president, and Dr. David Provenzano, current president, for the support of this initiative.

This work could not have been completed without the dedication and support of the Association of Pain Program Directors board who provided essential input and contribution to the manuscript.

About the Book

The evolution of pain medicine as a specialty is rooted in historical milestones, beginning with the introduction of ether anesthesia in the mid-nineteenth century and progressing through the establishment of multidisciplinary pain clinics and advanced educational frameworks. Formal pain medicine education emerged with the establishment of accredited fellowship programs, driven by the increasing complexity of pain management in mid-1970s and followed by first certification from American Board of Anesthesiologists in early 1990s. As pain medicine grows, challenges include ensuring uniform training not only in basics of pain medicine theoretical knowledge but also in advanced procedures and integrating novel technologies. Addressing these will be critical to maintaining the specialty's relevance and improving patient outcomes.

This book, emerged as a collaboration between the Association of pain program Directors (APPD) and American Society of Regional Anesthesia and Pain Medicine (ASRA PM), is organized in two essential parts: Part I explores the diagnosis and non-interventional treatment of chronic pain conditions while Part II addresses approaches to various interventions, procedures, and surgeries that can be used in treating chronic pain conditions as well as administrative topics such as contract negotiation, enhancing practice through research, and how to start a solo practice.

In the time where pain medicine is such a dynamic and innovation incubator, we need to ensure that next generations of pain practitioners speak the basic common language of our specialty. As such, we designed this book with the intention to be a comprehensive review to enhance pain fellowship curricula across the nation and worldwide, a massive reference for pain fellows preparing for the pain boards; it is also intended for pain Program Directors who need to ensure pain fellows are learning the latest developments in pain management, for junior practitioners in need of quick review of conditions that they have not seen often, as well as for more established practitioners that need to update their practice in a quick review

Contents

About the Editor

Magdalena Anitescu Professor of Anesthesia and Pain Medicine, is Section Chief of Pain Management Services and Program Director for the Multidisciplinary Pain Medicine Fellowship Program at the University of Chicago.

She has been involved in advancing the field of pain medicine for more than 20 years with her contributions to more than 40 peer-reviewed articles as well as numerous book chapters. She is the editor to several pain textbooks and the series editor for the Oxford University Press, Anesthesia Problem Based Learning, a series of 10 books, recently published.

Dr. Anitescu has been shaping the education in pain medicine for over 15 years. As program director for multidisciplinary pain medicine fellowship she was among the founding members for the Society of Academic Associations of Anesthesiology and Perioperative Medicine (SAAAPM) Association of Anesthesiology Subspecialty Program Directors (AASPD) organization. She participated to the reorganization of the Association of Pain Program Directors (APPD) on novel rules. To improve the collaboration among pain programs, Program Directors (PD) and their trainees, Dr. Anitescu initiated the Chicago pain summit, now at the 10th year anniversary, a scientific networking seminar that brings together alumni, current PD, fellows, and trainees from various specialties interested in a career in pain medicine, all from Midwest pain programs.

Dr. Anitescu is the past president of both APPD and AASPD; she served on those organizations' boards of directors and has been instrumental in introducing the pain medicine match. A founding member of Women in Neuromodulation, a committee under North American Neuromodulation Society (NANS) more than 10 years ago, she is its past Chair.

She holds leadership positions in American Society of Anesthesiologists (ASA) where she is the Chair of the Committee on Problem Based Learning Discussions, as well as in American Society of Regional Anesthesia and Pain Medicine (ASRA PM) where she was the Meeting Chair for the Fall Meeting 2020. She chaired the 30 year Anniversary North American Neuromodulation Society (NANS) Annual Meeting in 2024. She has been a member of Scientific Planning committees for the last 10 years in many professional organizations (ASA, ASRA, NANS, INS, SAAAPM).

She has been elected and serves as President Elect on the executive board of North America Neuromodulation Society (NANS), formerly being a Secretary and Director at large of the same organization as well as a board member of the International Neuromodulation Society (INS).

She is an accomplished educator and speaker to national and international meetings (ASRA, ASA, European Society of Regional Anesthesia (ESRA), NANS, INS, American Academy of Pain Medicine (AAPM), SAAAPM); during her career she mentored numerous generations of pain physicians.

Her research focuses on various mechanisms of action of neuromodulation devices in improving clinical outcomes of chronic pain and she is a PI for several clinical trials on this topic. Other research topics include infusion therapies in traumatic injuries and chronic pain of sickle cell disease as well as use of neuromodulation to improve vascular changes in diabetes. She has conducted successful research on the treatment of vertebral body metastases as well as evaluation and treatment of psychologic co-morbidities in chronic pain.

Part I

Educational Guidelines for Multidisciplinary Pain Medicine Fellowship: Pain Taxonomy, Chronic Pain Syndromes, Pain Assessment, Non-procedural Interventions for Chronic Pain, Opioid Management

Background and History of Pain Medicine Fellowship in the United States

1

Vinicius Tieppo Francio, Magdalena Anitescu,
Dalia Elmofty, Scott Brancolini, Boris Spektor,
Christopher Sobey, Puneet Mishra, Sayed Wahezi,
and Lynn Kohan

Abbreviations

ACGME	Accreditation Council of Graduate Medical Education
US	United States
ABA	American Board of Anesthesiologists
ABMS	American Board of Medical Specialties
RRC	Residency Review Committee

V. Tieppo Francio (✉)
Division of Pain Medicine, Department of Anesthesiology,
Washington University School of Medicine, St. Louis, MO, USA

M. Anitescu · D. Elmofty
Department of Anesthesia & Critical Care, University of Chicago Medicine, Chicago, IL, USA
e-mail: manitescu@bsd.uchicago.edu; delmofty@bsd.uchicago.edu

S. Brancolini
Department of Anesthesiology, University of Pittsburg, Pittsburg, PA, USA
e-mail: brancolinisa@upmc.edu

B. Spektor
Department of Anesthesiology, Emory University, Atlanta, GA, USA
e-mail: boris.spektor@emoryhealthcare.org

C. Sobey · P. Mishra
Department of Anesthesiology, Vanderbilt University, Nashville, TN, USA
e-mail: christopher.m.sobey@vumc.org; Puneet.mishra@vumc.org

S. Wahezi
Department of Physical Medicine & Rehabilitation, Montefiore Medical Center,
Bronx, NY, USA
e-mail: swahezi@montefiore.org

L. Kohan
Department of Anesthesiology, University of Virginia, Charlottesville, VA, USA
e-mail: LRK9G@uvahealth.org

© The Author(s), under exclusive license to Springer Nature Switzerland AG 2025
M. Anitescu (ed.), *Multidisciplinary Pain Medicine Fellowship*,
https://doi.org/10.1007/978-3-031-88357-6_1

3

ABPMR	American Board of Physical Medicine and Rehabilitation
ABPN	American Board of Psychiatry and Neurology
PM&R	Physical Medicine and Rehabilitation
ABPM	American Board of Pain Medicine
AAPM	American Academy of Pain Medicine
APPD	Association of Pain Program Directors
NRMP	National Resident Matching Program
GME	Graduate Medical Education
PC	Patient care
MK	Medical knowledge
PBLI	Practice-based learning and improvement
ICS	Interpersonal and communications skills
PROF	Professionalism
SBP	Systems-based practice
ABEM	American Board of Emergency Medicine
ABFM	American Board of Family Medicine
ABR	American Board of Radiology

Pain is the oldest and most complex medical problem. Pain is a symptom of numerous disease states that encompass nearly all medical specialties [1]. The required training to provide effective diagnosis and comprehensive treatment of pain necessitates a wide breadth of knowledge and skills that crosses medical specialties, which most effectively can be achieved with a multidisciplinary model. Pain medicine is interdisciplinary in nature and its evolution is parallel to core disciplines that contribute with shared knowledge and skills from the fields of anesthesiology, neurology, psychiatry, rheumatology, radiology, palliative care, emergency medicine, neurosurgery, and physical medicine and rehabilitation.

History of Pain Medicine

Pain became a relevant topic in medical discourses by mid-1800s with the introduction of ether and chloroform anesthesia; additionally, medical community began discussions on the relief of acute pain, control of severe intractable pain, and palliation of pain of those in dying states. By 1890, opium- and alcohol-based compounds were frequently utilized, and those situations raised addictive concerns; therefore, by 1914 the United States (US) narcotic control act was established. In the United States, by 1917, the leading tool to treat mild to moderate pain was aspirin, while opioids were utilized for severe pain, particularly during the First World War [1]. Between the First and Second World Wars, regional nerve blocks emerged as therapeutic use, in addition to with neurolytic/ablative procedures performed mainly for terminal cancer severe pain; surgical treatment of pain was also commonly practiced in this period [2]. The use of anesthetic nerve blocks enabled physicians to manage pain without having to resort to surgery immediately [3].

The first clinic in the United States to offer nerve blocks for pain relief was established in 1936; by 1947, a research-based pain clinic was founded at the University of Oregon to train students interested in the management of pain. Among them was a young Canadian psychologist named Robert Melzack [4]. Simultaneously, in 1953 a young anesthesiologist, John J. Bonica, practicing at Madigan Army Hospital in Washington during the war and immediately after found himself perplex with the vast magnitude of pain problems and the limited pain knowledge his colleagues and him had about treatment options. As such, aiming to promote evidence and shared knowledge of clinical decision-making for these challenging situations, the concept of multidisciplinary pain clinics and interdisciplinary pain field emerged and the formation of pain medicine as a specialty began [5].

In 1965, Melzack and Wall proposed the concept of the gate control theory, which transformed education and understanding of pain modulation and perception at the time [6]. By 1970, the International Association for the Study of Pain, the American Pain Society (its American chapter), and PAIN journal were established by the academic and scientific community [7]. Since then, Pain Medicine as a specialty, as well as its scholarly field, had experienced exponential growth, benefitting from advancements in research, technology, and an improved understanding of pain treatment opportunities [8].

History of Pain Medicine Fellowships

Pain Medicine education has evolved in parallel with the burgeoning field of pain medicine. Anesthesiologist John J. Bonica, author of the first comprehensive pain textbook in 1953, is credited as the father of our specialty; he created the first formalized training program in pain management at the University of Washington's multidisciplinary pain center in 1978 [5, 9, 10]. For the ensuing two decades, training was limited to several unaccredited notable academic anesthesiology programs across the United States.

Certification in the Specialty of Pain Medicine was originally developed in 1989 when the American Board of Anesthesiology (ABA) notified the American Board of Medical Specialties (ABMS) of its intent to offer a "Certificate of Added Qualifications in Pain Management." The ABMS approved the ABA pain management application in 1991. Starting in 1992, Pain Medicine programs could be accredited after the Accreditation Council of Graduate Medical Education (ACGME) approved the application from the Anesthesiology Residency Review Committee (RRC). The first certification examination was given in 1993. In 1998, the ABA supported a joint proposal by the American Board of Physical Medicine and Rehabilitation (ABPMR) and the American Board of Psychiatry and Neurology (ABPN) that allowed these boards to offer subspecialty certification in collaboration to optimize multidisciplinary training requirements and improve the quality of education. In 2002, the certificate title was changed to "Pain Medicine."

At present, six member boards of ABMS (anesthesiology, PM&R, psychiatry and neurology, family medicine, radiology, and emergency medicine) are approved as specialties that can acquire Pain Medicine certification, all using the ABA Pain Medicine examination. Although the American Board of Pain Medicine (ABPM) and the American Academy of Pain Management (AAPM) offer certification in pain management, the ABA subspecialty certificate is the only one recognized by the ABMS and the ACGME. After 2003, it is a requirement that all physicians must complete a fellowship in Pain Medicine (Multidisciplinary) accredited by the ACGME in order to take the ABA subspecialty certification in Pain Medicine exam to become Pain Medicine specialists [9, 11].

Multidisciplinary Pain Medicine fellowships are 1-year, multidisciplinary post-graduate training programs focused on the comprehensive diagnosis and management of chronic pain [12]. In 2004, there were 105 ACGME-accredited Pain Medicine fellowships in the United States, of which 94% were under Anesthesiology as primary specialty [11]. In 2006, regardless of the sponsoring activity, a more rigorous and unified set of requirements emphasizing specialty's multidisciplinary aspects, was adopted by the ACGME. This resulted in a 14.6% decline in the number of programs able to maintain accreditation; however, the remaining programs expanded the number of positions offered.

In 2013, the Association of Pain Program Directors (APPD) elected to establish a fellowship Match with the National Resident Matching Program (NRMP) for the 2014–2015 academic year. This led to a 14% growth in the number of ACGME-accredited Multidisciplinary Pain Medicine fellowship programs and a 19% increase in available positions over a 6-year interval available to multiple specialties (Table 1.1). The number of applicants per position has slowly decreased over the last 5 years from 1.3 in 2018 to 1.1 in 2022, translating into a steady increase in percent of applicants matched over the same 5-year time period, from 75.6% in 2018 to 84.6% in 2022 [13]. As Pain Medicine continues to be one of the most

Table 1.1 Total number of ACGME-accredited Pain Medicine fellowship programs and positions (2005–2021)

Year	Programs (N)	Fellow positions (N)
2023–2024	114	393
2022–2023	110	377
2021–2022	109	378
2020–2021	111	400
2019–2020	108	386
2018–2019	104	372
2017–2018	102	361
2016–2017	101	354
2015–2016	100	337
2014–2015	97	336
2013–2014	97	326
2012–2013	97	305
2011–2012	92	292
2010–2011	93	288
2009–2010	91	285
2008–2009	94	286
2007–2008	92	277
2006–2007	88	190
2005–2006	103	217

competitive fellowship programs in the United states, we noted an increased trend of more PM&R applicants matching into fellowships, while neurology and anesthesiology applicant's trend remained relatively stable within the past 3 years [12].

In 2024, the number of programs accredited by the ACGME was 117, which corresponded to a 12% increase in ACGME Pain Medicine fellowship programs within two decades with 393 available positions [12–15].

Evolution of Multidisciplinary Pain Medicine ACGME Milestones

Since the first certification of pain management issued in 1993, Pain Medicine education has naturally evolved to reflect a comprehensive curriculum with competency components in anesthesiology, neurology, PM&R, and psychiatry, given the multidisciplinary nature of the specialty [10, 11]. Pain Medicine Graduate Medical Education (GME) has evolved from a time- and structure-based model to a competency-based model [16]. Competency-based education is focusing on the acquisition of skill sets as opposed to time spent in training.

To achieve this goal, in 2001, the ACGME launched 6 core competencies that included patient care (PC), medical knowledge (MK), practice-based learning and improvement (PBLI), interpersonal and communication skills (ICS), professionalism (PROF), and systems-based practice (SBP). As training programs experienced difficulties in implementing these core competencies, the ACGME introduced the Milestones 1.0; in this initial set, the ACGME developed sub-competencies within each core competency that could be used to assess a trainee's skill acquisition over time from novice to expert [17]. As time passed and Milestone 1.0 was utilized by Pain Medicine Program Directors, it became apparent that there was a large degree of variability within the sub-competencies, and they lacked practicality; it was imperative that improvements could be made, and therefore, the ACGME began meeting with each base specialty to help develop Milestones 2.0. In 2020, the field of pain medicine began the process of developing our new milestones. The Milestones 2.0 working group, aimed to create less variability, combined certain sub-competencies, focused on use of positive language in each sub-competency, as well as created a supplemental guide that provides examples to better help users appropriately assess pain fellows. After a period provided for public comment, the Pain Medicine Milestones 2.0 were implemented in July 2022. Table 1.2 summarizes core ACGME competencies for Pain Medicine fellowship programs [18].

In 2020, the ACGME Program Requirements in Pain Medicine were revised and included the removal of minimum procedure numbers to be completed during Pain Medicine fellowship [19]. In response to this, the APPD elaborated a survey study to obtain basic information regarding procedural training and assess the differences within trainee's exposure across the spectrum of programs. Based on this unpublished data, out of 111 programs, 74 responses were received (66.7% response rate) with a mean fellowship size of four fellows. Fluoroscopic procedures were the most commonly completed procedures, with 93% of programs reporting that fellows

Table 1.2 ACGME core competencies in Pain Medicine fellowship education

Core competency	Description
Professionalism	Fellows must demonstrate a commitment to professionalism and adherence to ethical principles
Patient care and procedural skills	Fellows must be able to provide patient care that is patient and family centered, compassionate, equitable, appropriate, and effective
	Fellows must be able to perform all medical, diagnostic, and surgical procedures considered essential for the area of practice
	Fellows must be able to recognize risks, complications, and obtain informed consent
Medical knowledge	Fellows must demonstrate knowledge of established and evolving biomedical, clinical, epidemiological, and social-behavioral sciences, including scientific inquiry, as well as the application of this knowledge to patient care
Practice-based learning and improvement	Fellows must demonstrate the ability to investigate and evaluate their care of patient, to appraise and assimilate scientific evidence, and to continuously improve patient care based on constant self-evaluation and lifelong learning
Interpersonal and communication skills	Fellows must demonstrate interpersonal and communication skills that result in effective exchange of information and collaboration with patients, their families, and health professionals
Systems-based practice	Fellows must demonstrate an awareness of and responsiveness to the larger context and system of health care, including the structural and social determinants of health, as well as the ability to call effectively on other resources to provide optimal care

completed more than 50 procedures per year. In addition, 58% of programs reported fellows completed more than 50 landmark-based procedures and 63% reported more than 50 ultrasound-guided procedures per year. The most variability was noted in numbers of advanced/surgical interventions, with 4% reporting less than 5, 9% reporting between 5 and 10, 25% reporting between 11 and 20, 18% between 21 and 30, 13% reporting between 31 and 40, 6% reporting between 41 and 50, and 20% reporting more than 50 advanced procedures per fellow.

In summary, the survey conveyed valuable information to conclude that Pain Medicine trainees have a fairly similar and consistent distribution of procedure exposure regarding landmark-based, ultrasound-based, and fluoroscopic-based procedures during training. The variability in advanced procedures between training programs does demonstrate the limited exposure and inconsistency, which could limit trainees' proficiency.

According to the most recent ACGME Program Requirements for Pain Medicine, proficiency requirements for neuromodulation and other minimally invasive advanced procedures are not specifically defined; competency on these are delineated in "a range of direct, hands-on interventional pain techniques" [19]. Given the fast-paced evolution of the specialty with novel technologies and variability in neuromodulation and advanced procedures among Pain Medicine training programs, future consideration of updated education requirements or additional clarification with subsequent program requirement updates should be considered to bring more consistency across board certification and ensure adequate proficiency.

Multidisciplinary ACGME-Accredited Pain Medicine Fellowship Curriculum

Pain Medicine specialists are tasked with expertise in reducing pain and disability across a spectrum of disease states and pathological issues. These patients have typically been seen by multiple providers, in both primary care and other specialties before seeking treatment by a pain specialist. Given the diverse nature of painful conditions, trainees seeking Pain Medicine fellowship education may originate from different disciplines and will encounter a multidisciplinary training [18, 19].

ACGME-accredited fellowship programs in Pain Medicine must have a multidisciplinary educational curriculum, focused basic science knowledge of pain physiology, understanding of how these principles alter pain perception, and a comprehensive approach to diagnosis and management of chronic pain including pharmacological, non-pharmacological, and interventional treatments. Trainees in Pain Medicine must obtain a strong foundation of anatomy and physiology of pain, fluoroscopic and ultrasound-guided landmarks, understand proper patient selection for interventions, acquire technical proficiency, management of complications, and be competent with assessment of outcomes and quality of life [20].

ACGME-accredited fellowship programs are required to be conducted in an institution and/or its participating locations that possess ACGME-accredited residencies in at least one of four specialties (Anesthesiology, PM&R, Neurology, Psychiatry). There must be an institutional policy governing the educational resources committed to Pain Medicine that ensures cooperation of all the involved disciplines and a committee to regularly review the program's resource and its attainment of stated goals and objectives. ACGME-accredited programs must follow specific requirements that demonstrate their commitment to the multidisciplinary nature of the specialty, including core faculty members who completed an ACGME-accredited fellowship program, in at least two of the following specialties: anesthesiology, PM&R, and psychiatry and neurology [18, 19].

The educational components of ACGME-accredited Pain Medicine fellowship programs include competency-based goals and objectives designated to promote progress on a trajectory to autonomous Pain Medicine practice with gradual responsibility for patient management, supervision, and structured activities beyond patient care to include core didactic and research activities. The educational components of the curriculum must expand beyond the trainee's core specialty to include rotations in four required disciplines (neurology, anesthesiology, PM&R, psychiatry) and may embrace additional branches, such as palliative care, radiology, and addiction medicine. Table 1.3 summarizes these core competencies and required multidisciplinary rotations. The educational curriculum must include outpatient continuity clinic experience, acute pain, and cancer pain management, comprising of conservative, pharmacological, and interventional treatments [18, 19, 21–23].

Pain Medicine trainees must be able to perform both basic and advanced airway management, vascular access, and recognize how to administer and manage procedural sedation and physiological consequences of general anesthesia or conscious sedation. These are competencies covered by completing an Anesthesiology

Table 1.3 Summary of core competencies and required multidisciplinary rotations [19]

Rotation/discipline	Core competencies
Anesthesiology	Airway management
	Basic life support and advanced cardiac life support
	Vascular access
	General anesthesia
	Monitored anesthesia care (MAC/conscious sedation)
	Complications from anesthesia/sedation
	Regional nerve blocks
Physical Medicine & Rehabilitation	Musculoskeletal physical exam of the spine and appendicular skeleton
	Dynamic musculoskeletal ultrasonography assessment
	Prescription of comprehensive rehabilitation/therapy program and assisted devices to improve function
Neurology	Comprehensive neurological exam
	Neuroradiology imaging interpretation
	Electrodiagnostic evaluation
	Evaluation and management of spasticity
	Interdisciplinary management of neuromuscular pathologies
Psychiatry	Identification of psychosocial risk factors
	Patient education on pain psychology
	Cognitive behavioral therapies
	Identification and management of substance use disorders
Didactics and Scholarly activity	All fellows must complete a scholarly project that must be disseminated through a publication or presentation
	Journal article reviews
	Quality improvement projects
	Patient safety/morbidity and mortality (M&M) conferences
	Tumor boards/surgical planning conferences
	Grand rounds/research seminars
Radiology	Independent radiographic interpretation of commonly performed diagnostic studies (radiographs, computerized tomography/CT, magnetic resonance images, etc.)
	CT-guided interventional procedures
Palliative Care	End-of-life care
	Cancer pain

rotation. Musculoskeletal-based competencies include performing an appropriate comprehensive physical exam of the spine and appendicular skeleton involving dynamic ultrasonography and build an understanding on how to prescribe and develop an appropriate rehabilitation program along with the use of assistive equipment to help patients with chronic pain to reduce disability and return to function. Typically, obtaining these competencies involve rotations with PM&R. Neurology rotations aim to establish basic competence in core neurological concepts, such as optimizing a detailed neurological examination, neurological imaging interpretation, expanding trainee's exposure to electrodiagnostic evaluation, management of spasticity, and interpretation and exposing fellows to interdisciplinary assessment and management of neurological and neuromuscular pathologies. Radiology rotations may offer trainees a broader opportunity to enhance their ability to independently analyze imaging modalities that are relevant in Pain Medicine. Psychological competencies related to identifying pertinent psychiatric and psychosocial risk factors, explaining the importance of psychological therapies to patients, as well as understanding how to identify and manage substance use disorders are attained with rotations in psychology or psychiatry. In addition to these required rotations, programs have to ensure exposure to special populations, including pediatrics, pregnancy, end-of-life, and those with physical or cognitive disabilities. Inclusion of rotations in pediatrics, obstetrics, oncology, and acute/regional anesthesia may be needed to gain exposure related to these competency requirements [18, 19, 21–23]. The incorporation of simulation-based education provides a means of incorporating further exposure to unique situations, or advanced scenarios rarely encountered in clinical care [24]. Fellowship programs should provide didactic and clinical curricula designed to promote acquisition of competence in assessment, formulation, and coordination of a multidisciplinary treatment plan [18, 19].

ACGME-accredited Pain Medicine training encompasses a range of hands-on established interventional treatments, including neuraxial spinal injections, regional nerve blocks, and neuroablative and neuromodulation procedures. Nevertheless, over the past few years, the field has had a renaissance in new technologies beyond these established interventions and entered a realm of minimally invasive surgical pain management. These advancements expand the treatment algorithm and push the field to evolve. Concurrently, ACGME-accredited Pain Medicine training programs will have to adjust and balance trainee's learning with widely accepted evidence-based interventions, while fostering an environment of curiosity, eagerness, professional development, and continual self-improvement.

Although there have been significant improvements in training since the inception of Pain Medicine fellowship several decades ago, training programs have struggled to keep up with the exponential increase in educational content due to the fast-paced, evolving nature of the field and novel percutaneous surgical techniques. Several ideas have been discussed within the pain community regarding education in pain medicine, such as extending the fellowship length or recognizing it as an independent medical specialty [25, 26].

The future of Pain Medicine will continue to be bright as long as there are continuous efforts to expand funding for positions, advanced education and research, and as long as there is support from the ACGME and sponsoring institutions to maintain the highest quality of training, simultaneously with the advancements in the field [27]. Nevertheless, implementing significant changes in fellowship education is undeniably difficult, and there are numerous limitations, primarily budgetary restraints from institutions and the ACGME that may suppress proposed changes [25].

Pain Medicine Board Certification Options

The ABMS is the leading organization for physician to obtain board certification. The subspecialty certification in Pain Medicine is currently issued by six ABMS Member Boards, including Anesthesiology (ABA), PM&R (ABPMR), Psychiatry and Neurology (ABPN), Emergency Medicine (ABEM), Family Medicine (ABFM), and Radiology (ABR) [28]. Figure 1.1 illustrates the number of new Pain Medicine

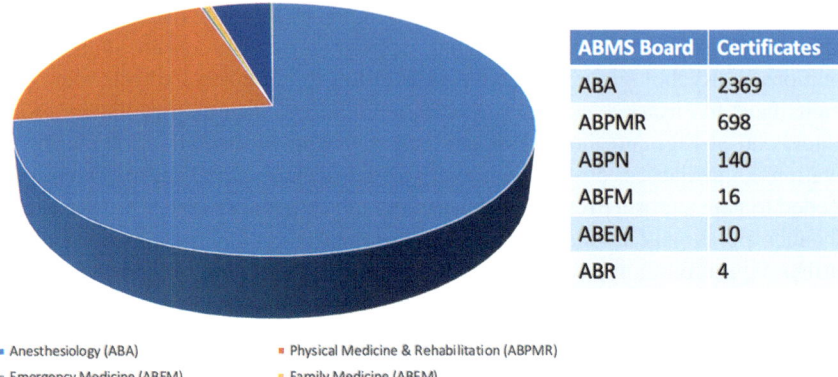

ABMS Board	Certificates
ABA	2369
ABPMR	698
ABPN	140
ABFM	16
ABEM	10
ABR	4

- Anesthesiology (ABA)
- Emergency Medicine (ABEM)
- Psychiatry & Neurology (ABPN)
- Physical Medicine & Rehabilitation (ABPMR)
- Family Medicine (ABFM)
- Radiology (ABR)

Fig. 1.1 New Pain Medicine certificates issued by ABMS Member Boards from 2011 to 2020

subspecialty certificates issued by ABMS Member Boards in the last decade. The process of attaining ABMS Pain Medicine board certification provides myriad benefits for pain physicians, hospitals, and patients. Physicians attain certification to demonstrate their competence and professionalism; hospitals and patients rely on ABMS Pain Medicine board certification to promote high quality care, enhance safety, and maintain confidence that the physicians providing care are committed to evidence-based, ethical pain management. ACGME-accredited Pain Medicine fellowships are the only nationwide recognized and federally sponsored training programs by which Pain Medicine is recognized as a subspecialty by the ABMS and Board Certification is available.

References[1]

1. Meldrum ML. A capsule history of pain management. JAMA. 2003;290(18):2470–5.
2. Leriche R. The surgery of pain. Young A, Trans. ed. London: Baillière Tindall & Cox; 1939.
3. Swerdlow M. Interview by Liebeskind JC. In: John C. Liebeskind history of pain collection. Los Angeles: Louise M. Darling Biomedical Library, University of California; 1996.
4. Livingston WK. Pain and suffering. Seattle: International Association for the Study of Pain Press; 1998.
5. Bonica JJ. The management of pain; with special emphasis on the use of analgesic block in diagnosis, prognosis, and therapy. Philadelphia: Lea & Febiger; 1953.
6. Melzack R, Wall PD. Pain mechanisms: a new theory. Science. 1965;150(3699):971–9. https://doi.org/10.1126/science.150.3699.971.
7. Collier R. A short history of pain management. CMAJ. 2018;190(1):E26–7. https://doi.org/10.1503/cmaj.109-5523.
8. Gallagher RM. Pain medicine 2008: past, present and future. Pain Med. 2008;9(3):267–70.

---

[1] (*) denotes essential references for additional reading.

9. Rathmell JP. American Society of Regional Anesthesia and Pain Medicine 2011. John J. Bonica Award Lecture: the evolution of the field of pain medicine. Reg Anesth Pain Med. 2012;37(6):652–6.
10. Owens WD, Abram SE. The genesis of pain medicine as a subspecialty in anesthesiology. J Anesth Hist. 2020;6(1):13–6.
11. Day M. Pain medicine: a medical specialty? Pain Pract. 2004;4:1–10.
12. *Tieppo Francio V, Gill B, Hagedorn JM, Pagan Rosado R, Pritzlaff S, Furnish T, Kohan L, Sayed D. Factors involved in applicant interview selection and ranking for chronic pain medicine fellowship. Reg Anesth Pain Med. 2022;47(10):592–7. https://doi.org/10.1136/rapm-2022-103538.
13. Fellowship Data & Reports [Internet]. NRMP. [cited 2022 May 20]. Available from: https://www.nrmp.org/match-data-analytics/fellowship-data-reports/
14. https://freida.ama-assn.org Accessed 5 Feb 2024.
15. https://www.nrmp.org/wp-content/uploads/2023/09/Anesthesiology-MRS-Report-2023.pdf. Accessed 5 Feb 2024.
16. Carraccio C, et al. Shifting paradigms: from Flexner to competencies. Acad Med. 2002;77(5):361–7.
17. Swing SR. The ACGME outcome project: retrospective and prospective. Med Teach. 2007;29(7):648–54.
18. The Accreditation Council for Graduate Medical Education. Pain Medicine Milestone. https://www.acgme.org/globalassets/pdfs/milestones/painmedicinemilestones.pdf. Accessed 23 Dec 2022.
19. *American Council for Graduate Medical Education. ACGME Program Requirements for Fellowship Education in Pain Medicine. Retrieved May 22, 2022 from https://www.acgme.org/globalassets/pfassets/programrequirements/530_pain-medicine_2020.pdf
20. *Pritzlaff SG, Goree JH, Hagedorn JM, Lee DW, Chapman KB, Christiansen S, Dudas A, Escobar A, Gilligan CJ, Guirguis M, Gulati A, Jameson J, Mallard CJ, Murphy MZ, Patel KV, Patel RG, Sheth SJ, Vanterpool S, Singh V, Smith G, Strand NH, Vu CM, Suvar T, Chakravarthy K, Kapural L, Leong MS, Lubenow TR, Abd-Elsayed A, Pope JE, Sayed D, Deer TR. Pain Education and Knowledge (PEAK) consensus guidelines for neuromodulation: a proposal for standardization in fellowship and training programs. J Pain Res. 2023;16:3101–17. https://doi.org/10.2147/JPR.S424589.
21. Rathmell JP. Next steps in improving subspecialty education in pain medicine. ASA Newslett. 2010;74:12–4.
22. Huntoon MA, Rathmell JP, Hidalgo NA. Update on interdisciplinary education in pain medicine. ASA Newslett. 2009;73:12–4.
23. Benzon HT, Zell C, Huntoon MA, Stock MC. The present stats of fellowships in pain medicine. ASA Newslett. 2009;72:8–12.
24. Singh N, Nielsen AA, Copenhaver DJ, Sheth SJ, Li CS, Fishman SM. Advancing simulation-based education in pain medicine. Pain Med. 2018;19(9):1725–36.
25. *Wahezi SE, Caparo M, Naeimi T, Kohan L. Fellowship education in a new era of pain medicine: concerns and commentary for change. Pain Med. 2024;25(1):3–4. https://doi.org/10.1093/pm/pnad116.
26. Dubois MY, Follett KA. Pain medicine: the case for an independent medical specialty and training programs. Acad Med. 2014;89(6):863–8. https://doi.org/10.1097/ACM.0000000000000265.
27. Mukhdomi TJ, Mukhdomi JJ. The changing pain medicine fellowship, potential for more disparities to come among training programs. Pain Med. 2021;22(9):2131–2.
28. About ABMS [Internet]. American Board of Medical Specialties. [cited 2022 May 15]. Available from: https://www.abms.org/about-abms/

Basic Medical Knowledge for the Pain Fellow

2

Vinicius Tieppo Francio, Magdalena Anitescu, Dalia Elmofty, Boris Spektor, and Lynn Kohan

Abbreviations

CNS	Central Nervous System
IASP	International Association for the Study of Pain
DRG	Dorsal Root Ganglion
NS	Nociceptive Specific
WDR	Wide Dynamic Range
GABA	Gamma-Aminobutyric Acid
VPL	Ventral Postero-lateral
IL	Interleukine
TNF	Tumor Necrosis Factor
EAA	Excitatory Amino Acids
NGF	Nerve Growth Factor
SST	Somatostatin
AMPA	Alpha Amino 3-hydroxy 5 methyl 4 isoxazelopropionic acid
NMDA	N-Methyl-D-Aspartate
mGluR	metabotropic G protein coupled receptor

V. Tieppo Francio (✉)
Division of Pain Medicine, Department of Anesthesiology, Washington University School of Medicine, St. Louis, MO, USA
e-mail: vtieppofrancio@wustl.edu

M. Anitescu · D. Elmofty
Department of Anesthesia & Critical Care, University of Chicago Medicine, Chicago, IL, USA
e-mail: manitescu@bsd.uchicago.edu; delmofty@bsd.uchicago.edu

B. Spektor
Department of Anesthesiology, Emory University, Atlanta, GA, USA
e-mail: boris.spektor@emoryhealthcare.org

L. Kohan
Department of Anesthesiology, University of Virginia, Charlottesville, VA, USA
e-mail: LRK9G@uvahealth.org

© The Author(s), under exclusive license to Springer Nature Switzerland AG 2025
M. Anitescu (ed.), *Multidisciplinary Pain Medicine Fellowship*,
https://doi.org/10.1007/978-3-031-88357-6_2

RVM   rostral ventromedial medulla
DLPT   dorsal pontine tegmentum
PAG   peri-aqueductal gray
AC   Adenylate Cyclase
PLC   Phospholipase C
cAMP   Cyclic adenosine monophosphate
PKA   protein kinase A
TRPV1   Transient receptor potential vanilloid
LTP   Long term potentiation

As the field of Pain Medicine continues to evolve, the required medical knowledge for pain fellows will concurrently expand. It is imperative for trainees in Pain Medicine to comprehend basic science knowledge on pathophysiological pain processes that can be applied in evaluating patients suffering from chronic pain and understand how these principles alter pain perception [1].

Anatomy, Physiology and Development of Pain Systems

The International Association for the Study of Pain (IASP) characterizes pain as "an unpleasant sensory and emotional experience associated with, or resembling that associated with, actual or potential tissue damage" [2]. This definition captures the essential intricacy of pain as a sensory experience colored through the lens of cognitive interpretation, which may be influenced by biological, psychological, and social factors [3]. The pain pathway initiates peripherally through the activation of nociceptors, where transduction processes take place. Subsequently, the transmission is facilitated by primary afferent neurons, culminating in synaptic connections within the dorsal horn of the spinal cord before entering the central nervous system (CNS) [4]. Four essential steps encompass the transformation of a noxious stimulus into the awareness of pain: transduction, transmission, modulation, and perception at higher cortical centers [5]. Figure 2.1 illustrates these pathways of pain perception.

Transduction It involves the conversion of peripheral noxious stimuli (mechanical, chemical, thermal) that evoked a chemical/electrical action potential into a nerve signal activating first-order neurons. These are specialized nociceptor fibers (Aδ and C fibers) that terminate at the dorsal horn lamina I and V and I-II, respectively. At 20 weeks of gestation, these nociceptors exist throughout skin and mucosal surfaces permitting the transduction phenomenon [6]. Inflammatory mediators such as bradykinin, serotonin, prostaglandins, leukotrienes, and cytokines are released from damaged tissues, which thereby stimulate these specialized receptors [4, 7]. Their properties are summarized in Table 2.1.

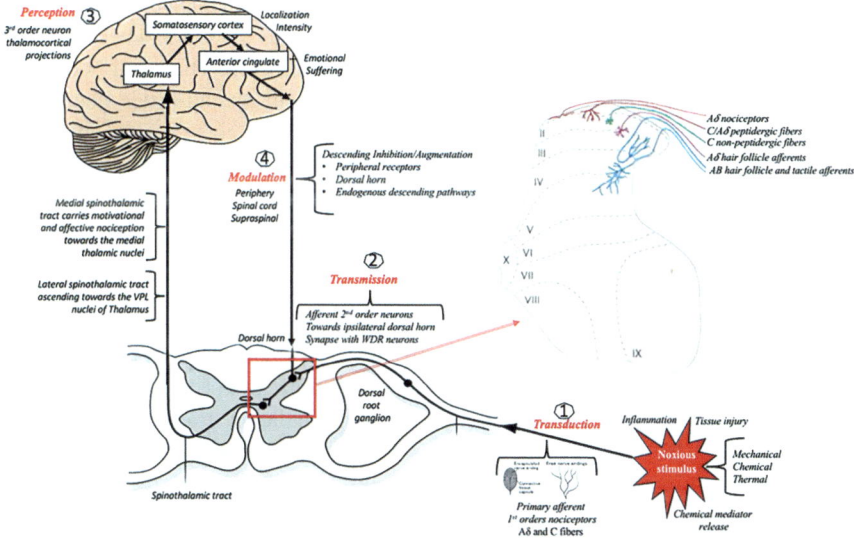

Fig. 2.1 Pathways of pain perception. (Created by/courtesy of Tieppo Francio, V)

Table 2.1 Fiber type and characteristics

Fiber type	Group	Characteristics	Function	Fiber diameter (microns)	Conduction velocity (m/s)
A-alpha (myelinated)	I	Primary muscle spindle afferent	Motor fibers to motoneurons	15	95
A-beta (myelinated)	II	Afferents from tendon organs, cutaneous mechanoreceptors	Cutaneous touch, pressure, vibration, proprioception	12–14	30–60
A-delta (myelinated)	n/a	Intrafusal fibers	Motor fiber to muscle spindles	6	20
A-gamma (myelinated)	III	Afferents from deep pressure receptors in muscles	Sharp fast pain, light touch, temperature	6–8	10–15
B (myelinated)	n/a	Small, lightly myelinated	Sympathetic pre-ganglionic autonomic fibers	3	7
C (unmyelinated)	IV	Unmyelinated nerve fibers; Sympathetic post-ganglionic fibers	Cutaneous pain afferents, dull, achy, burning pain, temperature	<1	<1.5

Courtesy of/created by Tieppo Francio, V

Transmission　This step involves the conveyance of peripheral nociceptor (Aδ-fibers and C-fibers) stimuli via afferent sensory neurons towards the CNS, where it terminates at the Rexed lamina I and V and I–II of the spinal cord. Their cell bodies are located within the dorsal root ganglion (DRG). Their second-order neurons is located in the ipsilateral dorsal horn and synapses with nociceptive specific (NS) and/or wide dynamic range (WDR) neurons. In these locations, complex interactions occur between these excitatory and inhibitory interneurons releasing glycine and gamma-aminobutyric acid (GABA) to modulate nociceptive transmission via pain pathways and by a spinal "gate control" mechanism.

Dorsal horn organization and myelination of spinothalamic tracts are complete by 30 weeks, with thalamocortical connections developing at 26–30 weeks' gestation to permit transmission and perception [6, 8]. From the dorsal horn, these neurons ascend contralaterally via the lateral spinothalamic tract to the ventral posterolateral (VPL) nuclei of the thalamus for pain discrimination/localization and via the medial spinothalamic tract to convey motivational and affective components of nociception towards the medial thalamic nuclei [5, 9, 10]. Table 2.2 describes the characteristics of these ascending pain pathways.

Modulation　Pain modulation is defined as an alteration in neural activity, either by inhibition or augmentation, along the pain pathways, which may occur in the periphery, spinal cord, and at higher centers [10]. In the periphery, ion channels and peripheral receptors (acid-sensing ion channels, purinergic P2X receptors, voltage-gated sodium, calcium, and potassium channels) at the peripheral terminal will detect noxious stimulus (changes in pH, chemical, thermal, or tissue destruction) and initiate a local inflammatory response (known as inflammatory soup). This results in the release of inflammatory mediators such as histamine, substance P, prostaglandins, leukotrienes, bradykinin, serotonin, nitric oxide, adenosine, cytokines (IL-1ß, IL-6, IL-8, TNF) excitatory amino acid (EAA), and nerve growth factor (NGF), which will enhance nociceptor sensitivity [11, 12]. Endogenous opioids, acetylcholine, which desensitize C-fibers nociceptors to mechanical and heat

Table 2.2 Characteristics of ascending pain pathways

	Lateral spinothalamic tract	Medial spinothalamic tract
Function	Sensory discriminative (localization) aspect of pain	Autonomic, affective, motivational components of pain
Structure	Neospinothalamic tract with somatotopic organization (caudal elements lateral, rostral elements medial)	Paleospinothalamic tract, little somatotopic organization
Origin	Neurons in lamina I and V	Neurons in lamina II and IV, VIII
2nd Order Neurons	Anterior white commissure	Anterior white commissure
3rd Order Neurons	Ventral posterior lateral (VPL) thalamic nucleus, ventral posterior inferior (VPI) nucleus and to post-central gyrus	Medial thalamic nuclei, periaqueductal gray matter (PAG), somatosensory cortex and limbic centers

Courtesy of/created by Tieppo Francio, V

stimuli, gamma-aminobutyric acid (GABA), and somatostatin (SST) can impair the synthesis, release, or effect of these pain-enhancing mediators, resulting in pain modulation [11–13]. At the spinal cord level, inhibitory pain modulation may occur by activating Aβ fibers with tactile, non-noxious stimuli towards inhibitory inter- neurons in the dorsal horn (lamina II), which once activated lead to inhibition of nociceptive C-fibers [14].

Specifically dorsal horn modulation occurs with NS neurons in lamina I and II in response to Aδ and C-fibers only, or in lamina V with WDR responding to all three sensory fibers, Aβ, Aδ and C-fibers in a graded manner depending on the intensity of the stimulation. This can lead to summation of potentials with repeated stimula- tion also known as the "wind-up phenomena" resulting in hyperalgesia, allodynia, and enhanced pain signaling. This is thought to involve excitatory neurotransmitter glutamate and membrane depolarization at the alpha amino 3-hydroxy 5-methyl-4- isoxazeloproprionic acid (AMPA), the N-methyl-D-aspartate (NMDA), and the G-protein coupled metabotropic (mGluR) receptors [15–17].

The endogenous inhibitory descending modulatory system originates from higher centers such as the hypothalamus, amygdala, rostral ventromedial medulla (RVM), dorsolateral pontine tegmentum (DLPT), and periaqueductal gray region (PAG) [5]. The prefrontal cortex and amygdala provide emotion-affective modula- tion of the cognitive functions in pain [18]. The PAG and RVM also communicate with noradrenergic, serotonergic, and dopaminergic systems to modulate pain by activating an endogenous opioid system [19, 20]. Three types of G-protein couple opioid receptors within the CNS (mu, delta, and kappa) that upon activation results in neurotransmitter inhibition, cell hyperpolarization, and reduction of cell excit- ability. Endogenous opioids, such as B-endorphins, predominately bind to mu opi- oid receptors; Dynorphins predominately bind to kappa opioid receptors, while Enkephalins predominately bind to delta opioid receptors [10]. Pain modulation via these descending inhibitory pain pathways develops after full-term birth, predispos- ing preterm infants to experience more pain [8].

Perception This is the final step in subjective sensation of pain involves an inter- play between nociception transduction, neural transmission, modulation, and cogni- tive interpretation. From the thalamus, nociceptive information projects via third-order neurons to the primary and secondary somatosensory cortices, pre- frontal and cingulate cortices, and limbic regions, where nociception is interpreted and processed [21]. Pain interpretation, perception, and awareness involve multiple cortical regions that are collectively defined as cortical pain matrix, which are cat- egorized into three different levels (primary, secondary, and tertiary). The primary and secondary matrices intercommunicate, while the third matrix integrates the input from the first and two region and reacts with a behavioral response [22, 23]. The primary matrix is composed by the somatosensory cortex, parietal operculum, and posterior insula, and it is responsible for pain perception, pain localization, pain quality, and pain intensity. The secondary cortical matrix is composed by the ante- rior cingulate cortex, anterior insula, amygdala, and hippocampus, and its main function is associated with the affective experience of pain, emotional processing, negative emotions, distress, and unpleasantness. Lastly, the tertiary cortical matrix involves the frontal cortex (orbitofrontal, anterolateral, prefrontal), medial cingulate, posterior cingulate gyrus and is responsible for the cognitive processing, cognitive meaning to pain, and influencing behavioral responses to pain [22, 23]. As such, pain perception may be influenced by emotional, social, environmental factors, as well as cultural and past experiences [2].

Types of Pain Syndromes

Pain can be classified into three major categories (acute, subacute, and chronic). Acute pain is a physiological response to a mechanical, chemical, or thermal stimuli [24]. There is no clear threshold of when acute pain becomes subacute, but it is generally recognized that when pain persists beyond the expected healing period (more than 3–6 months), it may be classified as a chronic pain [25, 26]. Furthermore, based on the International Association of the Study of Pain (IASP), pain can be subcategorized into particular types (nociceptive, neuropathic, and nociplastic), which can assist with differential diagnosis and treatment optimization to provide the best care for patients [27]. Table 2.3 summarizes their distinguished features. However, categorizing pain confined to one subtype is an oversimplification of real-life conditions, as most pain states represent a mixed pain pattern with substantial overlap [28, 29].

Nociceptive Pain The most common form of pain [28]. It is defined by the IASP as "pain that arises from actual or threatened damage to non-neural tissue and is due to activation of nociceptors" [27]. Nociceptive pain is subclassified into two main categories: somatic and visceral pain [28]. Further important definitions in somatic and visceral pain physiology includes referred pain and its distinctive clinical characters compared to neuropathic features such as radicular pain and radiculopathy [30].

- *Somatic pain*: Well-localized pain signals from joints, bones, muscles, skin, which follow the four-step neural pathway (transduction transmission, modulation, and perception), often described as intermittent, well-defined pain, aching, gnawing, throbbing, and cramping [28, 31]. Typically, nociceptive pain from soma has a clear and proportional relationship to movement-based factors and predictably occurs with specific activities or postures.
- *Visceral pain*: Described as diffuse and difficult to localize pain from internal organs/structures. It follows a similar pathway than somatic pain conveying at the dorsal horn, and it may be misinterpreted as somatic pain. However, uniquely visceral afferents traverse the prevertebral and paravertebral sympathetic ganglia when enroute to the dorsal horn [31].
- *Referred pain*: The etiology of referred pain may be somatic or visceral. Referred pain is defined as when pain is perceived in regions innervated by nerves other

Table 2.3 Distinguished features of nociceptive, neuropathic, and nociplastic pain

	Nociceptive pain	Neuropathic Pain	Nociplastic pain
Pathophysiology	Tissue or potential tissue damage resulting in peripheral nociceptor hyperactivity	Disease or injury to peripheral nerve or central nervous system (somatosensory system)	Abnormal processing of pain signals without any clear evidence of tissue damage involving the somatosensory system. Central or peripheral sensitization with augmented sensory processing and diminished inhibitory pathways resulting in hyper-responsiveness to pain
Clinical features	Throbbing, aching, pressure-like, non-dermatomal referral, often proximal > distal, infrequent sensory deficits. Typically, nociceptive pain has a clear and proportional relationship to movement-based factors and predictably occurs with specific activities or postures	Shooting, electrical-like, stabbing pain, frequently associated with sensory changes (numbness, tingling, allodynia) following a dermatomal pattern often distally. Weakness may be present. Typically, exacerbations are less-movement related	Diffuse, gnawing, aching, sharp pain. Non-dermatomal pattern. Non-linear and aberrant relationship with movement, often with disproportionate, non-mechanical, diffuse, unpredictable patterns of pain provocation or fear-avoidance
Examples	Degenerative (disc degeneration, facet arthropathy, primary osteoarthritis), inflammatory (discogenic pain, vertebrogenic pain), myofascial (multifidus dysfunction, muscle spasms)	Radiculopathy, spinal canal stenosis with neurogenic claudication, failed back surgery syndrome/post-laminectomy syndrome, complex regional pain syndrome	Chronic primary musculoskeletal pain, fibromyalgia, chronic widespread pain, chronic primary pelvic pain, complex regional pain syndrome

Adapted from Cohen et al. [28]

than those that innervate the site of noxious stimuli [30]. Visceral referred pain, also known as viscerosensory reflex, is regarded as a pathological combination of nociceptive processing pathways for visceral sensory afferents, and a classic example is the pathophysiological process of myocardial ischemia that concomitantly elicits left arm pain [32]. In contrast, somatic referred pain involves noxious stimulation of soma nerve endings from discs, zygapophyseal joints, sacroiliac joints, leading to a convergence of nociceptive afferents on second-order neurons in the dorsal horn where neural information from other structures converges. As such, the pattern is usually non-dermatomal (non-radicular) and follows the principle of same segmental innervation as the source. Since somatic referred pain is not caused by compression of nerve roots, there are no neurologi-cal signs upon examination. It can be often described as a dull, aching, gnawing, expanding pressure into an area that is wide, diffuse, and difficult to localize [30].

Neuropathic Pain It is defined by the IASP as "pain caused by a lesion or disease of the somatosensory nervous system," located either centrally or peripherally [27, 33]. It comprises approximately 15–25% of all pain conditions [28]. It is often described as electric like, shooting, or lancinating with an associated area of abnor-mal sensation or hypersensitivity, traditionally following a neural pattern and less-movement related [28, 34]. Neuropathic pain can either be spontaneous or secondary to a stimulus causing allodynia or hypersensitivity [35]. It is always considered maladaptive and often broken down into two subclasses: peripheral and central [28, 34].

- *Peripheral neuropathic pain* includes conditions such as radiculopathy, diabetic peripheral neuropathy, post-herpetic neuralgia, trigeminal neuralgia, and phan-tom limb pain [28, 34]. Radicular pain is a neuropathic type of pain evoked by ectopic discharges emanating from the dorsal nerve roots or ganglion, often caused by inflammation of the affected nerve, and elicits a distinctive pain, usu-ally of lancinating quality traveling along a radicular dermatomal distribution. Radiculopathy is yet another distinct entity defined as a neuropathic state in which conduction is blocked along a spinal nerve or its roots. Clinically, this dif-fers by the objective presence of neurological signs, such as diminished deep tendon reflexes, motor weakness following a myotomal patter, and sensory abnormalities along a dermatomal distribution. Although radicular pain and radiculopathy commonly occur together, these can present independently from each other [30].
- *Central neuropathic pain* includes traumatic, vascular, and autoimmune condi-tions. Specific examples include spinal cord injury, post-stroke pain, and multi-ple sclerosis, respectively [28].

Nociplastic Pain This is a third mechanistic pain category created to describe pain that does not fit into the classification of nociceptive or neuropathic pain [36, 37]. The IASP describes nociplastic pain as "pain that arises from altered nociception despite no clear evidence of actual or threatened tissue damage causing the activa-tion of peripheral nociceptors or evidence for disease or lesion of the somatosensory system causing the pain" [27]. Although mechanistically different from both neuro-pathic and nociceptive pain, the underlying mechanism of nociplastic pain is still poorly understood. It is thought to be related to an abnormal and augmented percep-tion and sensory processing of pain by the peripheral and/or central nervous system [28, 38, 39]. Nociplastic pain is often more diffuse and intense than one would expect from the underlying injury. It is also often related to altered mood, sleep, and memory [27]. Specific examples of nociplastic pain include chronic widespread pain, fibromyalgia, irritable bowel syndrome, complex regional pain syndrome [36,

38]. The IASP clinical criteria for nociplastic pain include: pain >3 months of duration, a regional pain distribution, no evidence of contributory nociceptive or neuropathic pain, and hypersensitivity [27, 40].

Mixed Pain Syndrome   Mixed pain syndrome is the term used to describe the continuum chronic pain cycle of an overlap in neuropathic, nociceptive, and/or nociplastic pain in the same area of the body [29]. It is important to note that this category has not yet been adapted by the IASP; however, it is increasingly recognized in the clinical and research realm. As of now, mixed pain is a clinical diagnosis based on overlap of pain categories without an explicit diagnostic criterion. The addition of the term syndrome acknowledges the presence of a constellation of symptoms with no single pathophysiological mechanism, but rather combined mechanisms that may occur concurrently [28, 38]. Figure 2.2 illustrates this important relation between different pain categories. Important examples of mixed pain syndromes include cancer pain, chronic post-surgical pain, and possibly non-specific low back pain [28, 29, 41, 42].

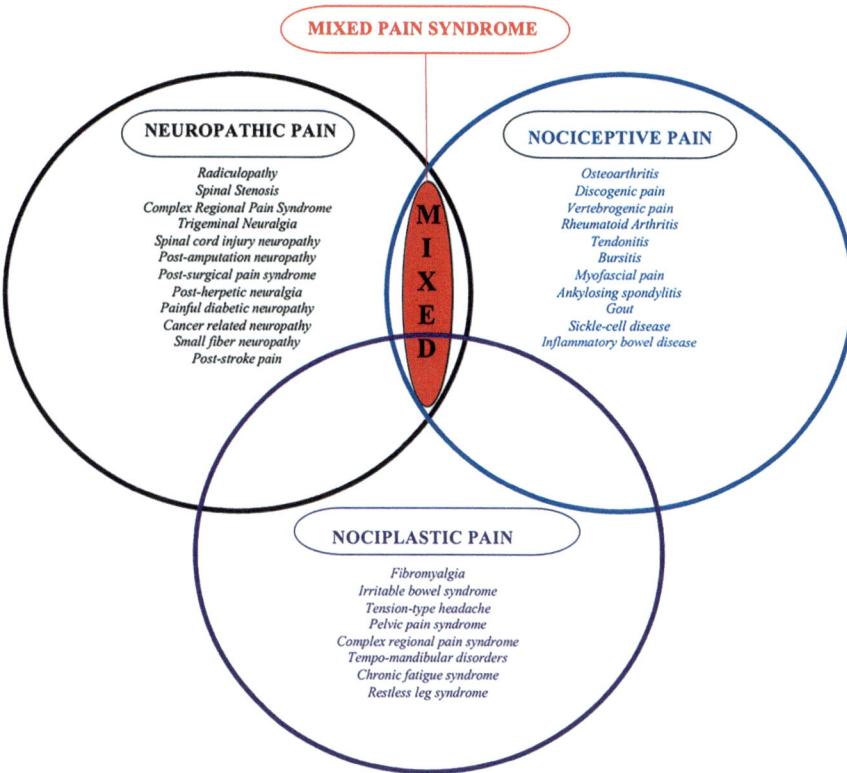

Fig. 2.2 Diagram displaying the complex interaction between nociceptive, neuropathic, nociplastic, and mixed pain syndromes

Common Pain Syndromes in Pain Medicine

Pathological pain syndromes such as peripheral sensitization or central sensitization may arise upon continued or recurrent release of inflammatory mediators that will sensitize the nociceptor and increase their rate of basal discharge (non-stimulated) with lowering of the stimulus threshold and increase in discharge rate with each increase in stimulus strength [3, 27]. Peripheral sensitization is a decrease in threshold and an increase in responsiveness of these peripheral nociceptors, often spontaneously, that occurs after tissue damage and inflammation, resulting from early post-translational changes with phosphorylation of ion channels (G-protein couple receptors or tyrosine kinase receptors) and altered gene expression leading to primary hyperalgesia [13]. In peripheral sensitization states, a gentle touch can elicit severe pain. The lowered threshold leads to more frequent firing and release of inflammatory mediators recruiting silent nociceptors that are not usually activated by painful stimuli [16]. These inflammatory mediators bind to the G-protein coupled receptors leading to the release of second messenger adenylate cyclase (AC) and phospholipase C (PLC). AC transforms adenosine triphosphate to cyclic adenosine monophosphate (cAMP) which in turn activates protein kinase A (PKA). PKA maintains the pain response and increased hyperalgesia [16]. PLC activates the transient receptor potential vanilloid (TRPV1) and, once sensitized, activates at temperatures below painful ranges [16]. Prolonged/increased peripheral activation from tissue injury may result in long-term changes at the level of the dorsal horn in the spinal cord and brain. Long-term potentiation (LTP) plays a role in memory and learning and is associated with pain sensitization. LTP can increase excitation at the level of the dorsal horn and intensify the pain response. Initiation of LTP is linked to the activation of the NMDA receptor, resulting in increased hyperalgesia at the site and surrounding areas. Long-term peripheral sensitization can lead to central sensitization over time [16].

In contrast to peripheral sensitization, central sensitization represents an outcome arising from the central nervous system contributing to altered sensory input interpretation and ultimately culminating in heightened synaptic transmission. This phenomenon is characterized by heterosynaptic potentiation, membrane hyperexcitability in microglia and astrocytes, alterations in gene transcription, and the induction of augmented action potentials output from dorsal horn neurons resulting in elevated calcium levels, glutamate, substance P, and calcitonin gene-related peptide (CGRP). This leads to an abnormal state of responsiveness or increased gain of the nociceptive system beyond the peripheral terminals and a state of facilitation, potentiation, and/or amplification within the CNS. Thereby, central sensitization represents a major functional shift in the somatosensory system from high-threshold nociception to low-threshold pain hypersensitivity, in which painful sensations may occur in the absence of noxious stimuli or peripheral injury [43]. Table 2.4 outlines the distinctive characteristics of peripheral and central sensitization.

Table 2.4 Characteristics of peripheral and central sensitization

Features	Peripheral sensitization	Central sensitization
Location	Peripheral nervous system (PNS)	Central nervous system (CNS)
Primary involvement	Peripheral nerve fibers and tissues	Central neurons and synapses
Mediators	Proinflammatory molecules, G-protein couple receptors, tyrosine kinase	Glutamate, Substance P, calcitonin gene-related peptide
Mechanism	Increased sensitivity of peripheral nociceptors	Amplification of pain signaling
Presentation	Heightened response to stimuli at the injury site	Widespread pain, hypersensitivity, heightened response to various stimuli not limited to the injury site
Duration/ Response	Temporary, adaptive response to pain	Chronic, may persist beyond the initial injury, may become a maladaptive response to pain

References[1]

1. Pritzlaff SG, Goree JH, Hagedorn JM, Lee DW, Chapman KB, Christiansen S, Dudas A, Escobar A, Gilligan CJ, Guirguis M, Gulati A, Jameson J, Mallard CJ, Murphy MZ, Patel KV, Patel RG, Sheth SJ, Vanterpool S, Singh V, Smith G, Strand NH, Vu CM, Suvar T, Chakravarthy K, Kapural L, Leong MS, Lubenow TR, Abd-Elsayed A, Pope JE, Sayed D, Deer TR. Pain Education and Knowledge (PEAK) consensus guidelines for neuromodulation: a proposal for standardization in fellowship and training programs. J Pain Res. 2023;16:3101–17. https://doi.org/10.2147/JPR.S424589.
2. *Raja SN, Carr DB, Cohen M, Finnerup NB, Flor H, Gibson S, et al. The revised International Association for the Study of Pain definition of pain: concepts, challenges, and compromises. Pain. 2020;161(9):1976–82.
3. *Elsenbruch S, Icenhour A, Enck P. Visceral pain: a biopsychological perspective. Neuroforum. 2017;23:105–10.
4. *Lee GI, Neumeister MW. Pain: pathways and physiology. Clin Plastic Surg. 2020;47:173–80.
5. *Bourne S, Machado AG, Nagel SJ. Basic anatomy and physiology of pain pathways. Neurosurg Clin N Am. 2014;25(4):629–38.
6. Taddio A, Katz J. Pain, opioid tolerance and sensitisation to nociception in the neonate. Best Pract Res Clin Anaesthesiol. 2004;18(2):291–302.
7. D'Mello R, Dickenson AH. Spinal cord mechanisms of pain. Br J Anaesth. 2008;101(1):8–16.
8. Van de Velde M, Jani J, De Buck F, Deprest J. Fetal pain perception and pain management. Semin Fetal Neonatal Med. 2006;11(4):232–6.
9. Steeds CE. The anatomy and physiology of pain. Surgery. 2009;27(12):507–11.
10. Reddi D, Curran N, Stephens R. An introduction to pain pathways and mechanisms. Br J Hosp Med (Lond). 2013;74(Suppl 12):C188–91. https://doi.org/10.12968/hmed.2013.74.sup12.c188.
11. Johnson AC, Greenwood-Van MB. The pharmacology of visceral pain. Adv Pharmacol. 2016;75:273–301.
12. Ossipov MH, Dussor GO, Porreca F. Central modulation of pain. J Clin Investig. 2010;120(11):3779–87.

---

[1](*) denotes essential references for additional reading.

13. Vardeh D, Mannion RJ, Woolf CJ. Toward a mechanism-based approach to pain diagnosis. J Pain. 2016;17(9 Suppl):T50–69. https://doi.org/10.1016/j.jpain.2016.03.001.
14. Melzack R, Wall PD. Pain mechanisms: a new theory. Science. 1965;150(3699):971–9. https://doi.org/10.1126/science.150.3699.971.
15. Wang M, Thyagarajan B. Pain pathways and potential new targets for pain relief. Biotechnol Appl Biochem. 2022;69(1):110–23.
16. Price D, Greenspan J, Dubner R. Neurons involved in the exteroceptive function of pain. Pain. 2003;106(3):215–9.
17. Russo CM, Brose WG. Chronic pain. Annual review of medicine. 1998;49:123.
18. Ji G, Fu Y, Ruppert KA, Neugebauer V. Pain-related anxiety-like behavior requires CRF1 receptors in the amygdala. Mol Pain. 2007;3:13.
19. Pertovaara A. Noradrenergic pain modulation. Prog Neurobiol. 2006;80(2):53–83.
20. Neugebauer V, Galhardo V, Maione S, Mackey SC. Forebrain pain mechanisms. Brin Res Rev. 2009;60(1):226–42.
21. Ringkamp M, Dougherty PM, Raja SN. Anatomy and physiology of the pain signaling process. In: Essentials of pain medicine. Elsevier; 2018. p. 3–10.e1.
22. Fenton BW, Shih E, Zolton J. The neurobiology of pain perception in normal and persistent pain. Pain Manag. 2015;5:297–317. https://doi.org/10.2217/pmt.15.27.
23. Xiang Y, Wang Y, Gao S, Zhang X, Cui R. Neural mechanisms with respect to different paradigms and relevant regulatory factors in empathy for pain. Front Neurosci. 2018 Jul;24(12):507. https://doi.org/10.3389/fnins.2018.00507.
24. Treede RD, Rief W, Barke A, Aziz Q, Bennett MI, Benoliel R, Cohen M, Evers S, Finnerup NB, First MB, Giamberardino MA. A classification of chronic pain for ICD-11. Pain. 2015;156(6):1003.
25. National Pharmaceutical Council and Joint Commission on Accreditation of Healthcare Organizations. Pain: current understanding of assessment, management, and treatments. Reston: National Pharmaceutical Council; 2001.
26. Banerjee S, Argáez C. Multidisciplinary treatment programs for patients with acute or subacute pain: a review of clinical effectiveness, cost-effectiveness, and guidelines [Internet]. Ottawa: Canadian Agency for Drugs and Technologies in Health; 2019.
27. IASP Terminology [Internet]. Washington DC, USA: International Association for the Study of Pain; 2021 [cited 2022 May 30].
28. *Cohen SP, Vase L, Hooten WM. Chronic pain: an update on burden, best practices and new advancements. Lancet. 2021:397P2082-97.
29. Freynhagen R, Parada HA, CalderonOspina CA, et al. Current understanding of the mixed pain concept: a brief narrative review. Curr Med Res Opin. 2019;35:1011–8.
30. Bogduk N. On the definitions and physiology of back pain, referred pain and radicular pain. PAIN. 2009;147:17–9.
31. Boezaart AP, Smith CR, Chembrovich S, Zasimovich Y, Server A, Morgan G, et al. Visceral versus somatic pain: an educational review of anatomy and clinical implications. Reg Anesth Pain Med. 2021;46(7):629–36.
32. Jin Q, Chang Y, Lu C, Chen L, Wang Y. Referred pain: characteristics, possible mechanisms, and clinical management. Front Neurol. 2023;14:1104817. https://doi.org/10.3389/fneur.2023.1104817.
33. Jensen TS, Baron R, Haanpaa M, Kalso E, Loeser JD, Rice AS, Treede RD. A new definition of neuropathic pain. PAIN. 2011;152:2204–5.
34. Baron R, Binder A, Wasner G. Neuropathic pain: diagnosis, pathophysiological mechanisms, and treatment. Lancet Neurol. 2010;9(8):807–19.
35. Treede RD, Rief W, Barke A, Aziz Q, Bennett MI, Benoliel R, Cohen M, Evers S, Finnerup NB, First MB, Giamberardino MA, Kaasa S, Korwisi B, Kosek E, Lavand'homme P, Nicholas M, Perrot S, Scholz J, Schug S, Smith BH, Svensson P, Vlaeyen JWS, Wang SJ. Chronic pain as a symptom or a disease: the IASP Classification of Chronic Pain for the International Classification of Diseases (ICD-11). Pain. 2019;160(1):19–27.

36. Kosek E, Cohen M, Baron R, et al. Do we need a third mechanistic descriptor for chronic pain states? Pain. 2016;157:1382–6.
37. Nijs J, Lahousse A, Kapreli E, Bilika P, Saraçoğlu İ, Malfliet A, Coppieters I, De Baets L, Leysen L, Roose E, Clark J, Voogt L, Huysmans E. Nociplastic pain criteria or recognition of central sensitization? Pain phenotyping in the past, present and future. J Clin Med. 2021;10(15):3203.
38. *Fitzcharles MA, Cohen SP, Clauw DJ, Littlejohn G, Usui C, Häuser W. Nociplastic pain: towards an understanding of prevalent pain conditions. Lancet. 2021;397(10289):2098–110.
39. Woolf CJ. Central sensitization: implications for the diagnosis and treatment of pain. Pain. 2011;152(3 Suppl):S2–S15.
40. Kosek E, Clauw D, Nijs J, Baron R, Gilron I, Harris RE, Mico JA, Rice AS, Sterling M. Chronic nociplastic pain affecting the musculoskeletal system: clinical criteria and grading system. Pain. 2021;
41. Freynhagen R, Rey R, Argoff C. When to consider "mixed pain"? The right questions can make a difference! Curr Med Res Opin. 2020;36(12):2037–46.
42. Caraceni A, Shkodra M. Cancer pain assessment and classification. Cancers (Basel). 2019;11(4):510.
43. Latremoliere A, Woolf CJ. Central sensitization: a generator of pain hypersensitivity by central neural plasticity. J Pain. 2009;10(9):895–926. https://doi.org/10.1016/j.jpain.2009.06.012.

Clinical States of Pain (Taxonomy)

3

W. Michael Hooten, Ryan S. D'Souza, and Ariana Nelson

Abbreviations

AIDS	Acquired immunodeficiency syndrome
BMS	Burning mouth syndrome
CALD	Culturally and linguistically diverse
CGRP	Calcitonin gene-related peptide
CPT	Current Procedural Terminology
CRPS	Complex regional pain syndrome
CT	Computer tomography
DSM	Diagnostic and statistical manual
EMG	Electromyography
HIV	Human immunodeficiency virus
HT	Hydroxytryptamine
IASP	International Association for the Study of Pain
MRI	Magnetic resonance imaging
NCV	Nerve conduction studies
NSAIDS	Nonsteroidal anti-inflammatory drugs
OUD	Opioid use disorder

W. M. Hooten
Department of Anesthesiology, Division of Pain Medicine, Mayo Clinic,
Rochester, MN, USA
e-mail: hooten.william@mayo.edu

R. S. D'Souza
Department of Anesthesiology and Perioperative Medicine, Mayo Clinic,
Rochester, MN, USA
e-mail: dsouza.ryan@mayo.edu

A. Nelson (✉)
Department of Anesthesiology, University of California, Irvine, CA, USA
e-mail: arianamn@hs.uci.edu

© The Author(s), under exclusive license to Springer Nature Switzerland AG 2025
M. Anitescu (ed.), *Multidisciplinary Pain Medicine Fellowship*,
https://doi.org/10.1007/978-3-031-88357-6_3

SUD	Substance use disorder
SUNCT	Short-lasting unilateral neuralgiform headache attacks with conjunctival injection and tearing
TMD	Temporomandibular disorder
TMJ	Temporomandibular joint
TRPV	Transient receptor potential vanilloid
TTH	Tension type headache

Introduction

Taxonomy is defined as an orderly system of nomenclature based on a set of rules and procedures. Disease taxonomy, otherwise referred to as disease classification, can be based on etiology, anatomical location, affected organ systems, pathophysiology, or a combination of these characteristics. The International Classification of Diseases 11th Revision [1] is the global standard for diagnostic health information, and it is used to support healthcare payment systems, safety and quality processes, and large-scale health services research. Another widely used classification system is Current Procedural Terminology (CPT®) [2] which is a set of codes used to report medical, surgical, and procedural services to health care organizations and insurance companies.

The Content Outline for the American Board of Anesthesiology's Pain Medicine Examination relies on the *Classification of Chronic Pain* system that was originally published by the International Association for the Study of Pain (IASP) in 1986. A second edition was published in 1994, and selected sections were updated in 2011 and 2012. In its current digital form, updates are incorporated on a continual basis and a print version of the book is no longer available. In this section, the IASP's *Classification of Chronic Pain* will be used as a template to organize and highlight key content regarding clinical pain conditions that are encountered in the daily practice of a pain medicine physician.

Tissue Pain

Tissue pain encompasses a broad range of acute and chronic pain states that can have characteristics of nociceptive, nociplastic, and neuropathic pain.

Acute Pain

Acute pain is a ubiquitous human experience, and it is one of the most widely cited indications for emergent, urgent, or outpatient medical assessments. In a multi-center study, 70% of patients in an emergency department setting were motivated to seek care due to the onset of acute pain [3], and a single center study found that 70% of inpatients report pain during hospital admission [4]. The high incidence and prevalence of pain in these settings impacts the outpatient chronic non-cancer pain population given the relatively high likelihood that symptoms will transition from acute to chronic pain.

Aside from major and minor trauma, acute inflammation and acute postoperative pain are highly prevalent conditions. Acute inflammation is initiated and propagated by a complex cascade of pro- and anti-inflammatory mediators [5]. Unresolved or chronic inflammation is associated with coronary artery disease, cerebral vascular disease, inflammatory bowel disease, a vast array of rheumatological disorders, and a wide range of cancer diagnoses [6].

The prevalence of moderate to severe acute postsurgical pain ranges up to 31–58% [7]. Predictors of poor acute postsurgical pain control include young age, female sex, symptoms of depression and anxiety, sleep disruption, higher body mass index, the presence of preoperative pain, and the use of preoperative analgesic medications [8]. Optimizing acute pain management is important because high levels of pain are associated with the development of persistent postsurgical pain [9, 10], which may develop in 10–40% of surgical patients [10, 11].

Other predictors of persistent postsurgical pain include tobacco smoking, presurgical pain, longer duration of surgery, and postsurgical complications (e.g., wound infection, cardiovascular, renal, gastrointestinal, thrombotic or neurologic adverse events) [10, 12]. A systematic review and component network meta-analysis found that serotonin-norepinephrine inhibitors and neural blockade were associated with a 10% reduction in the prevalence of persistent postsurgical pain. In addition, the combination of neural block (neuraxial, regional, or local infiltrate) and gabapentinoids or N-methyl-D-aspartate receptor antagonists were also effective, suggesting that treatment effect of multimodal interventions on prevention of persistent postsurgical pain is multiplicative [13].

Non-radicular Neck Pain

Non-radicular or axial neck pain is a common symptom with an estimated annual prevalence of 37.2% [14]. Risk factors for neck pain include genetic predisposition, sleep disturbance, mental health problems, obesity, tobacco smoking, sedentary lifestyle, trauma and whiplash, low back pain, and poor general health [15–18]. The clinical history, physical examination, and diagnostic testing should focus on identifying clinical signs of facet, intervertebral disc, muscle, and ligament involvement as sources of pain [19]. Neoplastic, inflammatory disease processes, trauma, atlantoaxial subluxation in Down syndrome and rheumatoid arthritis, infection, vascular abnormalities, and neurological disease should be considered "red flag" diagnoses warranting further diagnostic evaluation [19].

Pharmacological, interventional, and integrative treatments are available for axial neck pain. Although few trials have evaluated medications for neck pain, low levels of evidence support the use of topical nonsteroidal anti-inflammatory drugs (NSAIDs) (i.e., diclofenac) [20] and muscle relaxants (i.e., cyclobenzaprine) [21]. Facet-targeted injections, radiofrequency ablation of the cervical medial branches, epidural steroid injections, and trigger point injections are used to treat axial neck pain [19, 22]. The findings of multiple systematic reviews and meta-analyses suggest a broad range of integrative therapies are effective for neck pain including aerobic and strengthening exercises, spinal manipulation, and mindfulness meditation with structured movement and breath control (i.e., yoga, qigong) [19].

Myofascial pain, which can involve areas of discrete or diffuse sensitivity in one or more muscle groups, can be the primary source or an important contributing source of neck pain. The prevalence of myofascial pain in adults with chronic neck pain ranges up to 38% [23]. Although the origin of myofascial pain is not fully understood, sensitized muscles release excess acetylcholine, which can lead to sustained muscle contraction and sarcomere shortening, local ischemia, and release of inflammatory mediators [24]. A distinguishing characteristic of myofascial pain is the presence of trigger points, which are palpable bands of taut muscle that cause referred pain in a defined pattern spontaneously or after manual stimulation.

Radicular Neck Pain

The annual incidence of cervical radiculopathy is cited as 107.3 per 100,000 men and 63.5 per 100,000 women and the incidence peaks in the fifth decade of life [25]. Tobacco smoking, a history of lumbar radiculopathy, and strenuous lifting are risk factors, but a history of trauma or physical exertion immediately preceding symptom onset occurs in less than 15% of patients [25, 26]. In a retrospective, population-based study, 31.7% of patients reported a recurrence of symptoms, but 90.5% had minimal or no symptoms at a mean follow-up of 5.9 years [25]. In a systematic review involving eight studies, 83% of individuals reported complete recovery in two to three years [27].

Nerve root compression, spinal stenosis, and cervical myelopathy are important causes of cervical radiculopathy. The C7 and C6 nerve roots are most commonly involved. Disc herniation is associated with acute onset of symptoms, while insidious onset is associated with cervical spine spondylosis ((i.e., facet arthritis) [19]. Neck pain, upper extremity weakness, and diminished sensation (i.e., numbness) are key clinical signs. On physical examination, the specificity of the Spurling's test, shoulder abduction and neck distraction range from 80% to 90% but the sensitivity is less than 60% for the diagnosis of cervical radiculopathy. Although magnetic resonance imaging is widely used in the diagnostic evaluation of cervical radiculopathy, the false positive and false negative rates for diagnosing nerve root compression are 45% and 26%, respectively [28]. Electromyograph and nerve conduction studies can aid in the identification of nerve root dysfunction and identify the level or levels of nerve root involvement.

Cervical spine stenosis can involve the central spinal canal, lateral recesses, or intervertebral foramen. In the adult population, the estimated prevalence of cervical stenosis is 4.9%, but the prevalence increases with age; the prevalence is 6.8% among individuals 50 years or older and 9% among individuals older than 70 years [29]. Degenerative disc changes, facet joint and ligament hypertrophy, osteophyte formation, congenitally shortened pedicles, inflammatory disease processes, trauma, and previous spine surgery are potential causes of cervical spine stenosis. Clinical signs and symptoms include neck pain, upper extremity radicular pain in one or more dermatomes, reduced neck range of motion, and paraspinal tenderness. Magnetic resonance imaging, computerized tomography, and electrodiagnostic tests can aid in the diagnosis of cervical stenosis.

Cervical myelopathy results from compression of the spinal cord. The prevalence of cervical myelopathy is estimated to occur at a rate of 605 per million people [30]. Signs and symptoms are generally insidious in onset and include neck pain, upper extremity weakness, spasticity, hyperreflexia, impairments in fine motor function, and gait instability. Spinal cord compression and signal changes on T1 and T2 images are characteristic findings on MRI.

Treatments of the various causes of radicular neck pain overlap. For example, radicular pain can be treated with over the counter medications, analgesic antidepressants and anticonvulsants, muscle relaxants, and adjunct opioid therapy combined with physical modalities and integrative therapies [19]. Fluoroscopically guided interlaminar and CT-guided transforaminal epidural injections play an important role in treating cervical radicular pain and, when clinically indicated, some individuals may be candidates for spinal cord stimulation. Conservative management may only provide temporizing benefit for some individuals, and in the context of progressive pain or any symptoms of cervical myelopathy, referral for surgical management should be considered.

Non-radicular Low Back Pain

Non-radicular or axial low back pain is a leading cause of disability with a lifetime incidence of up to 84% [31]. Although approximately 30% of individuals will recover from a single episode of low back pain, at least 65% will continue to experience symptoms at 1-year follow-up [32]. Obesity, tobacco smoking, severe baseline disability, and a diagnosis of depression or anxiety are associated with development of chronic low back pain [33]. Intervertebral disc degeneration, facet joint and sacroiliac joint arthropathy, and several abdominal, paraspinal, and gluteal muscle groups are common sources of low back pain [34]. A stress fracture of the pars interarticularis, otherwise referred to as a pars defect, is a common source of low back pain in children and young adults. The incidence of pars defects is 6% to 8% and the vast majority involve the L5 vertebral body [35]. Neoplastic, inflammatory, and visceral disease processes, vascular, infectious, endocrine, and trauma are potential "red flag" causes of low back pain. Physical examination tests and imaging guidelines can aid in the evaluation and diagnosis of low back pain [34]. A vast array of physical modalities, structured exercise programs, integrative and psychological therapies, pharmacotherapies, image-guided spine injections including intraosseous basivertebral nerve ablation [36, 37], spinal cord stimulation and intrathecal drug therapy, and surgical management are used to treat low back pain [34].

Radicular Low Back Pain

Approximately 3% to 5% of adults experience symptoms of radicular low back pain [38]. At 1-month follow-up, 58% will report resolution of symptoms and 88% will be symptom free at 6 months [39]. In a systematic review that involved 38 studies, the incidence of symptomatic regression was 69% [40].

Nerve root compression and spinal stenosis are common causes of radicular back pain. Approximately 90% of cases are due to a herniated intervertebral disc of nerve roots at the L4-L5 or L5-S1 levels [41, 42]. Disc herniation is associated with acute onset of symptoms over 1 to 2 days, but an insidious onset is generally seen when nerve compression occurs in the context of foraminal stenosis associated with spondylosis. An important characteristic of nerve root compression is the distribution of pain, which should occur in dermatomal pattern, but up to one-third of patients may have multiple affected dermatomes [43]. Radicular pain is often described as sharp and burning, and pain can worsen with coughing and sneezing but is often improved with recumbency. Similar to non-radicular low back pain, the clinical evaluation should focus on identifying non-musculoskeletal or "red flag" causes of pain [34]. On physical examination, the sensitivity and specificity of the straight leg raise maneuver for identifying lumbar radiculopathy is 64% and 57%, respectively. The cross straight leg raise test, weakness in the great toe with dorsiflexion or extension, and impaired Achilles tendon reflexes all possess a sensitivity under 30%, but the specificities of these physical examination maneuvers exceed 93% in detecting lumbar radiculopathy [34].

Lumbar spine stenosis is often associated with both axial and radicular pain and is typically caused by a combination of disc protrusion, facet hypertrophy, and ligamentum flavum hypertrophy. The incidence of lumbar spine stenosis is estimated to be 5 cases per 100,000 people [44]. The hallmark symptom of lumbar spine stenosis is neurogenic claudication, which is also referred to as pseudoclaudication. Neurogenic claudication is typically associated with worsening radicular pain when standing or walking, but pain quickly dissipates in the seated position. The sensitivity and specificity of neurogenic claudication for lumbar spine stenosis is 88% and 34%, respectively [45]. In general, lumbar extension (i.e., reduction of lumbar spine cross-sectional area) worsens neural compression and pain, while lumbar flexion (i.e., increase in lumbar spine cross-sectional area) reduces compression and lessens pain [46, 47]. Other important distinguishing characteristics include age greater than 65 (sensitivity, 77%; specificity, 69%) and bilateral buttock or leg pain (sensitivity, 88%; specificity, 34%) [45, 48]. On physical examination, the presence of motor or sensory findings is generally useful in diagnosing lumbar spine stenosis, but the sensitivity and specificity of any specific physical examination maneuver vary widely [34]. Magnetic resonance imaging or computerized tomography of the lumbar spine can identify areas of stenosis, and electromyography (EMG) and nerve conduction testing (NCV) can be used to further localize specific nerve involvement.

Abrupt compression of the cauda equina due to massive disc herniation, a neoplastic process, or spine infection is characterized by rapid onset of radicular or low back pain, leg weakness, loss of perineal sensation, and bowel/bladder dysfunction. This constellation of symptoms is referred to as cauda equina syndrome and it is considered a surgical emergency.

Treatments of the various causes of radicular low back pain overlap. A broad range of medications are used to treat radicular low back pain including antidepressants, antiepileptics, NSAIDs, and acetaminophen. Fluoroscopically guided interlaminar or transforaminal epidural steroid injections are widely used, and spinal cord stimulation may provide long-term pain relief in carefully selected patients [34]. Physical and behavioral therapies, graded exercise, and a broad range of other integrative therapies are widely used to treat radicular low back pain [34]. A broad range of surgical techniques are available to treat radicular low back pain including spinal decompression, foraminotomies, discectomy, and disc prosthesis [34].

Musculoskeletal Pain

The prevalence of musculoskeletal pain affecting the upper extremities ranges from 8% to 28% [49], and the prevalence of hip and knee pain ranges from 14% to 25%, which increases in adults over 65 years of age [50, 51]. Sources of musculoskeletal pain can be generally categorized as involving soft tissues, joints, or both. Soft tissues comprise a broad range of recognized pain disorders [52] which are often associated with large and small joint pain. The most common cause of arthralgia is osteoarthritis, but inflammatory conditions such as rheumatological rheumatological disorders, injury, and infectious disease processes are important contributors. In addition to targeted imaging, which may include plain radiographs combined with MRI or CT, a broad range of physical examination maneuvers for specific joints and muscle groups are used in the diagnostic evaluation. Treatment options include medications, targeted physical therapy interventions, image-guided injections (e.g., corticosteroid, viscosupplementation, platelet-rich plasma), and surgical procedures (total joint arthroplasty, arthroscopy).

Myofascial Pain

Myofascial pain is a regional pain syndrome characterized by the presence of trigger points involving muscles or fascia. Trigger points are taut muscle bands that refer pain in a defined pattern either spontaneously or after stimulation such as manual palpation or needle insertion. The potential causes of myofascial pain are not fully elucidated. Tender or injured muscles release acetylcholine and inflammatory mediators which, in turn, can lead to motor endplate dysfunction, focal ischemia, sarcomere dysfunction, and localized pain [24]. The prevalence estimates of myofascial pain vary widely but range from 30% to 85% [23, 53, 54]. The diagnosis of myofascial pain is based on the presence of 5 major and 1 of 3 minor criteria [55]. The five major criteria include (1) localized spontaneous pain, (2) hyperalgesia in the referred area of a trigger point, (3) palpable taut band in the affected muscle, (4) localized tenderness, and (5) reduced range of motion [55]. Minor criteria included (1) reproduction of spontaneous pain with manual stimulation of the trigger point, (2) evocation of a local twitch response, and 3) pain relieved with muscle stretch or trigger point injection [55]. Muscle stretching, strengthening, and aerobic exercise are widely used to treat myofascial pain. Other treatments include medications (e.g., tricyclic antidepressants, serotonin norepinephrine reuptake inhibitors, muscle relaxants), trigger point injections, topical anesthetics, botulinum toxin type A injections, acupuncture, and transcutaneous electrical nerve stimulation [56].

Visceral Pain

Pain originating from internal organs is referred to as visceral pain. Commonly encountered syndromes can involve thoracic, abdominal, and pelvic organs. Clinical characteristics of visceral pain include poor localization with referral to somatic structures, sensitization of somatic tissues, prominent autonomic and affective responses, and nonspecific motor responses [57]. In general, viscera project afferent fibers to the central nervous system via autonomic and parasympathetic nerves, and these fibers have both sensory and autonomic regulatory functions. Visceral and somatic afferent fibers converge, which is, in part, responsible for referred visceral pain where visceral stimulation produces pain in a somatic structure (e.g., abdominal wall). Continued exposure of visceral nociceptors to noxious stimulation can produce hyperalgesia which can, in turn, lead to central sensitization [58]. Treatment of visceral pain depends upon the involved organs. Analgesic medications are widely used including analgesic antidepressants [59], anticonvulsants [60], over the counter analgesics, topical agents, and adjunct opioids. Fluoroscopically guided blocks of the celiac plexus, superior hypogastric plexus, and ganglion impar are commonly used to treat abdominal and pelvic visceral pain [61]. Visceral functions are highly influenced by cognitive and emotional centers of the brain, and psychological therapy should be considered when high levels of negative affect or emotional dysregulation are evident [62, 63]. Implantation of an intrathecal drug delivery system [64] or spinal cord stimulator [65] may be warranted for visceral pain that is recalcitrant to conventional treatment.

Urogenital Pain

Pain localized to the pelvis, genitalia, or perineal regions often originates from pelvic viscera. One in seven women [66] and one in 13 men [67] will be affected by some form of chronic urogenital pain. Conditions common to both sexes include chronic interstitial cystitis and bladder pain syndrome. Sex-specific conditions include endometriosis, dysmenorrhea, and vulvodynia in women and prostatitis, orchialgia and proctodynia in men. Neurological (e.g., pudendal neuralgia, genitofemoral neuralgia, iliohypogastric neuralgia, ilioinguinal neuralgia), musculoskeletal (e.g. levator ani spasm, osteitis pubis, piriformis syndrome, sacroiliac joint disorders), gastrointestinal [68, 69] (e.g., chronic constipation, hemorrhoids, proctalgia fugax, proctitis, diverticulitis), oncological (e.g., neoplasm, cystic mesothelioma), and rheumatological (e.g., fibromyalgia, rheumatoid arthritis, spondylopathies) systems are other potential sources of urogenital pain. A goal of physical examination is to localize the source of pain by carefully reproducing the patients' symptoms. Diagnostic imaging (e.g., MRI, CT, plain roentgenograms), laboratory evaluations (e.g., urinalysis and culture, testing for sexually transmitted infections, assessing inflammatory and autoimmune markers), and urological testing (e.g., voiding cystourethrogram) can help establish the diagnosis. Medications used to treat urogenital pain include NSAIDs [70], alpha-blockers [70, 71], analgesic antidepressants [71–73] (e.g., tricyclic antidepressants, norepinephrine serotonin reuptake inhibitors), muscle relaxants (e.g. baclofen suppositories) and antiepileptics in some [73, 74] but not all studies [68, 69, 75] (e.g., pregabalin, gabapentin). Depending on the underlying diagnosis, surgery may be indicated, but other procedural interventions are available including diagnostic and therapeutic image-guided nerve blocks [76], trigger point injections [77, 78], botulinum toxin A [79–81], and neuromodulation [65, 82, 83] (e.g., dorsal root ganglion stimulation, dorsal column spinal cord stimulation). Interdisciplinary rehabilitation [84–86] and psychological therapies [63, 87] are often indicated due to impairments in emotional and physical functioning.

Pain During Pregnancy and Labor

The estimated incidence of pain during pregnancy is 55% [88] and the most frequently affected body regions include the low back (41%), hips (28%), and feet (22%) [88]. Migraine headache, fibromyalgia, pelvic pain, and autoimmune diseases are commonly occurring chronic pain conditions that are frequently encountered during pregnancy. Although migraine and autoimmune disease-related symptoms often improve during pregnancy, low back, and pelvic pain frequently worsen due, in part, to the effects of estrogen and progesterone on musculoskeletal structures. Magnetic resonance imaging and ultrasound are the imaging modalities of choice during pregnancy because avoiding ionizing radiation is critically important. When indicated, nonpharmacologic treatments (e.g., physical therapy, psychological therapies), including ultrasound-guided injections (e.g., sacroiliac injections, trigger point injections), are preferred in order to minimize the risks of pharmacotherapy to the neonate. However, commonly used analgesic medications include acetaminophen, NSAIDs, low dose opioids, and local anesthetics.

Analgesia during labor and delivery is dependent, in part, on the stage of labor [89]. Visceral pain predominates during the first stage of labor due to cervical dilation and distention of the lower uterine segments. Afferent nerve fibers from these structures travel with the sympathetic chain and enter the dorsal root ganglia at the T10-L1 level. Somatic pain predominates during the second stage due to distention of the pelvic floor, perineum, and pelvic structures surrounding the vagina. The pudendal nerve carries nociceptive impulses from these structures to the dorsal root ganglia at the S2-S4 levels. Neuraxial analgesia (e.g., epidural, spinal, combined spinal epidural) is widely used for labor analgesia but to be effective during the first stage of labor, T10-L1 level must be blocked, and the S2-S4 levels must be blocked to provide analgesia during the second stage [90]. Other interventions for labor analgesia include systemic opioids, nitrous oxide, and nonpharmacologic techniques such as acupuncture, acupressure, massage, relaxation, hydrotherapy, and incorporation of a support person [91, 92].

Headache and Orofacial Pain

Headache

Headache disorders are one of the most prevalent and disabling conditions worldwide [93]. Approximately 95% of the general population experience headaches at some point in life. Data from the Global Burden of Disease Study reveal an estimated global prevalence of 14.0% for migraines and 26.0% for tension-type headaches [94].

Headaches are stratified into primary headaches and secondary headaches. Primary headache, which constitutes the vast majority of all headaches (98%), is defined as a headache that is unrelated to an underlying medical condition [95]. Primary headache disorders commonly include tension-type headache (TTH), migraine with or without aura, and trigeminal autonomic cephalalgias. Trigeminal autonomic cephalalgias consist of cluster headaches, paroxysmal hemicrania, short-lasting unilateral neuralgiform headache attacks with conjunctival injection and tearing (SUNCT), and hemicrania continua. Secondary headache is due to an underlying medical condition, which can include a space-occupying lesion such as malignancy, infection such as meningitis or encephalitis, subarachnoid hemorrhage, vascular disease such as giant-cell arteritis or cerebral venous thrombosis, and idiopathic intracranial hypertension [95].

A thorough history and physical examination including a focused neurological exam is critical for establishing the correct headache diagnosis. Details should be obtained on headache location and laterality, character, frequency, duration, chronicity, and other accompanying symptoms such as autonomic symptoms, nausea, photophobia, and phonophobia [93]. Further, the clinician should investigate the presence of notable red flag signs and symptoms including sudden onset of a thunderclap headache, new-onset headache in a patient older than 50 or younger than 10 years of age, the presence of systemic symptoms (e.g. fever), history of malignancy or compromised immunity, neurological deficits, changes in the pattern of pain, pregnancy, and progressive worsening of headache over several weeks [96]. The presence of a red flag sign or symptom may prompt the need for further evaluation with a headache specialist and diagnostic testing with neuroimaging [96].

Tension-type headache presents with a bilateral pressure-like sensation in the frontal and/or temporal regions [93]. Chronic TTH is defined as 15 or more headache-days per month for at least three months. First-line abortive treatment includes NSAIDs, while first-line preventive treatment includes a tricyclic antidepressant (e.g., amitriptyline) [97].

Migraine headache manifests with unilateral or bilateral throbbing pain along any part of the head and is frequently accompanied by nausea, vomiting, photophobia, and phonophobia [93]. Premonitory symptoms, aura, and postdromal symptoms may also occur. Abortive pharmacotherapy for acute migraine includes acetaminophen, NSAIDs, triptans, ergot derivatives, ditans, and gepants [93]. Although triptans are commonly used abortive agents, this class of medication should be avoided in patients with coronary artery disease, stroke, and peripheral arterial disease given their vasoconstrictive effects via the 5-HT_{1B} serotonin subtype receptor [98]. Caution is recommended if triptans are prescribed to patients on concomitant antidepressants that may increase the risk for serotonin syndrome [99]. Ditans (e.g., lasmiditan) were initially developed in 2019 and are a class of abortives with serotonin activity that is more highly selective for the 5-HT_{1F} receptor subtype, resulting in lower risk for vasoconstrictive adverse events compared to triptans [98]. Gepants (e.g., rimegepant, ubrogepant) are calcitonin gene-related peptide (CGRP) inhibitors with high efficacy but can cause nausea and dizziness [100]. Preventive pharmacotherapy for migraines includes antihypertensives (e.g., propranolol), antidepressants (e.g., amitriptyline), and antiepiletic drugs (e.g., topiramate). In patients with refractory symptoms, monoclonal antibodies to calcitonin gene-related peptide (CGRP) (e.g., galcanezumab) or its receptor (e.g., erenumab) may be offered as prophylactic pharamacotherapy [100]. Neuromodulation may also be used to treat migraine and includes either non-invasive vagal nerve stimulators, transcranial magnetic stimulators, and transcutaneous supraorbital neurostimulators [101]. Advanced interventional options include injection therapy with onabotulinum toxin A, sphenopalatine ganglion block, implantable peripheral nerve stimulation of the trigeminal nerve or vagus nerve, and high-cervical dorsal column spinal cord stimulation [93, 102–104].

Cluster headache presents with sharp, unilateral pain in the orbital and/or frontal areas accompanied by ipsilateral autonomic symptoms of conjunctival injection, ptosis, miosis, and rhinorrhea [105]. Cluster headaches last between 30 minutes to 3 hours and have a circadian periodicity and circannual attack periods [105]. Abortive therapy includes triptans, high-flow oxygen administration, vagus nerve stimulation, and sphenopalatine ganglion block [106]. Preventive treatment consists of verapamil, lithium, CGRP monoclonal antibodies, and vagus nerve stimulation [106].

In primary headaches with atypical features or refractory cases of primary headache, alternative diagnoses due to secondary causes should be investigated. Cervicogenic headache may occur due to pathology in various anatomical structures of the cervical spine. A common occurrence is cervical spine facet joint osteoarthritis with referred headaches in the occipital region that can be treated with intra-articular facet steroid injection therapy or radiofrequency ablation of cervical medial branch nerves [107]. Occipital neuralgia is another common cause of headaches localized to the occiput and can be treated with steroid injection therapy targeting the occipital nerves at the level of the occiput or C2 nerve root, as well as implantable peripheral nerve stimulation [103, 108].

Orofacial Pain

Orofacial pain is defined as pain located in the face, head, or neck and may result from musculoskeletal, neurovascular, and neuropathic etiologies. The prevalence of orofacial pain is 17% to 26% in the general population and the prevalence is greater in females [109, 110]. Toothache is the most prevalent facial pain complaint followed by temporomandibular disorder (TMD) which frequently involves the temporomandibular joint (TMJ), masticatory muscles, and other musculoskeletal structures of the head and neck [111]. Accompanying symptoms may include otalgia, tinnitus, and dizziness [111]. Trauma to the ligaments, cartilage, disc, or bone in the TMJ may lead to oxidative stress and pro-inflammatory cytokines, which can adversely modulate TMJ function and lead to sensitization [112]. Genetic polymorphisms may increase the risk of abnormal pain responsiveness and processing, which may contribute to the development of chronic TMD [113]. Although anatomical and pathological mechanisms play a role in TMD, the etiology is often multifactorial involving behavioral, environmental, emotional, and social factors [114]. Furthermore, an association exists between chronic TMDs and mental health conditions (e.g., depression, anxiety, posttraumatic stress disorder, childhood abuse) [115].

Osteoarthritis and disc-condyle pathology affecting the TMJ are the most common anatomical abnormalities associated with TMJ pain [116]. Several types of disc-condyle pathology have been described including varying combinations of disc displacement with reduction, intermittent locking, and limitation in opening. Additional anatomical sources of TMJ pain include neoplasms (e.g., chondroma, osteochondroma, malignancy) [117], disorders in masticatory muscles involving overuse and muscle tissue ischemia, and myofascial pain [118].

Treatment options for TMDs are dependent on the underlying etiology [119]. First-line treatment involves conservative therapy with a combination of physical therapy, acupuncture, massage therapy, and cognitive behavioral therapy [119]. Application of oral appliances such as oral orthotics or occlusal appliances, changes to oral parafunction habits, and changes in dietary habits such as avoidance of hard and highly viscous foods may facilitate reduction in stress to the TMJ [119]. Pharmacotherapeutic options include NSAIDs, muscle relaxants, systemic steroids, and neuromodulating agents such as antidepressants and anticonvulsants [119, 120]. Injection therapy with botulinum toxin A is particularly helpful for masticatory muscle disorders and bruxism [121]. Surgical options to correct structural pathology may include arthrocentesis, arthroscopy, arthrotomy, and reconstructive jaw surgery [119, 120].

Neurovascular orofacial pain refers to pain in the intraoral region without head pain [122]. This condition manifests with toothache-like sensations or pulsatile pain. This disorder does not respond to dental treatment but responds to abortive and preventive anti-migraine pharmaceuticals such as triptans [122].

Cranial neuralgia is defined as pain originating from cervical or craniofacial nerves, which may include trigeminal, glossopharyngeal, vagus, or occipital nerves [123]. The quality of pain from cranial neuralgia is described as paroxysmal, lancinating, and lighting-type quality exacerbated by tactile triggers or physical stimuli to the face. Cranial neuralgia may be a primary disorder or the result of an underlying secondary disease process. In addition to conservative therapy and pharmacotherapy mentioned above for other headache disorders, additional options may include nerve blocks with steroid and local anesthetic, pulsed radiofrequency ablation, and implantable peripheral nerve stimulation [103, 124, 125]. Peripheral nerve stimulation is typically offered for occipital neuralgia [103]. Additional interventional and surgical options for trigeminal neuralgia include microvascular decompression, glycerol rhizotomy, and gamma knife radiosurgery [126].

Less frequently encountered facial pain conditions [127] include persistent idiopathic facial pain, idiopathic dentoalveolar pain, and burning mouth syndrome (BMS) [128], which presents with intraoral burning and dysesthesias without oral structural pathology. Burning mouth syndrome is a diagnosis of exclusion and treatment is restricted to topical therapies, analgesic antidepressants, and antiepileptics [128]. Other infrequently encountered conditions include giant cell arteritis [129], myocardial ischemia [130], oropharyngeal carcinomas, and brain tumors involving the middle cranial fossa or cerebellopontine angle [131].

Nerve Damage

Neuropathic Pain

Neuropathic pain is defined as pain arising from a lesion or disease process involving the peripheral or central nervous system [127]. The estimated prevalence of neuropathic pain in the general population ranges from 7% to 15% [132, 133], but in adults with diabetes the estimated prevalence is 21% [134]. Neuropathic pain generally results from injury to unmyelinated C fibers and myelinated $A\beta$ and $A\delta$ fibers [135]. The pathophysiology of neuropathic pain is related, in part, to the increase in density of voltage-gated sodium channels at the site of injury producing ectopic discharges and hyperexcitability [136]. Other contributing pathophysiological mechanisms include alterations in the distribution of transient receptor potential vanilloid type 1 ($TRPV_1$) channels, extension of sympathetic fibers into the region of the dorsal root ganglion, and reductions in spinal cord inhibitory controls [136, 137].

Abnormalities in sensation and pain perception characterize neuropathic pain and common clinical signs, and symptoms include paresthesias, dysesthesia, hyperalgesia, and allodynia [135]. Pain is often described as a burning, tingling, pins and needles, or shooting sensation [135, 136]. Although the majority of painful peripheral neuropathies involve the lower extremities, particularly the feet, upper extremity involvement can also occur. Common findings on physical examination include reduced tactile, thermal, and vibratory sensation; loss of deep tendon reflexes in the involved body regions; and reduced muscle strength. Electrodiagnostic testing (e.g., EMG, NCV) can be useful for localizing the level of nerve dysfunction (e.g., nerve root vs. plexus vs. peripheral nerve) and for identifying the presence of active demyelination [138]. Electrodiagnostic testing may be within normal limits if the peripheral neuropathy only involves small fibers; if a painful small-fiber neuropathy is suspected, reduced density of small-fibers on skin biopsy may help establish the diagnosis [139]. Laboratory testing is also essential to identify any underlying disease process or reversible cause of painful neuropathy. Although the differential diagnosis is broad, general diagnostic categories include autoimmune, infectious, nutritional deficiencies, toxic, oncological, or metabolic disease processes.

Treatment of painful neuropathies is dependent on etiology. Any reversible causes or identified disease process should be treated, which may require referral to the appropriate medical specialist. Antiepileptics (e.g., gabapentin, pregabalin, valproate), serotonin-norepinephrine reuptake inhibitors (e.g., duloxetine, venlafaxine), and tricyclic antidepressant medications (nortriptyline, amitriptyline) are effective treatments [140]. Simple analgesics (e.g., acetaminophen, NSAIDS), herbal remedies (e.g., alpha lipoic acid, acetyl-L-carnitine), low dose opioids, and topical agents (e.g., lidocaine 5% patch) can be used solely or combined with other agents to develop a multimodal pharmacologic treatment plan [141]. Aerobic exercise, acupuncture, and psychological interventions including cognitive behavioral therapy may also be indicated [142, 143]. Spinal cord [144, 145] or dorsal root ganglion [146] stimulation and intrathecal drug therapy [147, 148] should be considered for painful neuropathies recalcitrant to conventional treatments.

Complex Regional Pain Syndrome

Signs and symptoms of complex regional pain syndrome (CRPS) predominately occur following fracture (up to 48.5% of incident cases [149]), trauma, or surgery. Two CRPS subtypes have been described based on the absence or presence of nerve injury; (1) type 1 occurs in the absence of identifiable nerve injury, and (2) type 2 occurs in the setting of nerve injury. The estimated incidence of CRPS 1 and CRPS 2 in a US population-based study was 5.46 and 0.82 per 100,000 person-years, respectively [150], while the overall incidence of CRPS in a European population-based study was 26.2 per 100,000 person-years [151]. The female to male ratio ranges from 3:1 to 4:1, and the peak age of onset ranges from 46 to 70 years of age [150, 151].

Upregulation of sympathetic activity, proinflammatory changes contributing to peripheral sensitization, development of autoantibodies, and development of central sensitization have been implicated in the pathogenesis of CRPS [152]. The diagnostic criteria for CRPS, commonly referred to as the Budapest criteria, have a sensitivity and specificity of 99% and 69%, respectively [153]. The Budapest criteria are based on signs and symptoms from four categories: (1) sensory (e.g., allodynia, hyperalgesia), (2) vasomotor (e.g., skin color and temperature changes), (3) sudo-motor/edema (e.g., altered sweating, edema), and (4) motor/tropic (e.g., reduced range of motion, trophic change affecting skin, hair, and nails). The diagnostic criteria also require the presence of pain disproportionate to the inciting event and the absence of any other disease process that could better explain the constellation of symptoms. Triple-phase bone scan [154], plain radiographs, quantitative sensory testing to assess sudomotor function [155], and EMG/NCV [156] may support the diagnosis of CRPS and aid in identifying other contributing disease processes, but CRPS remains a clinical diagnosis.

Physical therapy, exercise, mirror therapy, and graded motor imagery are widely used to treat CRPS-related pain and impairments in functioning [157]. Multiple medications are used including antiepileptics, analgesic antidepressants, NSAIDs, and topical agents [158, 159]. Intravenous ketamine and bisphosphonates may also contribute to the analgesic effects of a multimodal pharmacologic treatment plan [158, 159]. Fluoroscopically guided or ultrasound-guided [160, 161] lumbar sympathetic [162] and stellate ganglion [163] blocks are widely used for lower and upper extremity CRPS, respectively, and spinal cord [164] and dorsal root ganglion [165, 166] stimulation are associated with improvements in pain and functionality. A combination of psychological, behavioral, and psychopharmacologic therapies should be considered when comorbid mental health conditions are identified [167, 168].

Special Cases

Pain in Infants, Children, Adolescents, and Older Adults

In children, pain assessment is dependent on developmental stage and age. Neonates (age less than 4 weeks) and infants (age up to 1 year) are preverbal, and pain assessment is based on assessing behaviors and physiologic parameters. The Neonatal Infant Pain Scale quantifies the severity of procedural pain by assessing facial expression, intensity of crying, breathing patterns, arm and leg position, and state of arousal [169]. The CRIES Scale assesses postoperative pain in infants using information collected across five domains: (1) severity of crying, (2) oxygen requirements, (3) increased heart rate and blood pressure, (4) expression (e.g., grimace, grunt), and (5) level of Sleeplessness [170]. In children 2 to 7 years of age, the FLACC Scale assesses pain using signs and symptoms from five categories: (1) face, (2) legs (e.g., position and movement), (3) activity level, (4) cry level, and (5) Consolability [171]. A revised FLACC Scale has been developed for use in children with cognitive impairments [172]. In children 8 to 12 years of age, the verbal numeric pain scale [173] or the FACES Pain Rating Scale [174] can be used to accurately assess pain.

Assessment of pain in older adults can be confounded by cognitive deficits due to a broad range of neurodegenerative and cerebrovascular disorders. The Pain

Assessment in Advanced Dementia assesses pain using signs and symptoms from five domains: (1) breathing with no vocalization, (2) distressed vocalizations, (3) facial expressions, (4) body posture, and (5) consolability [175]. Other assessment instruments include the Pain Assessment in Impaired Cognition [176] and the Pain Assessment Checklist for Seniors with Limited Ability to Communicate [177].

Pain Issues in Individuals with Limited Ability to Communicate Due to Neurocognitive Impairments

Aphasia is a neurocognitive impairment in expressive or receptive language processing that can affect the ability to communicate by speaking, reading, writing, and listening. Aphasia is an acquired disorder generally occurring in the context of an acute left hemispheric stroke, but other causes include head trauma, tumor, encephalitis, or neurodegenerative disorders. Word-finding difficulties, slurred speech, difficulties interpreting language, and frustration when attempting to produce speech are common signs of aphasia. Subtypes of aphasia are generally categorized based on the ability to formulate intelligible speech (e.g., expressive aphasia), impairments in the production of understandable speech (e.g., motor aphasia characterized by dysarthria or dysphonia), or impairments in the ability to comprehend speech, which may involve other modalities of communication (e.g., writing, reading, auditory). In clinical practice, the subtypes of aphasia often overlap. Knowledge about pain assessment in adults with aphasia or compromised ability to communicate represents an unmet need [178]. The Pain Assessment in the Communicatively Impaired tool has been validated for use in patients residing in long-term care facilities [179, 180] but not in patients with aphasia. In a systematic review, the vertical visual analog scale and Faces Pain Scale were recommended for use in patients with aphasia, but a reliable and valid pain rating instrument for patients with aphasia is not currently available [181].

Pain Relief in Persons with Substance Use and Addiction Disorders

Addiction is defined by the American Society of Addiction Medicine as a complex interaction between brain circuits, genetics, the environment, and individual life experiences resulting in compulsive behaviors that persist despite harmful consequences [182]. The term *addiction* has been preferentially replaced in nomenclature by *substance use disorder* (SUD) to reduce stigma and encourage patients to access healthcare to aid in symptom management. SUDs are diagnosed using the *Diagnostic and Statistical Manual, fifth edition* (DSM-5) [183] where diagnostic criteria are applied to identify patterns of maladaptive substance use leading to physical or mental impairments in functioning. Neurobiologically, substance use is reinforced, or rewarded, by amplifying dopaminergic activity in the striatum, globus pallidus, thalamus, and nucleus accumbens [184].

The estimated prevalence of any SUD in adults with chronic pain ranges from 3% to 48% [185], and the estimated prevalence of opioid use disorder (OUD) in adults receiving long-term opioid therapy ranges from 21% to 36% [186, 187]. Although SUD screening instruments are widely used in clinical practice, scores should be interpreted cautiously with awareness of the sensitivity and specificity of the recommended cutoff score for each individual screening tool. For example, the Current Opioid Misuse Measure cutoff score of 10 has a sensitivity and specificity of 85% and 82%, respectively [188], and the CAGE questionnaire cutoff score of 8 for identifying alcohol misuse has a sensitivity and specificity of 71% and 90%, respectively [189].

The most effective therapy for OUD includes medication assisted treatment (MAT) (e.g., buprenorphine combined with naloxone methadone, or naltrexone) [190, 191] but patients also benefit from a variety of psychosocial interventions with or without concomitant MAT [191–194]. When opioid tapering is under consideration or clinically indicated, clinicians should use a patient-centered approach [34, 195]. Treatment of chronic pain in the context of SUDs, including OUD, should focus on optimizing non-opioid analgesic medications [196], incorporating behavioral and psychological therapies [197, 198], and ensuring access to advanced procedural interventions [199, 200]. Considerations for managing acute pain include incorporating a multimodal approach and careful management of concomitant use of medications for OUD (e.g., buprenorphine) [201–203]. Patients with SUD on buprenorphine should continue this medication in the pre-operative and perioperative period [204].

Pain Relief in Areas of Deprivation and Conflict

In the developing world and regions of the world embroiled in conflict, unique barriers limit delivering analgesic care to people with cancer-related pain [205], HIV/AIDS [206], neuropathic pain related to environmental exposures [207, 208], and trauma including trauma stemming for torture [209–211]. Poorly functioning pharmaceutical delivery processes [212] including legal barriers limiting access to opioids [213], lack of effective healthcare polices, and limited access to healthcare education and training are critical barriers to deploying comprehensive pain care in the developing world [214–216]. Proposed solutions towards improving pain care include increasing awareness of the importance of pain care among political and healthcare leaders, increasing the availability of low-cost educational materials (e.g., internet-based materials, prior-edition print textbooks), on-site teaching and mentorship, and increasing access to real time video-based clinical teaching [214, 217, 218].

Pain Relief in Culturally and Linguistically Diverse People

The burden of chronic pain is influenced by a complex array of cultural and linguistic factors. In defined populations, culturally and linguistically diverse (CALD) community members experience a greater prevalence of pain [219, 220] and are at greater risk of receiving inadequate pain care [221–223]. Beliefs about pain causation, approaches to pain management, and the differences in attitudes about patient autonomy influence physiotherapy-based pain care in people with chronic pain from CALD communities [224]. Furthermore, the intersection of social identities may contribute to the unequal burden of chronic pain in communities of CALD people [225]. More specifically, ethnocultural, social class, gender, and migration status coalesce to create and sustain health disparities in people from CALD communities [225]. Effective clinical and educational interventions aimed at chronic disease management and prevention include (1) use of bi-lingual community-based health care workers, (2) deployment of cultural competency training for health care workers, (3) use of interpreter services for CALD people, (4) distribution of culturally sensitive multimedia health promotion materials for CALD communities, and (5) the creation of community-based point-of-care services for CALD patients [226].

Summary

Pain is a complex process originating in real or perceived injury to tissues or viscera but is always overlaid by the patient psychological experience of the pain. Multiple treatment modalities exist to treat these acute or chronic symptoms, and typically a multi-modal approach achieves the best outcomes, especially when accounting for special cases such as patients with substance use disorders. Other challenging populations include pediatric patients, patients living in resource limited areas, and patients with communication barriers (organic or linguistic/cultural). A patient-centered approach should always be prioritized when treating pain of any duration in any patient population as this is the hallmark of an empathetic and successful pain physician.

References[1]

1. International Classification of Diseases, Eleventh Revision (ICD-11), World Health Organization (WHO) 2019/2021.
2. American Medical Association. CPT (Current Procedural Terminology. https://www.ama-assn.org/amaone/cpt-current-procedural-terminology
3. Todd KH, Ducharme J, Choiniere M, Crandall CS, Fosnocht DE, Homel P, Tanabe P, Group PS. Pain in the emergency department: results of the pain and emergency medicine initiative (PEMI) multicenter study. J Pain. 2007;8(6):460–6.

---

[1](*) denotes essential references for additional reading.

4. *Wu CL, Hung YL, Wang YR, Huang HM, Chang CH, Wu CC, Hung CJ, Yeh TF. Pain prevalence in hospitalized patients at a tertiary academic medical center: exploring severe persistent pain. PLoS One. 2020;15(12):e0243574.
5. Medzhitov R. The spectrum of inflammatory responses. Science. 2021;374(6571):1070–5.
6. Nathan C. Nonresolving inflammation redux. Immunity. 2022;55(4):592–605.
7. *Park R, Mohiuddin M, Arellano R, Pogatzki-Zahn E, Klar G, Gilron I. Prevalence of postoperative pain after hospital discharge: systematic review and meta-analysis. Pain Rep. 2023;8(3):e1075. https://doi.org/10.1097/PR9.0000000000001075. PMID: 37181639; PMCID: PMC10168527.
8. Yang MMH, Hartley RL, Leung AA, Ronksley PE, Jette N, Casha S, Riva-Cambrin J. Preoperative predictors of poor acute postoperative pain control: A systematic review and meta-analysis. BMJ Open. 2019;9(4):e025091.
9. Sharma LR, Schaldemose EL, Alaverdyan H, Nikolajsen L, Chen D, Bhanvadia S, Komen H, Yaeger L, Haroutounian S. Perioperative factors associated with persistent postsurgical pain after hysterectomy, cesarean section, prostatectomy, and donor nephrectomy: a systematic review and meta-analysis. Pain. 2022;163(3):425–35.
10. Johansen A, Romundstad L, Nielsen CS, Schirmer H, Stubhaug A. Persistent postsurgical pain in a general population: prevalence and predictors in the tromso study. Pain. 2012;153(7):1390–6.
11. Glare P, Aubrey KR, Myles PS. Transition from acute to chronic pain after surgery. Lancet. 2019;393(10180):1537–46.
12. Willingham M, Rangrass G, Curcuru C, Ben Abdallah A, Wildes TS, McKinnon S, Kronzer A, Sharma A, Helsten D, Hall B, Avidan MS, Haroutounian S. Association between postoperative complications and lingering post-surgical pain: an observational cohort study. Br J Anaesth. 2020;124(2):214–21.
13. Allen C, Walker AM, Premji ZA, Beauchemin-Turcotte ME, Wong J, Soh S, Hawboldt GS, Shinkaruk KS, Archer DP. Preventing persistent postsurgical pain: a systematic review and component network meta-analysis. Eur J Pain. 2022;26(4):771–85.
14. Fejer R, Kyvik KO, Hartvigsen J. The prevalence of neck pain in the world population: a systematic critical review of the literature. Eur Spine J. 2006;15(6):834–48.
15. Croft PR, Lewis M, Papageorgiou AC, Thomas E, Jayson MIV, Macfarlane GJ, Silman AJ. Risk factors for neck pain: a longitudinal study in the general population. Pain. 2001;93(3):317–25.
16. Linton SJ. A review of psychological risk factors in back and neck pain. Spine (Phila Pa 1976). 2000;25(9):1148–56.
17. Nilsen TI, Holtermann A, Mork PJ. Physical exercise, body mass index, and risk of chronic pain in the low back and neck/shoulders: longitudinal data from the Nord-Trondelag health study. Am J Epidemiol. 2011;174(3):267–73.
18. Yabe Y, Hagiwara Y, Sekiguchi T, Sugawara Y, Tsuchiya M, Yoshida S, Tsuji I. Sleep disturbance is associated with neck pain: a 3-year longitudinal study after the great East Japan earthquake. BMC Musculoskelet Disord. 2022;23(1):459.
19. Cohen SP, Hooten WM. Advances in the diagnosis and management of neck pain. BMJ. 2017;358:j3221.
20. Haroutiunian S, Drennan DA, Lipman AG. Topical NSAID therapy for musculoskeletal pain. Pain Med. 2010;11(4):535–49.
21. Borenstein DG, Korn S. Efficacy of a low-dose regimen of cyclobenzaprine hydrochloride in acute skeletal muscle spasm: results of two placebo-controlled trials. Clin Ther. 2003;25(4):1056–73.
22. Hurley RW, Adams MCB, Barad M, Bhaskar A, Bhatia A, Chadwick A, Deer TR, Hah J, Hooten WM, Kissoon NR, Lee DW, McCormick Z, Moon JY, Narouze S, Provenzano DA, Schneider BJ, van Eerd M, Van Zundert J, Wallace MS, Wilson SM, Zhao Z, Cohen SP. Consensus practice guidelines on interventions for cervical spine (facet) joint pain from a multispecialty international working group. Reg Anesth Pain Med. 2022;47(1):3–59.

23. Chiarotto A, Clijsen R, Fernandez-de-Las-Penas C, Barbero M. Prevalence of myofascial trigger points in spinal disorders: a systematic review and meta-analysis. Arch Phys Med Rehabil. 2016;97(2):316–37.
24. Kuan TS. Current studies on myofascial pain syndrome. Curr Pain Headache Rep. 2009;13(5):365–9.
25. Radhakrishnan K, Litchy WJ, O'Fallon WM, Kurland LT. Epidemiology of cervical radiculopathy. A population-based study from Rochester, Minnesota, 1976 through 1990. Brain. 1994;117(Pt 2):325–35.
26. Woods BI, Hilibrand AS. Cervical radiculopathy: epidemiology, etiology, diagnosis, and treatment. J Spinal Disord Tech. 2015;28(5):E251–9.
27. Wong JJ, Cote P, Quesnele JJ, Stern PJ, Mior SA. The course and prognostic factors of symptomatic cervical disc herniation with radiculopathy: a systematic review of the literature. Spine J. 2014;14(8):1781–9.
28. Kuijper B, Tans JT, van der Kallen BF, Nollet F, Lycklama ANGJ, de Visser M. Root compression on MRI compared with clinical findings in patients with recent onset cervical radiculopathy. J Neurol Neurosurg Psychiatry. 2011;82(5):561–3.
29. Lee MJ, Cassinelli EH, Riew KD. Prevalence of cervical spine stenosis. Anatomic study in cadavers. J Bone Joint Surg Am. 2007;89(2):376–80.
30. Nouri A, Tetreault L, Singh A, Karadimas SK, Fehlings MG. Degenerative cervical myelopathy: epidemiology, genetics, and pathogenesis. Spine (Phila Pa 1976). 2015;40(12):E675–93.
31. Henschke N, Kamper SJ, Maher CG. The epidemiology and economic consequences of pain. Mayo Clin Proc. 2015;90(1):139–47.
32. Itz CJ, Geurts JW, van Kleef M, Nelemans P. Clinical course of non-specific low back pain: a systematic review of prospective cohort studies set in primary care. Eur J Pain. 2013;17(1):5–15.
33. Stevans JM, Delitto A, Khoja SS, Patterson CG, Smith CN, Schneider MJ, Freburger JK, Greco CM, Freel JA, Sowa GA, Wasan AD, Brennan GP, Hunter SJ, Minick KI, Wegener ST, Ephraim PL, Friedman M, Beneciuk JM, George SZ, Saper RB. Risk factors associated with transition from acute to chronic low back pain in us patients seeking primary care. JAMA Netw Open. 2021;4(2):e2037371.
34. Hooten WM, Cohen SP. Evaluation and treatment of low back pain: a clinically focused review for primary care specialists. Mayo Clin Proc. 2015;90(12):1699–718.
35. Leone A, Cianfoni A, Cerase A, Magarelli N, Bonomo L. Lumbar spondylolysis: a review. Skeletal Radiol. 2011;40(6):683–700.
36. Fischgrund JS, Rhyne A, Franke J, Sasso R, Kitchel S, Bae H, Yeung C, Truumees E, Schaufele M, Yuan P, Vajkoczy P, Depalma M, Anderson DG, Thibodeau L, Meyer B. Intraosseous basivertebral nerve ablation for the treatment of chronic low back pain: 2-year results from a prospective randomized double-blind sham-controlled multicenter study. Int J Spine Surg. 2019;13(2):110–9.
37. Khalil JG, Smuck M, Koreckij T, Keel J, Beall D, Goodman B, Kalapos P, Nguyen D, Garfin S, Investigators IT. A prospective, randomized, multicenter study of intraosseous basivertebral nerve ablation for the treatment of chronic low back pain. Spine J. 2019;19(10):1620–32.
38. Tarulli AW, Raynor EM. Lumbosacral radiculopathy. Neurol Clin. 2007;25(2):387–405.
39. Hakelius A. Prognosis in sciatica. A clinical follow-up of surgical and non-surgical treatment. Acta Orthop Scand Suppl. 1970;129:1–76.
40. Wang Y, Dai G, Jiang L, Liao S. The incidence of regression after the non-surgical treatment of symptomatic lumbar disc herniation: a systematic review and meta-analysis. BMC Musculoskelet Disord. 2020;21(1):530.
41. Bartleson J, Deen GH. Spine disorders: medical and surgical management. Cambridge: Cambridge university Press; 2009.
42. Koes BW, van Tulder MW, Peul WC. Diagnosis and treatment of sciatica. BMJ. 2007;334(7607):1313–7.

43. Vroomen PC, de Krom MC, Knottnerus JA. Diagnostic value of history and physical examination in patients suspected of sciatica due to disc herniation: a systematic review. J Neurol. 1999;246(10):899–906.
44. Melancia JL, Francisco AF, Antunes JL. Spinal stenosis. Handb Clin Neurol. 2014;119:541–9.
45. Katz JN, Dalgas M, Stucki G, Katz NP, Bayley J, Fossel AH, Chang LC, Lipson SJ. Degenerative lumbar spinal stenosis. Diagnostic value of the history and physical examination. Arthritis Rheum. 1995;38(9):1236–41.
46. Katz JN, Harris MB. Clinical practice. Lumbar spinal stenosis. N Engl J Med. 2008;358(8):818–25.
47. Kobayashi S. Pathophysiology, diagnosis and treatment of intermittent claudication in patients with lumbar canal stenosis. World J Orthop. 2014;5(2):134–45.
48. Suri P, Rainville J, Kalichman L, Katz JN. Does this older adult with lower extremity pain have the clinical syndrome of lumbar spinal stenosis? JAMA. 2010;304(23):2628–36.
49. Walker-Bone KE, Palmer KT, Reading I, Cooper C. Soft-tissue rheumatic disorders of the neck and upper limb: prevalence and risk factors. Semin Arthritis Rheum. 2003;33(3):185–203.
50. Christmas C, Crespo CJ, Franckowiak SC, Bathon JM, Bartlett SJ, Andersen RE. How common is hip pain among older adults? Results from the third national health and nutrition examination survey. J Fam Pract. 2002;51(4):345–8.
51. Nguyen US, Zhang Y, Zhu Y, Niu J, Zhang B, Felson DT. Increasing prevalence of knee pain and symptomatic knee osteoarthritis: survey and cohort data. Ann Intern Med. 2011;155(11):725–32.
52. Hubbard MJ, Hildebrand BA, Battafarano MM, Battafarano DF. Common soft tissue musculoskeletal pain disorders. Prim Care. 2018;45(2):289–303.
53. Skootsky SA, Jaeger B, Oye RK. Prevalence of myofascial pain in general internal medicine practice. West J Med. 1989;151(2):157–60.
54. Vazquez-Delgado E, Cascos-Romero J, Gay-Escoda C. Myofascial pain syndrome associated with trigger points: a literature review. (i): epidemiology, clinical treatment and etiopathogeny. Med Oral Patol Oral Cir Bucal. 2009;14(10):e494–8.
55. Simons DG, Travell JG. Myofascial origins of low back pain. 1. Principles of diagnosis and treatment. Postgrad Med. 1983;73(2):66. 68–70, 73 passim
56. Urits I, Charipova K, Gress K, Schaaf AL, Gupta S, Kiernan HC, Choi PE, Jung JW, Cornett E, Kaye AD, Viswanath O. Treatment and management of myofascial pain syndrome. Best Pract Res Clin Anaesthesiol. 2020;34(3):427–48.
57. Sikandar S, Dickenson AH. Visceral pain: the ins and outs, the ups and downs. Curr Opin Support Palliat Care. 2012;6(1):17–26.
58. Cervero F. Visceral hyperalgesia revisited. Lancet. 2000;356(9236):1127–8.
59. Ballou S, Iturrino J, Rangan V, Cheng V, Kelley JM, Lembo A, Kaptchuk TJ, Nee J. Improving medication tolerance: a pilot study in disorders of gut-brain interaction treated with tricyclic antidepressants. J Clin Gastroenterol. 2022;56(5):452–6.
60. Olesen SS, Graversen C, Olesen AE, Frokjaer JB, Wilder-Smith O, van Goor H, Valeriani M, Drewes AM. Randomised clinical trial: Pregabalin attenuates experimental visceral pain through sub-cortical mechanisms in patients with painful chronic pancreatitis. Aliment Pharmacol Ther. 2011;34(8):878–87.
61. Vorenkamp K, Yi P, Kemp A. Sympathetic blocks for visceral pain. Phys Med Rehabil Clin N Am. 2022;33(2):475–87.
62. Herati AS, Moldwin RM. Alternative therapies in the management of chronic prostatitis/chronic pelvic pain syndrome. World J Urol. 2013;31(4):761–6.
63. Urits I, Callan J, Moore WC, Fuller MC, Renschler JS, Fisher P, Jung JW, Hasoon J, Eskander J, Kaye AD, Viswanath O. Cognitive behavioral therapy for the treatment of chronic pelvic pain. Best Pract Res Clin Anaesthesiol. 2020;34(3):409–26.
64. Chaiban G, Abdallah RT, Abd-Elsayed A, Kalia H, Malinowski M, Bhatia A, Burkey A, Carayannopoulos A, Christiansen S, Karri J, Lee E, Malik T, Meacham K, Orhurhu VJE, Raskin JS, Sivanesan E, Tolba R, Raslan AM. North American neuromodulation society

educational curriculum for intrathecal drug delivery systems implantation and management. Neuromodulation. 2022;26:1208.

65. Hunter C, Dave N, Diwan S, Deer T. Neuromodulation of pelvic visceral pain: review of the literature and case series of potential novel targets for treatment. Pain Pract. 2013;13(1):3–17.

66. Mathias SD, Kuppermann M, Liberman RF, Lipschutz RC, Steege JF. Chronic pelvic pain: prevalence, health-related quality of life, and economic correlates. Obstet Gynecol. 1996;87(3):321–7.

67. Ferris JA, Pitts MK, Richters J, Simpson JM, Shelley JM, Smith AM. National prevalence of urogenital pain and prostatitis-like symptoms in Australian men using the national institutes of health chronic prostatitis symptoms index. BJU Int. 2010;105(3):373–9.

68. He Y, Zhuang X, Ma W. Is gabapentin effective and safe in the treatment of chronic pelvic pain in women: a systematic review and meta-analysis. Int Urogynecol J. 2022;33(5):1071–81.

69. Horne AW, Vincent K, Hewitt CA, Middleton LJ, Koscielniak M, Szubert W, Doust AM, Daniels JP, Ga PPc. Gabapentin for chronic pelvic pain in women (gapp2): a multicentre, randomised, double-blind, placebo-controlled trial. Lancet. 2020;396(10255):909–17.

70. Anothaisintawee T, Attia J, Nickel JC, Thammakraisorn S, Numthavaj P, McEvoy M, Thakkinstian A. Management of chronic prostatitis/chronic pelvic pain syndrome: a systematic review and network meta-analysis. JAMA. 2011;305(1):78–86.

71. Giannantoni A, Porena M, Gubbiotti M, Maddonni S, Di Stasi SM. The efficacy and safety of duloxetine in a multidrug regimen for chronic prostatitis/chronic pelvic pain syndrome. Urology. 2014;83(2):400–5.

72. Zhang M, Li H, Ji Z, Dong D, Yan S. Clinical study of duloxetine hydrochloride combined with doxazosin for the treatment of pain disorder in chronic prostatitis/chronic pelvic pain syndrome: an observational study. Medicine (Baltimore). 2017;96(10):e6243.

73. Sator-Katzenschlager SM, Scharbert G, Kress HG, Frickey N, Ellend A, Gleiss A, Kozek-Langenecker SA. Chronic pelvic pain treated with gabapentin and amitriptyline: a randomized controlled pilot study. Wien Klin Wochenschr. 2005;117(21–22):761–8.

74. Agarwal MM, Elsi Sy M. Gabapentenoids in pain management in urological chronic pelvic pain syndrome: gabapentin or pregabalin? Neurourol Urodyn. 2017;36(8):2028–33.

75. Pontari MA, Krieger JN, Litwin MS, White PC, Anderson RU, McNaughton-Collins M, Nickel JC, Shoskes DA, Alexander RB, O'Leary M, Zeitlin S, Chuai S, Landis JR, Cen L, Propert KJ, Kusek JW, Nyberg LM Jr, Schaeffer AJ, Chronic Prostatitis Collaborative Research N. Pregabalin for the treatment of men with chronic prostatitis/chronic pelvic pain syndrome: a randomized controlled trial. Arch Intern Med. 2010;170(17):1586–93.

76. Peng PW, Tumber PS. Ultrasound-guided interventional procedures for patients with chronic pelvic pain – a description of techniques and review of literature. Pain Physician. 2008;11(2):215–24.

77. Baltazar M, Russo JAO, De Lucca V, Mitidieri AMS, da Silva APM, Gurian MBF, Poli-Neto OB, Rosa ESJC. Therapeutic ultrasound versus injection of local anesthetic in the treatment of women with chronic pelvic pain secondary to abdominal myofascial syndrome: a randomized clinical trial. BMC Womens Health. 2022;22(1):325.

78. Weinschenk S, Benrath J, Kessler E, Strowitzki T, Feisst M. Therapy with local anesthetics to treat vulvodynia. A pilot study. Sex Med. 2022;10(2):100482.

79. Karp BI, Tandon H, Vigil D, Stratton P. Methodological approaches to botulinum toxin for the treatment of chronic pelvic pain, vaginismus, and vulvar pain disorders. Int Urogynecol J. 2019;30(7):1071–81.

80. Panunzio A, Tafuri A, Mazzucato G, Cerrato C, Orlando R, Pagliarulo V, Antonelli A, Cerruto MA. Botulinum toxin-a injection in chronic pelvic pain syndrome treatment: a systematic review and pooled meta-analysis. Toxins (Basel). 2022;14(1):25.

81. Parsons BA, Goonewardene S, Dabestani S, Pacheco-Figueiredo L, Yuan Y, Zumstein V, Cottrell AM, Borovicka J, Dinis-Oliveira P, Berghmans B, Elneil S, Hughes J, Messelink BEJ, de C Williams AC, Baranowski AP, Engeler DS. The benefits and harms of botulinum toxin-a in the treatment of chronic pelvic pain syndromes: a systematic review by the European association of urology chronic pelvic pain panel. Eur Urol Focus. 2022;8(1):320–38.

82. Tate JL, Stauss T, Li S, Rotte A, Subbaroyan J. A prospective, multi-center, clinical trial of a 10-khz spinal cord stimulation system in the treatment of chronic pelvic pain. Pain Pract. 2021;21(1):45–53.
83. Kapural L, Narouze SN, Janicki TI, Mekhail N. Spinal cord stimulation is an effective treatment for the chronic intractable visceral pelvic pain. Pain Med. 2006;7(5):440–3.
84. Baranowski AP, Mandeville AL, Edwards S, Brook S, Cambitzi J, Cohen M. Male chronic pelvic pain syndrome and the role of interdisciplinary pain management. World J Urol. 2013;31(4):779–84.
85. Twiddy H, Lane N, Chawla R, Johnson S, Bradshaw A, Aleem S, Mawdsley L. The development and delivery of a female chronic pelvic pain management programme: a specialised interdisciplinary approach. Br J Pain. 2015;9(4):233–40.
86. Allaire C, Williams C, Bodmer-Roy S, Zhu S, Arion K, Ambacher K, Wu J, Yosef A, Wong F, Noga H, Britnell S, Yager H, Bedaiwy MA, Albert AY, Lisonkova S, Yong PJ. Chronic pelvic pain in an interdisciplinary setting: 1-year prospective cohort. Am J Obstet Gynecol. 2018;218(1):114.e111–2.
87. Till SR, As-Sanie S, Schrepf A. Psychology of chronic pelvic pain: prevalence, neurobiological vulnerabilities, and treatment. Clin Obstet Gynecol. 2019;62(1):22–36.
88. Munro A, George RB, Chorney J, Snelgrove-Clarke E, Rosen NO. Prevalence and predictors of chronic pain in pregnancy and postpartum. J Obstet Gynaecol Can. 2017;39(9):734–41.
89. Irani RA, Foster S. Overview of the mechanisms of induction of labor. Semin Perinatol. 2015;39(6):426–9.
90. Halliday L, Nelson SM, Kearns RJ. Epidural analgesia in labor: a narrative review. Int J Gynaecol Obstet. 2022;159(2):356–64.
91. Arendt KW, Tessmer-Tuck JA. Nonpharmacologic labor analgesia. Clin Perinatol. 2013;40(3):351–71.
92. Hodnett ED, Gates S, Hofmeyr GJ, Sakala C. Continuous support for women during childbirth. Cochrane Database Syst Rev. 2012;10:CD003766.
93. Robbins MS. Diagnosis and management of headache: a review. JAMA. 2021;325(18):1874–85.
94. Stovner LJ, Hagen K, Linde M, Steiner TJ. The global prevalence of headache: an update, with analysis of the influences of methodological factors on prevalence estimates. J Headache Pain. 2022;23(1):34.
95. Ahmed F. Headache disorders: differentiating and managing the common subtypes. Br J Pain. 2012;6(3):124–32.
96. Do TP, la Cour Karottki NF, Ashina M. Updates in the diagnostic approach of headache. Curr Pain Headache Rep. 2021;25(12):80.
97. Jackson JL, Mancuso JM, Nickoloff S, Bernstein R, Kay C. Tricyclic and tetracyclic antidepressants for the prevention of frequent episodic or chronic tension-type headache in adults: a systematic review and meta-analysis. J Gen Intern Med. 2017;32(12):1351–8.
98. Qubty W, Patniyot I. Migraine pathophysiology. Pediatr Neurol. 2020;107:1–6.
99. Dodick DW, Shewale AS, Lipton RB, Baum SJ, Marcus SC, Silberstein SD, Pavlovic JM, Bennett NL, Young WB, Viswanathan HN, Doshi JA, Weintraub H. Migraine patients with cardiovascular disease and contraindications: an analysis of real-world claims data. J Prim Care Community Health. 2020;11:2150132720963680.
100. Chiang CC, Schwedt TJ. Calcitonin gene-related peptide (CGRP)-targeted therapies as preventive and acute treatments for migraine-the monoclonal antibodies and gepants. Prog Brain Res. 2020;255:143–70.
101. Tiwari V, Agrawal S. Migraine and neuromodulation: a literature review. Cureus. 2022;14(11):e31223.
102. Al-Kaisy A, Palmisani S, Carganillo R, Wesley S, Pang D, Rotte A, Santos A, Lambru G. Safety and efficacy of 10 kHz spinal cord stimulation for the treatment of refractory chronic migraine: a prospective long-term open-label study. Neuromodulation. 2022;25(1):103–13.
103. Strand N, D'Souza RS, Hagedorn JM, Pritzlaff S, Sayed D, Azeem N, Abd-Elsayed A, Escobar A, Huntoon MA, Lam CM, Deer TR. Evidence-based clinical guidelines from the

American society of pain and neuroscience for the use of implantable peripheral nerve stimulation in the treatment of chronic pain. J Pain Res. 2022;15:2483–504.

104. Yuan H, Chuang TY. Update of neuromodulation in chronic migraine. Curr Pain Headache Rep. 2021;25(11):71.

105. Wei DY, Yuan Ong JJ, Goadsby PJ. Cluster headache: epidemiology, pathophysiology, clinical features, and diagnosis. Ann Indian Acad Neurol. 2018;21(Suppl 1):S3–8.

106. Gooriah R, Buture A, Ahmed F. Evidence-based treatments for cluster headache. Ther Clin Risk Manag. 2015;11:1687–96.

107. Grandhi RK, Kaye AD, Abd-Elsayed A. Systematic review of radiofrequency ablation and pulsed radiofrequency for management of cervicogenic headaches. Curr Pain Headache Rep. 2018;22(3):18.

108. Cohen SP, Peterlin BL, Fulton L, Neely ET, Kurihara C, Gupta A, Mali J, Fu DC, Jacobs MB, Plunkett AR, Verdun AJ, Stojanovic MP, Hanling S, Constantinescu O, White RL, McLean BC, Pasquina PF, Zhao Z. Randomized, double-blind, comparative-effectiveness study comparing pulsed radiofrequency to steroid injections for occipital neuralgia or migraine with occipital nerve tenderness. Pain. 2015;156(12):2585–94.

109. Lipton JA, Ship JA, Larach-Robinson D. Estimated prevalence and distribution of reported orofacial pain in the United States. J Am Dent Assoc. 1993;124(10):115–21.

110. Slade GD, Bair E, Greenspan JD, Dubner R, Fillingim RB, Diatchenko L, Maixner W, Knott C, Ohrbach R. Signs and symptoms of first-onset TMD and sociodemographic predictors of its development: the OPPERA prospective cohort study. J Pain. 2013;14(12 Suppl):T20–32.e21–23.

111. Murphy MK, MacBarb RF, Wong ME, Athanasiou KA. Temporomandibular disorders: a review of etiology, clinical management, and tissue engineering strategies. Int J Oral Maxillofac Implants. 2013;28(6):e393–414.

112. Cairns BE. Pathophysiology of TMD pain--basic mechanisms and their implications for pharmacotherapy. J Oral Rehabil. 2010;37(6):391–410.

113. Nackley AG, Tan KS, Fecho K, Flood P, Diatchenko L, Maixner W. Catechol-o-methyltransferase inhibition increases pain sensitivity through activation of both beta2- and beta3-adrenergic receptors. Pain. 2007;128(3):199–208.

114. Maixner W, Diatchenko L, Dubner R, Fillingim RB, Greenspan JD, Knott C, Ohrbach R, Weir B, Slade GD. Orofacial pain prospective evaluation and risk assessment study–the OPPERA study. J Pain. 2011;12(11 Suppl):T4–11.e11–12.

115. Auerbach SM, Laskin DM, Frantsve LM, Orr T. Depression, pain, exposure to stressful life events, and long-term outcomes in temporomandibular disorder patients. J Oral Maxillofac Surg. 2001;59(6):628–33. discussion 634

116. Kalladka M, Quek S, Heir G, Eliav E, Mupparapu M, Viswanath A. Temporomandibular joint osteoarthritis: diagnosis and long-term conservative management: a topic review. J Indian Prosthodont Soc. 2014;14(1):6–15.

117. Yibulayin F, Yu CX, Feng L, Wang M, Lu MM, Luo Y, Liu H, Yang ZC, Wushou A. Malignant tumours of temporomandibular joint. BMC Cancer. 2020;20(1):967.

118. Cho GH, Lee Y. Analysis of masticatory muscle activity based on presence of temporomandibular joint disorders. Med Sci Monit. 2020;26:e921337.

119. Gil-Martínez A, Paris-Alemany A, López-de-Uralde-Villanueva I, La Touche R. Management of pain in patients with temporomandibular disorder (TMD): challenges and solutions. J Pain Res. 2018;11:571–87.

120. Wu M, Cai J, Yu Y, Hu S, Wang Y. Therapeutic agents for the treatment of temporomandibular joint disorders: progress and perspective. Front Pharmacol. 2020;11:596099.

121. Shehri ZG, Alkhouri I, Hajeer MY, Haddad I, Abu Hawa MH. Evaluation of the efficacy of low-dose botulinum toxin injection into the masseter muscle for the treatment of nocturnal bruxism: a randomized controlled clinical trial. Cureus. 2022;14(12):e32180.

122. Romero-Reyes M, Uyanik JM. Orofacial pain management: current perspectives. J Pain Res. 2014;7:99–115.

123. Gadient PM, Smith JH. The neuralgias: diagnosis and management. Curr Neurol Neurosci Rep. 2014;14(7):459.
124. Chua NH, Halim W, Beems T, Vissers KC. Pulsed radiofrequency treatment for trigeminal neuralgia. Anesth Pain Med. 2012;1(4):257–61.
125. Manolitsis N, Elahi F. Pulsed radiofrequency for occipital neuralgia. Pain Physician. 2014;17(6):E709–17.
126. Obermann M. Treatment options in trigeminal neuralgia. Ther Adv Neurol Disord. 2010;3(2):107–15.
127. Vaegter HB, Andersen PG, Madsen MF, Handberg G, Enggaard TP. Prevalence of neuropathic pain according to the IASP grading system in patients with chronic non-malignant pain. Pain Med. 2014;15(1):120–7.
128. Aravindhan R, Vidyalakshmi S, Kumar MS, Satheesh C, Balasubramanium AM, Prasad VS. Burning mouth syndrome: a review on its diagnostic and therapeutic approach. J Pharm Bioallied Sci. 2014;6(Suppl 1):S21–5.
129. Thomas DC, Thomas P, Pillai DP, Joseph D, Lingaiah U, Mathai BC, Ravi A, Chhabra S, Pitchumani PK. Giant cell arteritis: a case-based narrative review of the literature. Curr Pain Headache Rep. 2022;26:725.
130. López-López J, Garcia-Vicente L, Jané-Salas E, Estrugo-Devesa A, Chimenos-Küstner E, Roca-Elias J. Orofacial pain of cardiac origin: review literature and clinical cases. Med Oral Patol Oral Cir Bucal. 2012;17(4):e538–44.
131. Romero-Reyes M, Salvemini D. Cancer and orofacial pain. Med Oral Patol Oral Cir Bucal. 2016;21(6):e665–71.
132. DiBonaventura MD, Sadosky A, Concialdi K, Hopps M, Kudel I, Parsons B, Cappelleri JC, Hlavacek P, Alexander AH, Stacey BR, Markman JD, Farrar JT. The prevalence of probable neuropathic pain in the us: results from a multimodal general-population health survey. J Pain Res. 2017;10:2525–38.
133. van Hecke O, Austin SK, Khan RA, Smith BH, Torrance N. Neuropathic pain in the general population: a systematic review of epidemiological studies. Pain. 2014;155(4):654–62.
134. Abbott CA, Malik RA, van Ross ER, Kulkarni J, Boulton AJ. Prevalence and characteristics of painful diabetic neuropathy in a large community-based diabetic population in the U.K. Diabetes Care. 2011;34(10):2220–4.
135. Baron R, Binder A, Wasner G. Neuropathic pain: diagnosis, pathophysiological mechanisms, and treatment. Lancet Neurol. 2010;9(8):807–19.
136. *Gilron I, Baron R, Jensen T. Neuropathic pain: principles of diagnosis and treatment. Mayo Clin Proc. 2015;90(4):532–45.
137. Rosenbaum T, Morales-Lazaro SL, Islas LD. TRP channels: a journey towards a molecular understanding of pain. Nat Rev Neurosci. 2022;23(10):596–610.
138. Ross MA. Electrodiagnosis of peripheral neuropathy. Neurol Clin. 2012;30(2):529–49.
139. Lauria G, Hsieh ST, Johansson O, Kennedy WR, Leger JM, Mellgren SI, Nolano M, Merkies IS, Polydefkis M, Smith AG, Sommer C, Valls-Sole J, European Federation of Neurological S, Peripheral Nerve S. European federation of neurological societies/peripheral nerve society guideline on the use of skin biopsy in the diagnosis of small fiber neuropathy. Report of a joint task force of the European federation of neurological societies and the peripheral nerve society. Eur J Neurol. 2010;17(7):903–12. e944–909
140. Finnerup NB, Attal N, Haroutounian S, McNicol E, Baron R, Dworkin RH, Gilron I, Haanpaa M, Hansson P, Jensen TS, Kamerman PR, Lund K, Moore A, Raja SN, Rice AS, Rowbotham M, Sena E, Siddall P, Smith BH, Wallace M. Pharmacotherapy for neuropathic pain in adults: a systematic review and meta-analysis. Lancet Neurol. 2015;14(2):162–73.
141. Balanaser M, Carley M, Baron R, Finnerup NB, Moore RA, Rowbotham MC, Chaparro LE, Gilron I. Combination pharmacotherapy for the treatment of neuropathic pain in adults: systematic review and meta-analysis. Pain. 2022;164(2):230–51.
142. Baute V, Zelnik D, Curtis J, Sadeghifar F. Complementary and alternative medicine for painful peripheral neuropathy. Curr Treat Options Neurol. 2019;21(9):44.

143. Rowin J. Integrative neuromuscular medicine: neuropathy and neuropathic pain: consider the alternatives. Muscle Nerve. 2019;60(2):124–36.
144. de Vos CC, Meier K, Zaalberg PB, Nijhuis HJ, Duyvendak W, Vesper J, Enggaard TP, Lenders MW. Spinal cord stimulation in patients with painful diabetic neuropathy: a multicentre randomized clinical trial. Pain. 2014;155(11):2426–31.
145. Petersen EA, Stauss TG, Scowcroft JA, Brooks ES, White JL, Sills SM, Amirdelfan K, Guirguis MN, Xu J, Yu C, Nairizi A, Patterson DG, Tsoulfas KC, Creamer MJ, Galan V, Bundschu RH, Mehta ND, Sayed D, Lad SP, DiBenedetto DJ, Sethi KA, Goree JH, Bennett MT, Harrison NJ, Israel AF, Chang P, Wu PW, Argoff CE, Nasr CE, Taylor RS, Caraway DL, Mekhail NA. Durability of high-frequency 10-khz spinal cord stimulation for patients with painful diabetic neuropathy refractory to conventional treatments: 12-month results from a randomized controlled trial. Diabetes Care. 2022;45(1):e3–6.
146. D'Souza RS, Kubrova E, Her YF, Barman RA, Smith BJ, Alvarez GM, West TE, Abd-Elsayed A. Dorsal root ganglion stimulation for lower extremity neuropathic pain syndromes: an evidence-based literature review. Adv Ther. 2022;39(10):4440–73.
147. Hayek SM, Sweet JA, Miller JP, Sayegh RR. Successful management of corneal neuropathic pain with intrathecal targeted drug delivery. Pain Med. 2016;17(7):1302–7.
148. Karri J, Doan J, Vangeison C, Catalanotto M, Nagpal AS, Li S. Emerging evidence for intrathecal management of neuropathic pain following spinal cord injury. Front Pain Res (Lausanne). 2022;3:933422.
149. Beerthuizen A, Stronks DL, Van't Spijker A, Yaksh A, Hanraets BM, Klein J, Huygen F. Demographic and medical parameters in the development of complex regional pain syndrome type 1 (CRPS1): prospective study on 596 patients with a fracture. Pain. 2012;153(6):1187–92.
150. Sandroni P, Benrud-Larson LM, McClelland RL, Low PA. Complex regional pain syndrome type I: incidence and prevalence in Olmsted county, a population-based study. Pain. 2003;103(1–2):199–207.
151. de Mos M, de Bruijn AG, Huygen FJ, Dieleman JP, Stricker BH, Sturkenboom MC. The incidence of complex regional pain syndrome: a population-based study. Pain. 2007;129(1–2):12–20.
152. Shim H, Rose J, Halle S, Shekane P. Complex regional pain syndrome: a narrative review for the practising clinician. Br J Anaesth. 2019;123(2):e424–33.
153. Harden NR, Bruehl S, Perez R, Birklein F, Marinus J, Maihofner C, Lubenow T, Buvanendran A, Mackey S, Graciosa J, Mogilevski M, Ramsden C, Chont M, Vatine JJ. Validation of proposed diagnostic criteria (the "Budapest criteria") for complex regional pain syndrome. Pain. 2010;150(2):268–74.
154. Moon JY, Park SY, Kim YC, Lee SC, Nahm FS, Kim JH, Kim H, Oh SW. Analysis of patterns of three-phase bone scintigraphy for patients with complex regional pain syndrome diagnosed using the proposed research criteria (the 'Budapest criteria'). Br J Anaesth. 2012;108(4):655–61.
155. Lee HJ, Kim SE, Moon JY, Shin JY, Kim YC. Analysis of quantitative sudomotor axon reflex test patterns in patients with complex regional pain syndrome diagnosed using the Budapest criteria. Reg Anesth Pain Med. 2019;44:1026.
156. Bank PJ, Peper CL, Marinus J, Beek PJ, van Hilten JJ. Deficient muscle activation in patients with complex regional pain syndrome and abnormal hand postures: an electromyographic evaluation. Clin Neurophysiol. 2013;124(10):2025–35.
157. Smart KM, Ferraro MC, Wand BM, O'Connell NE. Physiotherapy for pain and disability in adults with complex regional pain syndrome (CRPS) types I and II. Cochrane Database Syst Rev. 2022;5(5):CD010853.
158. Mangnus TJP, Bharwani KD, Dirckx M, Huygen F. From a symptom-based to a mechanism-based pharmacotherapeutic treatment in complex regional pain syndrome. Drugs. 2022;82(5):511–31.

159. *Fassio A, Mantovani A, Gatti D, Rossini M, Viapiana O, Gavioli I, Benini C, Adami G. Pharmacological treatment in adult patients with CRPS-I: a systematic review and meta-analysis of randomized controlled trials. Rheumatology (Oxford). 2022;61(9):3534–46.
160. Ryu JH, Lee CS, Kim YC, Lee SC, Shankar H, Moon JY. Ultrasound-assisted versus fluoroscopic-guided lumbar sympathetic ganglion block: a prospective and randomized study. Anesth Analg. 2018;126(4):1362–8.
161. Imani F, Hemati K, Rahimzadeh P, Kazemi MR, Hejazian K. Effectiveness of stellate ganglion block under fluoroscopy or ultrasound guidance in upper extremity CRPS. J Clin Diagn Res. 2016;10(1):UC09–12.
162. Yoo Y, Lee CS, Kim J, Jo D, Moon JY. Botulinum toxin type a for lumbar sympathetic ganglion block in complex regional pain syndrome: a randomized trial. Anesthesiology. 2022;136(2):314–25.
163. Yucel I, Demiraran Y, Ozturan K, Degirmenci E. Complex regional pain syndrome type I: efficacy of stellate ganglion blockade. J Orthop Traumatol. 2009;10(4):179–83.
164. Ho E, Yazdanpanah N, Ho J, Drukman B, Chang A, Agarwal S. Parameters of spinal cord stimulation in complex regional pain syndrome: systematic review and meta-analysis of randomized controlled trials. Pain Physician. 2022;25(8):521–30.
165. Graca MJ, Lubenow TR, Landphair WR, McCarthy RJ. Efficacy and safety of cervical and high-thoracic dorsal root ganglion stimulation therapy for complex regional pain syndrome of the upper extremities. Neuromodulation. 2022;26:1781.
166. Deer TR, Levy RM, Kramer J, Poree L, Amirdelfan K, Grigsby E, Staats P, Burton AW, Burgher AH, Obray J, Scowcroft J, Golovac S, Kapural L, Paicius R, Kim C, Pope J, Yearwood T, Samuel S, McRoberts WP, Cassim H, Netherton M, Miller N, Schaufele M, Tavel E, Davis T, Davis K, Johnson L, Mekhail N. Dorsal root ganglion stimulation yielded higher treatment success rate for complex regional pain syndrome and causalgia at 3 and 12 months: a randomized comparative trial. Pain. 2017;158(4):669–81.
167. Kessler A, Yoo M, Calisoff R. Complex regional pain syndrome: an updated comprehensive review. NeuroRehabilitation. 2020;47(3):253–64.
168. Scarff JR. Managing psychiatric symptoms in patients with complex regional pain syndrome. Innov Clin Neurosci. 2022;19(1–3):56–9.
169. Lawrence J, Alcock D, McGrath P, Kay J, MacMurray SB, Dulberg C. The development of a tool to assess neonatal pain. Neonatal Netw. 1993;12(6):59–66.
170. Krechel SW, Bildner J. Cries: a new neonatal postoperative pain measurement score. Initial testing of validity and reliability. Paediatr Anaesth. 1995;5(1):53–61.
171. Merkel SI, Voepel-Lewis T, Shayevitz JR, Malviya S. The FLACC: a behavioral scale for scoring postoperative pain in young children. Pediatr Nurs. 1997;23(3):293–7.
172. Malviya S, Voepel-Lewis T, Burke C, Merkel S, Tait AR. The revised FLACC observational pain tool: improved reliability and validity for pain assessment in children with cognitive impairment. Paediatr Anaesth. 2006;16(3):258–65.
173. Page MG, Katz J, Stinson J, Isaac L, Martin-Pichora AL, Campbell F. Validation of the numerical rating scale for pain intensity and unpleasantness in pediatric acute postoperative pain: sensitivity to change over time. J Pain. 2012;13(4):359–69.
174. Garra G, Singer AJ, Taira BR, Chohan J, Cardoz H, Chisena E, Thode HC Jr. Validation of the Wong-Baker faces pain rating scale in pediatric emergency department patients. Acad Emerg Med. 2010;17(1):50–4.
175. Warden V, Hurley AC, Volicer L. Development and psychometric evaluation of the pain assessment in advanced dementia (PAINAD) scale. J Am Med Dir Assoc. 2003;4(1):9–15.
176. Corbett A, Achterberg W, Husebo B, Lobbezoo F, de Vet H, Kunz M, Strand L, Constantinou M, Tudose C, Kappesser J, de Waal M, Lautenbacher S, EU-COST action td Pain Assessment in Patients with Impaired Cognition eDChwc-tn. An international road map to improve pain assessment in people with impaired cognition: the development of the pain assessment in impaired cognition (PAIC) meta-tool. BMC Neurol. 2014;14:229.

177. Fuchs-Lacelle S, Hadjistavropoulos T. Development and preliminary validation of the pain assessment checklist for seniors with limited ability to communicate (PACSLAC). Pain Manag Nurs. 2004;5(1):37–49.
178. Soares CD, Panuganti PK, Shrivastava A, Aroor S, Keinath KM, Bromagen MC, Howard ME, Carlson C, Smith JH. Experimental pain assessment in patients with poststroke aphasia. Neurology. 2018;91(9):e793–9.
179. Kaasalainen S, Stewart N, Middleton J, Knezacek S, Hartley T, Ife C, Robinson L. Development and evaluation of the pain assessment in the communicatively impaired (PACI) tool: part II. Int J Palliat Nurs. 2011;17(9):431–8.
180. Kaasalainen S, Stewart N, Middleton J, Knezacek S, Hartley T, Ife C, Robinson L. Development and evaluation of the pain assessment in the communicatively impaired (PACI) tool: part I. Int J Palliat Nurs. 2011;17(8):387–91.
181. de Vries NJ, Sloot PH, Achterberg WP. Pain and pain assessment in stroke patients with aphasia: a systematic review. Aphasiology. 2017;31(6):703–19.
182. American Society of Addiction Medicine. Definition of Addiction. September 15, 2019. https://www.asam.org/docs/default-source/quality-science/asam's-2019-definition-of-addiction-(1).pdf?sfvrsn=b8b64fc2_2
183. American Psychiatric Association. Diagnostic and statistical manual of mental disorders. 5th ed. Arlington: American Psychiatric Association; 2013.
184. Koob GF, Volkow ND. Neurobiology of addiction: a neurocircuitry analysis. Lancet Psychiatry. 2016;3(8):760–73.
185. Morasco BJ, Gritzner S, Lewis L, Oldham R, Turk DC, Dobscha SK. Systematic review of prevalence, correlates, and treatment outcomes for chronic non-cancer pain in patients with comorbid substance use disorder. Pain. 2011;152(3):488–97.
186. Jantarada C, Silva C, Guimaraes-Pereira L. Prevalence of problematic use of opioids in patients with chronic noncancer pain: a systematic review with meta-analysis. Pain Pract. 2021;21(6):715–29.
187. *Vowles KE, McEntee ML, Julnes PS, Frohe T, Ney JP, van der Goes DN. Rates of opioid misuse, abuse, and addiction in chronic pain: a systematic review and data synthesis. Pain. 2015;156(4):569–76.
188. Smith SM, Paillard F, McKeown A, Burke LB, Edwards RR, Katz NP, Papadopoulos EJ, Rappaport BA, Slagle A, Strain EC, Wasan AD, Turk DC, Dworkin RH. Instruments to identify prescription medication misuse, abuse, and related events in clinical trials: an ACTTION systematic review. J Pain. 2015;16(5):389–411.
189. Dhalla S, Kopec JA. The cage questionnaire for alcohol misuse: a review of reliability and validity studies. Clin Invest Med. 2007;30(1):33–41.
190. SAMHSA: Medications for Opioid Use Disorder. Treatment Improvement Protocol (TIP) Series 63. 2020. Substance Abuse and Mental Health Services Administration, Rockville, MD. https://store.samhsa.gov/sites/default/files/SAMHSA_Digital_Download/PEP21-02-01-002.pdf
191. The ASAM national practice guideline for the treatment of opioid use disorder: 2020 focused update. J Addict Med. 2020;14(2S Suppl 1):1–91.
192. Dugosh K, Abraham A, Seymour B, McLoyd K, Chalk M, Festinger D. A systematic review on the use of psychosocial interventions in conjunction with medications for the treatment of opioid addiction. J Addict Med. 2016;10(2):93–103.
193. Rice D, Corace K, Wolfe D, Esmaeilisaraji L, Michaud A, Grima A, Austin B, Douma R, Barbeau P, Butler C, Willows M, Poulin PA, Sproule BA, Porath A, Garber G, Taha S, Garner G, Skidmore B, Moher D, Thavorn K, Hutton B. Evaluating comparative effectiveness of psychosocial interventions adjunctive to opioid agonist therapy for opioid use disorder: a systematic review with network meta-analyses. PLoS One. 2020;15(12):e0244401.
194. Ii T, Sato H, Watanabe N, Kondo M, Masuda A, Hayes SC, Akechi T. Psychological flexibility-based interventions versus first-line psychosocial interventions for substance use disorders: systematic review and meta-analyses of randomized controlled trials. J Contextual Behav Sci. 2019;13:109–20.

195. Merlin JS, Young SR, Starrels JL, Azari S, Edelman EJ, Pomeranz J, Roy P, Saini S, Becker WC, Liebschutz JM. Correction to: managing concerning behaviors in patients prescribed opioids for chronic pain: a Delphi study. J Gen Intern Med. 2018;33(9):1587.

196. Agency for Healthcare Research and Quality. Systematic Review on Nonopioid Pharmacologic Treatments for Chronic Pain: Surveillance Report 3. Literature update period: January 2022 through April 1, 2022. https://effectivehealthcare.ahrq.gov/sites/default/files/related_files/surveillance-report-3-nonopioid-pharm-chronic-pain.pdf

197. Ilgen MA, Coughlin LN, Bohnert ASB, Chermack S, Price A, Kim HM, Jannausch M, Blow FC. Efficacy of a psychosocial pain management intervention for men and women with substance use disorders and chronic pain: a randomized clinical trial. JAMA Psychiatry. 2020;77(12):1225–34.

198. Garland EL, Hanley AW, Riquino MR, Reese SE, Baker AK, Salas K, Yack BP, Bedford CE, Bryan MA, Atchley R, Nakamura Y, Froeliger B, Howard MO. Mindfulness-oriented recovery enhancement reduces opioid misuse risk via analgesic and positive psychological mechanisms: a randomized controlled trial. J Consult Clin Psychol. 2019;87(10):927–40.

199. Hatheway JA, Bansal M, Nichols-Ricker CI. Systemic opioid reduction and discontinuation following implantation of intrathecal drug-delivery systems for chronic pain: a retrospective cohort analysis. Neuromodulation. 2020;23(7):961–9.

200. Pollard EM, Lamer TJ, Moeschler SM, Gazelka HM, Hooten WM, Bendel MA, Warner NS, Murad MH. The effect of spinal cord stimulation on pain medication reduction in intractable spine and limb pain: a systematic review of randomized controlled trials and meta-analysis. J Pain Res. 2019;12:1311–24.

201. Burns SL, Majdak P, Urman RD. Perioperative and periprocedural anesthetic management of opioid tolerant patients and patients with active and medically treated opioid use disorder. Curr Opin Anaesthesiol. 2022;35(4):514–20.

202. Ward EN, Quaye AN, Wilens TE. Opioid use disorders: perioperative management of a special population. Anesth Analg. 2018;127(2):539–47.

203. Warner NS, Warner MA, Cunningham JL, Gazelka HM, Hooten WM, Kolla BP, Warner DO. A practical approach for the management of the mixed opioid agonist-antagonist buprenorphine during acute pain and surgery. Mayo Clin Proc. 2020;95(6):1253–67.

204. Kohan L, Potru S, Barreveld AM, Sprintz M, Lane O, Aryal A, Emerick T, Dopp A, Chhay S, Viscusi E. Buprenorphine management in the perioperative period: educational review and recommendations from a multisociety expert panel. Reg Anesth Pain Med. 2021;46(10):840–59.

205. Li Z, Aninditha T, Griene B, Francis J, Renato P, Serrie A, Umareddy I, Boisseau S, Hadjiat Y. Burden of cancer pain in developing countries: a narrative literature review. Clinicoecon Outcomes Res. 2018;10:675–91.

206. Wahab KW, Salami AK. Pain as a symptom in patients living with HIV/AIDS seen at the outpatient clinic of a Nigerian tertiary hospital. J Int Assoc Physicians AIDS Care (Chic). 2011;10(1):35–9.

207. Haroun OMO, Hietaharju A, Bizuneh E, Tesfaye F, Brandsma WJ, Haanpaa M, Rice ASC, Lockwood DNJ. Investigation of neuropathic pain in treated leprosy patients in Ethiopia: a cross-sectional study. Pain. 2012;153(8):1620–4.

208. Lasry-Levy E, Hietaharju A, Pai V, Ganapati R, Rice AS, Haanpaa M, Lockwood DN. Neuropathic pain and psychological morbidity in patients with treated leprosy: a cross-sectional prevalence study in Mumbai. PLoS Negl Trop Dis. 2011;5(3):e981.

209. de C Williams AC, Baird E. Special considerations for the treatment of pain from torture and war. Curr Anesthesiol Rep. 2016;6(4):319–26.

210. Williams ACC, Amris K. Treatment of persistent pain from torture: review and commentary. Med Confl Surviv. 2017;33(1):60–81.

211. Teodorescu DS, Heir T, Siqveland J, Hauff E, Wentzel-Larsen T, Lien L. Chronic pain in multi-traumatized outpatients with a refugee background resettled in Norway: a cross-sectional study. BMC Psychol. 2015;3(1):7.

212. Kamerman PR, Wadley AL, Davis KD, Hietaharju A, Jain P, Kopf A, Meyer AC, Raja SN, Rice ASC, Smith BH, Treede RD, Wiffen PJ. World health organization essential medicines lists: where are the drugs to treat neuropathic pain? Pain. 2015;156(5):793–7.

213. Vranken MJ, Mantel-Teeuwisse AK, Junger S, Radbruch L, Lisman J, Scholten W, Payne S, Lynch T, Schutjens MH. Legal barriers in accessing opioid medicines: results of the ATOME quick scan of national legislation of Eastern European countries. J Pain Symptom Manag. 2014;48(6):1135–44.

214. Lohman D, Schleifer R, Amon JJ. Access to pain treatment as a human right. BMC Med. 2010;8:8.

215. Makhlouf SM, Ahmed S, Mulvey M, Bennett MI. Attitudes, knowledge, and perceived barriers towards cancer pain management among healthcare professionals in Libya: a national multicenter survey. J Cancer Educ. 2022;38:789.

216. Dharsee N, Haule M, Mlawa G, Lwanga T. Identifying training needs in pain management—a survey of staff at a tertiary cancer care centre. Pain Stud Treatmtent. 2022;10:9–20.

217. Ahmed A, Khan RA, Yasir M, Siddiqui S, Abbasi S, Asad V, Rozina K, Aamir R, Afshan G. A course on acute pain management for nurses: an endeavour to improve acute pain relief in a developing country. Med Ed Publish 2016. https://doi.org/10.15694/mep.12016.000021.

218. Nia S, Epstein JH. Pain relief in areas of deprivation and conflict. In: Academic pain medicine; 2019. p. 365–9.

219. Kurita GP, Sjogren P, Juel K, Hojsted J, Ekholm O. The burden of chronic pain: a cross-sectional survey focussing on diseases, immigration, and opioid use. Pain. 2012;153(12):2332–8.

220. Nahin RL. Estimates of pain prevalence and severity in adults: United States, 2012. J Pain. 2015;16(8):769–80.

221. Allen-Watts K, Sims AM, Buchanan TL, DeJesus DJB, Quinn TL, Buford TW, Goodin BR, Rumble DD. Sociodemographic differences in pain medication usage and healthcare provider utilization among adults with chronic low back pain. Front Pain Res (Lausanne). 2021;2:806310.

222. Johnson AJ, Sibille KT, Cardoso J, Terry EL, Powell-Roach KL, Goodin B, Staud R, Redden D, Fillingim RB, Booker SQ. Patterns and correlates of self-management strategies for osteoarthritis-related pain among older non-hispanic black and non-hispanic white adults. Arthritis Care Res (Hoboken). 2021;73(11):1648–58.

223. Fuentes M, Hart-Johnson T, Green CR. The association among neighborhood socioeconomic status, race and chronic pain in black and white older adults. J Natl Med Assoc. 2007;99(10):1160–9.

224. Yoshikawa K, Brady B, Perry MA, Devan H. Sociocultural factors influencing physiotherapy management in culturally and linguistically diverse people with persistent pain: a scoping review. Physiotherapy. 2020;107:292–305.

225. *Brady B, Veljanova I, Chipchase L. The intersections of chronic noncancer pain: culturally diverse perspectives on disease burden. Pain Med. 2019;20(3):434–45.

226. Henderson S, Kendall E, See L. The effectiveness of culturally appropriate interventions to manage or prevent chronic disease in culturally and linguistically diverse communities: a systematic literature review. Health Soc Care Community. 2011;19(3):225–49.

Pain Assessment and Evaluation

4

Anuj Aggarwal, Meredith Barad, Stephanie Jones,
Scott Pritzlaff, Alpana Gowda, and Ameet Nagpal

Abbreviations

ACEs	Adverse childhood experiences
BPQ	Brief Pain Questionnaire
BPS	biopsychosocial model of pain
CCK	Choleycystokinin
CMAP	Compound muscle action potential
COMM	Current opioid misuse measure
CPS-NAID	Pediatric Pain Profile, Chronic Pain Scale for Nonverbal Adults with Intellectual Disabilities
CT	Computed tomography
DLPFC	Dorsolateral prefrontal cortex
EEG	Electroencephalography
EMG	Electromyography

A. Aggarwal · M. Barad (✉) · A. Gowda
Department of Anesthesiology, Perioperative Medicine and Pain, Stanford Hospital and Clinics, Stanford, CA, USA
e-mail: akaggarw@stanford.edu; mbarad@stanford.edu; agowda@stanford.edu

S. Jones
Department of Anesthesiology and Pain Management, University of Texas Southwestern Medical Center, Dallas, TX, USA
e-mail: stephanie.jones@utsouthwestern.edu

S. Pritzlaff
Department of Anesthesiology and Pain Medicine, University of California Davis, Sacramento, CA, USA
e-mail: spritzlaff@ucdavis.edu

A. Nagpal
Department of Orthopaedics and Physical Medicine & Rehabilitation, Medical University of South Carolina, Charleston, SC, USA
e-mail: nagpal@musc.edu

FCE	Functional capacity evaluation
FLACC	Consolability Scale
fMRI	Functional magnetic resonance Image
FPS	Faces Pain Scale
FR	Radiofrequency
IASP	The International Association for the Study of Pain
IME	Independent Medical Evaluation
IMMPACT	Initiative on Methods, Measurement, and Pain Assessment in Clinical Trials
MCC	Mid cingulate cortex
MEG	Magnetoencephalography
MFAPS	Muscle fiber action potentials
MPI	Multidimensional Pain Inventory
MRI	Magnetic resonance imaging
MRS	Magnetic Resonance Spectroscopy
MUP	Motor unit potential
NIDA	National Institute
NIH	National Institutes of Health
NM-ASSIST	Modified Alcohol, Smoking and Substance Involvement Screening Test
NMJ	stimulus to neuromuscular junction 2) time delay across the NM
NRS	Numerical rating scale
ORT	Opioid Risk Tool
PAG	Periaqueductal gray
PCA	Patient Controlled Analgesia
PCC	Posterior cingulate cortex
PCL-5	PTSD Checklist for DSM-5
PCS	Pain Catastrophizing Scale
PET	Positron Emission Tomography
PHQ-9	Patient Health Questionnaire
PMQ	Pain medication questionnaire
PROMIS	Patient-Reported Outcomes Measurement Information System
PSIS	Posterior Superior Iliac Crest
PTSD	Post Traumatic Stress Disorder
rACC	Rostral anterior cingulate cortex
SI	Suprailiac Joint
SOAPP	Screener and opioid assessment for patients with pain
SPECT	Single photon emission computed tomography
T	Tesla
VAS	Visual analog scale
VDS	Verbal Descriptor Scale
VRS	Verbal rating scale
WCE	Work capacity evaluation
WHO	World Health Organization

Introduction

Pain, originally derived from the Latin word for "penalty," has seen its definition evolve over time. The International Association for the Study of Pain (IASP) updated its definition in 2020, expanding it to include six key insights, such as its personal nature and the distinction between pain and nociception. Assessing pain remains challenging, primarily relying on self-reporting through scales, and these can be influenced by various factors, including cultural differences and language barriers. Special scales are designed for children, nonverbal patients, and patients with dementia. Assessment of pain is complicated by placebo, which plays a significant role in pain perception and treatment, influenced by factors like patient expectations and the provider-patient relationship.

The biopsychosocial model offers a comprehensive approach to evaluating and assessing pain. This model underpins the importance of considering diverse factors such as race, ethnicity, gender, and age in pain assessment and treatment, reflecting the complexity of pain and the challenges in its management across different patient populations. This chapter serves to provide the reader with a discussion and summary of the rationale and history of how pain is assessed as well as the techniques we use to examine pain through the physical examination, patient-reported outcomes, psychological evaluation, and imaging modalities.

The Description of Pain

Pain is derived from Latin for "penalty" (poena). The definition and understanding of pain have also varied with time among cultural groups. In 2020, the International Association for the Study of Pain (IASP) revised the original 1970s definition of pain. They defined pain as "an unpleasant sensory and emotional experience associated with, or resembling that associated with actual or potential tissue damage." The definition was further expanded by noting six aspects regarding pain:

1. Pain is a personal experience.
2. Pain and nociception are different phenomena.
3. Individuals learn the concept of pain through life experiences.
4. Self-report of pain should be respected.
5. Pain, while adaptive, can adversely affect the function and social/psychological well-being.
6. The inability to communicate does not negate the possibility of a painful experience.

The IASP maintains a list of commonly used terminology, allowing researchers and clinicians to use a shared vocabulary to describe painful conditions and states. Common descriptive terms include *allodynia, dysesthesia, hyperalgesia, hyperpathia, hypoesthesia, and paresthesia*. These terms refer to a specific response to a stimulus threshold. The IASP also defines types of pain conditions, including

Table 4.1 Select IASP definitions [1]

Term	Definition
Allodynia	Pain due to a stimulus that does not normally provoke pain
Dysesthesia	An unpleasant abnormal sensation
Hyperalgesia	Increased pain from a stimulus that normally provokes pain
Hyperesthesia	Increased sensitivity to stimulation, excluding special senses
Hyperpathia	A painful syndrome characterized by an abnormally painful reaction to a stimulus, especially a repetitive stimulus, as well as an increased threshold
Neuropathic pain	Pain caused by a lesion or disease of the somatosensory nervous system
Nociceptive pain	Pain that arises from actual or threatened damage to non-neuronal tissue and is due to the activation of nociceptors
Nociplastic pain	Pain that arises from altered nociception despite no clear evidence for disease or lesion of the somatosensory system causing the pain
Paresthesia	An abnormal sensation, whether spontaneous or evoked

neuralgia, neuropathic pain, neuropathy, central neuropathic pain, peripheral neu-ropathic pain, nociplastic pain, nociceptive pain, spontaneous pain, and evoked pain. In addition, the IASP defines chronic pain as pain that persists or recurs for more than three months (Table 4.1) [1–3].

The Measurement of Pain

Despite extensive efforts, self-reporting pain remains the best way to directly evaluate a patient's current state for research/clinical purposes. To self-report, patients must be able to assess and describe their pain experience. Various factors can influence pain reporting, including how an individual appraises pain, perceived control over pain, and pain catastrophizing. Unidimensional scales are the most common way to report pain and include the verbal rating scale (VRS), visual analog scale (VAS), and numerical rating scale (NRS), among others. These scales are invalid if a patient engages in conscious or unconscious misrepresentation, if there are cultural disparities in description/self-evaluation of pain, or if impacted by language barriers. Multidimensional measures are based on patient-reported information but measure multiple domains. They provide greater information but take longer to administer and utilize. Examples include the Brief Pain Inventory, McGill Pain Questionnaire, West Haven Yale Multidimensional Pain Inventory, Oswestry Disability Index, etc. [4–9].

Special scales have been developed for specific populations. Of note, for children, the colored analog scale, Baker FACES, and FACES Pain Scale Revisited are commonly used and adjusted for developmental needs. Specific scales exist for nonverbal adults and infants, including Face, Legs, Activity, Cry, Consolability Scale (FLACC), Pediatric Pain Profile, Chronic Pain Scale for Nonverbal Adults with Intellectual Disabilities (CPS-NAID), and Pain Assessment in Patients with Dementia. In the research setting, Patient-Reported Outcomes Measurement Information System (PROMIS) and Initiative on Methods, Measurement, and Pain

Assessment in Clinical Trials (IMMPACT) are commonly utilized and assist in understanding responses compared to large population sets [10–13].

Placebo in Pain

Placebo is a neuro-psycho-physiological interaction with data suggesting that placebo analgesia is mediated by endogenous opioid and non-opioid mechanisms (cholecystokinin (CCK), dopamine). Several factors have been found to influence the placebo response, including patient expectation, patient conditioning, learned behaviors, and provider-patient interactions; in certain cases, these are additive. Neuroimaging studies demonstrate activation with placebo in the dorsolateral prefrontal cortex (DLPFC), the rostral anterior cingulate cortex (rACC), and the periaqueductal gray (PAG) regions involved in the descending pain modulating network. Significant interactions suggest that the descending rACC/PAG/RVM pain-modulating circuit is involved in placebo analgesia. This network then inhibits regions involved in pain processing, such as the mid and posterior cingulate cortex (MCC, PCC), insula, and thalamus [14–17].

While placebo plays an important role in clinical trials, it presents several challenges. Firstly, several phenomena that influence results/data are sometimes misattributed to placebo in research and clinical practice. This includes regression to the mean, natural history of the disease, response bias, reporting bias, and the Hawthorne effect. Secondly, research suggests that patient factors may influence placebo, including age, sex, genetics, etc. There have been calls to eliminate placebo for clinical research, primarily arguing that treatment should be compared to standard of care and not placebo, as well as that placebo involves deception and thus violates patient autonomy [18]. The ethics of placebo in clinical trials and clinical practice continue to be debated, with a principle guiding factor being protecting placebo recipients from harm. Given the widespread use of placebo in clinical research, patients must express an understanding of the potential to receive a placebo before starting the trial. While it is considered unethical to deceive a patient knowingly, the placebo effect is likely ubiquitous in healthcare. This concept is highlighted by the open-hidden paradigm, in which a treatment is less effective when given covertly. The increased effectiveness of open treatment suggests that patient understanding of treatment and the patient-provider relationship are crucial in treatment delivery [16].

In contrast to placebo, the nocebo effect refers to negative side effects expected only for active treatment but experienced by placebo recipients. It can also refer to negative effect when something is not done. Research has shown that there are likely nocebo responders similar to how there are placebo responders, with CCK, dopamine, and opioid systems likely playing roles [19].

Epidemiology of Pain

It remains challenging to study the epidemiology of pain due to its subjective nature and lack of consensus on how to define and measure pain. Incidence and prevalence are complex for chronic pain; the Institute of Medicine, as part of the 2010 Patient Protection and Affordable Care Act, performed an econometric study that estimated 100 million American adults are affected by chronic pain [20]. In noting the epidemiology of pain, it is important to differentiate mild impact from high-impact chronic pain. High-impact chronic pain is associated with substantial restriction of participation in work, social, and self-care activities for six months or more; the economic burden is estimated at >500 billion dollars/year. However, there is a need for better data on the prevalence, incidence, and treatment of chronic pain. Data suggest that pain is more prevalent in individuals with limited access to health care services, in certain racial/ethnic minorities, in certain geographic regions, and in certain occupational roles. When looking at specific populations, such as children or adolescents, the data becomes even less precise and highlights areas for further research [21, 22].

Assessment of Pain as a Biopsychosocial Experience

The original biopsychosocial model (BPS) of pain, developed by Engel [23], proposed that biological, psychological, and social factors are involved in determining when patients are viewed as sick by themselves or by others. Adapted by Gatchel and colleagues [24–26], the BPS model of chronic pain suggests that biological and psychological factors consist of central (i.e., biological, cognitive, somatic, affective) and peripheral (i.e., autonomic, endocrine, immune) processes. Social factors (e.g., social support, culture) interact with the biological and psychological factors to influence a person's experience of chronic pain. This conceptual model has been adapted to guide research in a variety of chronic pain conditions [27–30] and has been widely accepted as the most inclusive model for assessing chronic pain and formulating effective, comprehensive treatment plans.

The biopsychosocial-spiritual model recognizes the impact of religious factors in modulating a patient's pain experience, and patients' spiritual backgrounds should be noted in a comprehensive pain assessment. A 2021 review evaluated the relationship between religious beliefs and attitudes and clinical outcomes, including patients' perceived pain intensity, pain interference, disability, physical functioning, and coping among patients with chronic musculoskeletal pain syndromes. There was weak evidence that religiosity is positively associated with worse pain-related beliefs and worse pain-related emotions, but with positive impacts on coping strategies and pain acceptance [31].

Race and Ethnicity in Pain

Despite increased awareness and focus on improving disparities in healthcare, disparities in pain treatment continue to be prevalent. Evidence shows that racial and ethnic minorities have disproportionately unrelieved pain. African Americans report higher pain levels from medical conditions including AIDS, glaucoma, migraine headaches, and postoperative pain [32]. Across multiple clinical settings, evidence has shown that racial and ethnic minorities, compared to Caucasian patients, are less likely to be prescribed analgesics [33, 34]. Disparities in pain management decisions when treating minorities have been reported across various conditions and clinical scenarios, including emergency care, cancer pain treatment, and acute postoperative pain treatment. Studies show that African American and Hispanic patients are more likely to be undertreated for pain than their Caucasian counterparts [35]. Non-white patients seen in the emergency department are 22–30% less likely to receive analgesic medications, 17–30% less likely to receive opioids, and tend to have longer wait times compared to their white counterparts [36]. Several factors are proposed to contribute to disparities in pain care. Patient factors contributing to differences in pain treatment outcomes include racial and ethnic differences in the patient's experience of pain. Some studies show that African American patients report a greater pain-related disability, suffering, and psychological symptoms related to pain, which may influence these patients' pain experiences negatively, contributing to disparities in care [35, 37]. Racial and ethnic disparities in pain treatment also heavily contribute to disparities in pain relief. Because the primary means to assess pain remains the patient's subjective and the provider's impression of the patient's pain severity, implicit stereotypes may impact the observer's perception. Examples of physician bias include evidence that negative stereotypes have been documented for racial and ethnic minorities that experience pain [38, 39]. African-Americans and Hispanics have been shown to receive more scrutiny for potential drug abuse, despite evidence showing no increased rate of aberrant drug use amongst these populations [40, 41]. Evidence shows that primary care providers are more likely to underestimate pain intensity in African American patients than in other racial groups [42].

Special Populations and Pain

Special populations, such as pregnant women, older adults, those with mental health disorders, those with active or past substance abuse, and opioid-tolerant patients, often have unique characteristics and experiences. Due to their unique circumstances, certain populations may be more prone to specific pain syndromes. For instance, 45% of women develop pelvic girdle or low back pain during pregnancy, and up to 25% develop these pain syndromes in the postpartum period. Pelvic girdle pain describes pain in the regions of one or both sacroiliac (SI) joints and the gluteal region. Patients may also report pain in the pubic symphysis region. In contrast, low back pain of pregnancy is defined as pain in the lumbar region. Risk factors include strenuous work, previous low back pain, or pain syndromes in a previous pregnancy, and these factors should be considered when performing the initial assessment of pain in the pregnant patient [43].

A full psychological history and review of affective symptoms should be included in a comprehensive pain assessment. Systematic reviews indicate that chronic pain patients show elevations in all indices of self-reported negative affect, which include depression, anxiety, and emotional distress [44–46]. These psychological factors should be assessed in patients with persistent pain. Historically, psychological distress was often interpreted to be a consequence of chronic pain. Still, many studies now suggest that premorbid psychological dysfunction increases the risk of developing chronic pain. Therefore, psychological distress may be a predisposing risk factor for developing chronic pain syndromes [47–50]. Research has well established the role of emotional distress in the pain experience, and research in the last three decades has shown that adverse childhood experiences (ACEs), defined as potentially traumatic events, are associated with higher rates of pain in adulthood, and adults with chronic pain are much more likely to report ACEs, even suggesting a cumulative effect. Research is looking into mechanisms, treatment options, and differentiating between types of ACEs and their impact on chronic pain.

Older Adults and Pain

Older adults are less likely to have pain assessment documented in various clinical scenarios, contributing to undertreatment of pain in the older adult population [51–53]. Multiple factors influence which pain assessment tools are most appropriate for the aging population. In acute pain scenarios, abnormalities in blood pressure, heart rate, or respiratory rate are common and can be used as surrogates to assess the severity of pain. However, these variabilities in a patient's vitals are not present in chronic pain situations. Healthcare providers need to rely on comprehensive assessment, including self-reported measurements, cognitive assessments, and collateral sources.

For those older adults who are cognitively intact, and even those with mild dementia, self-reported instruments such as the NRS (numerical rating scale) and VDS (verbal descriptor scale) are commonly used and validated [54]. Various assessment tools may be utilized according to older individuals' unique disabilities. In older patients with language impediments and cognitive impairment, which impacts their ability to conceptualize the VAS and NRS when quantifying pain severity, the Faces Pain Scale (FPS) has been successfully utilized as a more appropriate alternate tool [55]. Assessment of pain intensity in older adults should include an assessment of functional status. Screening for mobility impairments should be routine in the older population, as a change in mobility may be an early sign of pain. Gait speed is a good predictor of disability and, therefore, may be a useful measure when assessing functionality [56]. Studies show that older adults may under report pain because of the belief that pain is a "normal part of aging." Thus, gathering collateral information from loved ones or caregivers may give the healthcare provider improved insight into the true nature of a patient's pain experience. In cases where patients have significant cognitive impairment, caregivers or healthcare providers are encouraged to use behavioral clues to gauge pain severity.

Sex and Gender Issues in Pain

Per the World Health Organization, "Gender is used to describe the characteristics of women and men that are socially constructed, while sex refers to those that are biologically determined." [57] In examining the role of sex and gender in pain we will first look at the influence of sex. Sex hormones influence pain response, affecting men and women differently. Sex hormones and their receptors are present and impact both areas of the central and peripheral nervous systems associated with nociceptive transmission [58, 59]. Estradiol and progesterone effects on pain sensitivity are relatively complex. Both estradiol and progesterone exert pro-nociceptive and anti-nociceptive effects on pain, however, testosterone is anti-nociceptive and therefore protective in the pain response [60]. There may be sex-related differences in the endogenous opioid system. Smith and colleagues found that women in high estradiol and low progesterone states exhibited decreased pain sensitivity than those women in low estradiol states. In a review of experimental pain differences amongst children, most experiments showed no differences in pain sensitivity. However, the difference was more pronounced with older children (greater than 12 years of age), with girls tending to be more sensitive and less tolerant to painful stimuli than boys. This difference in older children but not in younger children suggests a hormonal influence on pain sensitivity [61]. Certain pain syndromes seem to have hormonal influences. Sex differences in response to pain interventions may exist. One review of 18 studies showed that female patients had lower opioid use in postoperative pain settings [62]. However, these findings have not been consistent. A recent meta-analysis reported mixed results for sex differences in opioid analgesic efficacy [63]. While the authors found no sex-specific effects for mu-opioid analgesia across clinical studies evaluating mu-opioids, there did appear to be a greater 'analgesic' effect for female patients when restricting analyses to patient-controlled analgesia (PCA) usage.

Some evidence suggests psychosocial factors influence the pain response amongst the different sexes, though the available literature does focus primarily on heteronormative gender differences. Catastrophizing is associated with increased pain and pain-related disability, and cisgender women tend to engage in catastrophizing more often than their male counterparts. These differences thereby influence treatment outcomes amongst men and women [64]. A lower degree of self-efficacy has been found to be associated with higher levels of pain and physical symptomatology and evidence shows that cisgender men demonstrate greater self-efficacy. This difference in self-efficacy was subsequently related to lower cold pressor pain sensitivity amongst male participants [65].

Large-scale epidemiological studies across multiple different regions find that women report pain more frequently than men [66]. Sociocultural beliefs about femininity and masculinity appear to impact pain responses among the different sexes, as pain expression is generally more socially acceptable amongst women. This difference in social acceptance may lead to a bias in pain reporting in women and thus treatment-seeking. One study revealed that both men and women believed that men report pain less than women due to it being less socially acceptable [67]. Review of pain responses across multiple painful stimuli and various pain measures remains highly consistent. Women have higher pain sensitivity when compared to men [68]. Unfortunately, much of the literature on these gender and sex differences does not adequately differentiate between sex and gender roles, and future studies should hopefully differentiate the different impacts gender and sex make on pain sensitivity and individuals' chronic pain experience. The vast majority of the available literature on these impacts focuses primarily on the heteronormative experience.

Language Barriers and Pain

Physician/patient communication can also lead to disparities in healthcare. Factors including language barriers for those patients who are not primarily English-speaking, including lack of access to interpreting services, contribute to poor outcomes. Cultural differences in communication styles and health literacy, shown to impact African-American populations as well as other minority groups, impact patient/provider communication. Poor communication impacts the patient/physician therapeutic relationship, the patient's trust in their healthcare provider, and ultimately treatment outcomes [42, 69].

Assessment of Pain

Multiple factors outside of the biomedical context contribute to a patient's pain experience. Cultural influences, comorbid mood disorders, including present or prior history of substance dependence, sexual abuse, previous trauma, older age, chronic disease, and economic disparity are all examples of psychosocial factors which contribute to a patient's pain experience. An important aspect of the pain assessment is acknowledgment of the influence of various comorbidities and psychosocial determinants of health that impact pain perception and experience.

Comprehensive pain assessment should include review of the patient's social situation. Social forces impact pain experience, assessment, and pain-related outcomes in treatment. In a review by Jensen et al., it was found that increased perceived social support was associated with better outcomes, including less pain and improved overall functioning in patients with pain and disability related to spinal cord injury, multiple sclerosis, and acquired amputation [70]. There is also substantial literature illustrating the important role of social support in the pain experience caused by cancer and its treatments [30, 71]. Other important social interactions, such as relationships at work, impact pain assessment and treatment outcomes. Lack of social support at work, work dissatisfaction, and interactions with the disability compensation system are significant predictors of pain-related work disability [72–74].

Assessment of nutritional status, sleep function, sexual function, general health, past treatments, and pharmacological management are all important when evaluating patients with complex chronic pain syndromes. Sleep hygiene can impact not only patient function but also pain sensitivity. Insomnia and other sleep disorders are highly prevalent among those experiencing chronic pain. Sleep disorders, including non-restorative sleep, are closely related to the manifestation of central sensitization, are characterized by low-grade neuroinflammation, and commonly associated with affective disturbance, including anxiety and stress [75]. Nutritional status may also contribute to the patient's pain severity and should be considered in a comprehensive pain assessment. Muscular pain and myalgias have been associated with deficiencies in amino acids, magnesium, selenium, and vitamins B and D. Research also shows that those deficient in certain essential nutrients may develop dysfunction of pain inhibitory mechanisms. These deficiencies may contribute to fatigue and other chronic pain symptoms, including severity of pain in fibromyalgia [76].

Physical Examination in Chronic Pain Syndrome

The pain examination is a close second to history as a diagnostic tool in the assessment of pain (Table 4.2). While there are many ways to think about the elements of the physical examination required for pain assessment, a hybrid model known as the "comprehensive neuromusculoskeletal evaluation" combines key elements of both the neurologic and musculoskeletal exams and is geared for the pain physician [77] and will be presented here. Regardless of the order, this is a key element in working with the chronic pain patient. A survey of 120 chronic pain patients showed that 97% felt that a physical exam allowed the doctor to find useful information, 92% felt that the physical exam showed that the doctor cares for them, and 87% felt that the exam was as important as an MRI [78].

The general observation of the patient includes vital signs, pain behaviors, observation of gait, mannerisms, coordination, interaction with others, and appearance. During this initial discussion, a basic mental status examination determining the patient's level of consciousness and alertness, general understanding of why they are seeing you, and orientation to person, place, and time can be added on. The

Table 4.2 Elements of the chronic pain physical exam

Physical exam elements
Observation of patient
Basic mental status examination
Inspection and palpation
Range of motion/strength testing
Reflexes/tone
Sensory testing
Coordination/gait
Provocative maneuvers

inspection of the patient specifically looks at the affected region, looking for cutaneous landmarks (scars, rashes, etc.), symmetry, temperature, trauma, muscle bulk, posture, or alignment if applicable. After inspection, palpation/percussion serves to further narrow the cause of pain and identifies areas that could serve as pain generators, such as lymph nodes, trigger points, and nerve entrapments (Tinel sign).

Focusing on the affected area range of motion, both active and passive, can be used to identify soft tissue restrictions, laxity, and hypermobility. Strength testing is then used to assess motor function. The standard muscle grading system to assess strength over a 0–5 scale is an effort-dependent scale [79]. For a full discussion on the evolution of this scale and the controversies that surround it, please see Dyck et al. [80]. This presents challenges for many pain patients who are limited in effort due to pain. This should be recognized and noted on the exam so as not to misrepresent the level of weakness. It is ideal to test the muscle on one side more than the other to achieve a comparison, remembering, though, that the dominant side should always be stronger, although this difference may be subtle. Patterns of muscle weakness can help make the diagnosis; for example, proximal muscle weakness may suggest a myopathy, whereas distal muscle weakness can suggest a polyneuropathy. Muscle tone can also be examined during this process, looking for hypotonia or spasticity [77].

The goal of the sensory exam is to determine which fibers and tracks are involved. An initial description of the pain can be very helpful with localization with "sharp, shooting" pain transmitted by fast A-delta fibers and dull, poorly localized burning pain transmitted by C fibers. Allodynia, should be very easy to pick up on the initial gross sensory exam. If a deficit or an area of allodynia is discovered, then a more detailed exam can occur. Pinprick and temperature are mediated by A-delta (cold) and C fibers (warm). Hyperalgesia, a severe pain in response to a mild noxious stimulus is often assessed with pinprick. Vibration, proprioception, and fine touch are mediated by A-beta fibers. Higher cortical sensory testing, such as graphesthesia and stereognosis may also be used. These tools can be used to form a "lesion map." [77, 81]

Once a sensory lesion is detected, it needs to be understood in the context of the injury—is it a peripheral sensory nerve fitting the distribution of a cutaneous innervation map, or is it a radicular pattern fitting the distribution of the dermatome map? A broader area of involvement may suggest a plexopathy vs. a central pathology involving the brain and/or spinal cord.

Deep tendon reflexes can assist in localizing the lesion to upper or lower motor neurons and have a standardized grading system of 0 to 4+. They can also be helpful in distinguishing poor effort from true weakness. If the reflex testing is eliciting hypoactive reflexes, consider distraction techniques—or voluntary contraction of muscles not being tested. The Jendrassik maneuver is a classic distraction technique and entails hooking the digits of both hands and forcibly trying to separate them while the examiner is testing reflexes. Several reflexes are referred to as "pathologic" for their ability to suggest an upper motor neuron abnormality. Clonus (more than several beats), Babinski (also referred to as a positive plantar reflex testing), and the Hoffman sign are examples [77, 81]. Coordination and gait are helpful for assessing cerebellar function as well as sensory. The traditional finger-nose-finger and heel-knee-shin assess cerebellar function. Balance or equilibrium can be observed in the heel-toe walk in a straight line. A Romberg test is performed; however, a failed test can indicate a problem in the sensory (proprioceptive), cerebellar, or vestibular system. Gait assessment should be performed in a hallway where the patient has space to walk. This can be useful to detect certain gaits, such as a high steppage gait or a neuropathic gait due to weakness in the foot dorsiflexors and an attempt to prevent them from dragging.

The last parts of the physical exam are the special tests and provocative tests that can further hone in on the diagnosis. While there are many, we have compiled a list of the key ones for pain physicians (see Table 4.3) [97–100].

Tests to identify functional behaviors can also be employed. Waddell signs are a series of 8 tests developed by Gordon Waddell in 1980 as a method to identify patients with low back pain who were likely to experience a poor surgical outcome after surgery. The signs were used by other clinicians to detect psychogenic, sometimes inappropriately labeled "non-organic," manifestations of low back pain in patients and further expanded to identify malingering in patients. Two systematic reviews [101, 102] to evaluate the evidence concluded that Waddell signs do not correlate with psychological distress, do not discriminate organic from non-organic problems, and the underlying pathology may represent an organic issue as well as fail to demonstrate an association between Waddell signs and secondary gain or malingering [103]. Furthermore, there is no randomized study that has determined its sensitivity or specificity for low back pain. As Main and Waddell propose, positive Waddell signs in a patient offer only a psychological alert that may warrant a complete psychological evaluation [104].

Psychological Evaluation

Psychological evaluation is a key component of comprehensive management strategies, and advertising it as such can reduce possible feelings of stigma associated with psychological assessment. The evaluation consists of the clinical interview and patient-reported outcome measures. The assessment is structured to assess key domains. Depression and anxiety are the most common mental health conditions that co-occur with chronic pain. Furthermore, individuals with chronic pain are more likely to acquire a mood or anxiety disorder as a consequence of having pain and life changes that pertain to chronic pain, such as sleep impairment, disability, and social isolation. Additionally, mental health conditions increase the risk of developing future chronic pain. Thus, this bi-directional relationship makes it imperative to assess and to continue to assess the psychological state of the patient. Psychological assessment in pain medicine is also critically important for understanding underlying mood disorders, adverse childhood experiences, expectations of therapy, and ongoing life stressors. The roles of depression and anxiety in the experience of pain have long been established, and it is understood that they can contribute to and worsen the overall experience of pain. These psychological

Table 4.3 Provocative Maneuvers Except when noted, pain evoked by the maneuver is indicative of a positive test

Joint	Test	Indication	Specificity and sensitivity	Technique
Cervical	Distraction	Cervical radiculopathy Symptoms with gentle traction are considered positive.	Sensitivity 44% Specificity 90% [82]	With the patient in supine, the examiner stands at the head and places hands at the patient's mastoid processes and pulls the head gently towards the examiner's torso.
Cervical	Spurling test	Cervical radiculopathy	Sensitivity 92% Specificity 95% [83]	The examiner assists the patient in gently extending and rotating the cervical spine, resulting in narrowing of the cervical neural foramina.
Shoulder	Empty can sign	Supraspinatus tendinopathy/tear	Sensitivity 88% Specificity 62% [84]	The patient attempts to elevate the arms against resistance while the elbows are extended, the arms are abducted and the thumbs are pointing downward.
Shoulder		Infraspinatus/teres minor examination		The patient attempts to externally rotate the arms against resistance while the arms are at the sides and the elbows are flexed to 90°
Shoulder	Lift off test	Assessment of the subscapularis function	Sensitivity 22% Specificity 94% [84]	The patient rests the dorsum of the hand on the back in the lumbar area. Inability to move the hand off the back by further internal rotation of the arm suggests injury to the subscapularis muscle.
Shoulder	Appley scratch test	Acromioclavicular joint	Sensitivity 83.7% specificity 71.4% [85]	Touch superior and inferior aspect of opposite scapula

(continued)

Table 4.3 (continued)

Joint	Test	Indication	Specificity and sensitivity	Technique
Shoulder	Neer test	Subacromial impingement	Sensitivity 72% Specificity 60% [86]	Stabilize the patient's scapula with one hand, while passively flexing the arm while it is internally rotated. Pain in the testing position is positive.
Shoulder	Hawkins Maneuver	Supraspinatus tendon impingement	Sensitivity 79% Specificity 59% [86]	The examiner forcefully moves the patient's shoulder into internal rotation or to the end of range of motion or until reports of pain. Pain reported in the superolateral shoulder in testing is considered positive.
Shoulder	Drop arm	Rotator cuff tear	Sensitivity 73% Specificity 77% [87]	Stand behind the seated patient and while supporting the arm at the elbow, passively abduct the patient's arm to 90° and full external rotation. Then release the elbow support and ask patient to slowly lower the arm to neutral. Sudden dropping of the arm or weakness in maintaining position is considered positive.
Shoulder	Yergason test	Biceps tendonitis	Sensitivity 43% Specificity 79% [88]	Elbow fixed to 90° degrees with forearm pronated. Ask patient to perform supination while palpating the bicipital groove. Pain or tenderness in biceps tendon is positive.
Shoulder	Clunk sign	Labral disorder	Sensitivity 44% Specificity 68% [89]	With patient in supine, and elbow fixed to 90°, provider stabilizes back of shoulder joint and externally rotates shoulder. The feeling of a "clunk" at the glenohumeral joint and patient discomfort is positive.

(continued)

Table 4.3 (continued)

Joint	Test	Indication	Specificity and sensitivity	Technique
Elbow	Cozen test	Lateral epicondylitis		The patient resists supination or wrist dorsiflexion with the arm in full extension. Pain is typically located just distal to the lateral epicondyle over the extensor tendon mass.
Elbow		Medial epicondylitis: Tennis elbow		On palpation, pain is present from the tip of the medial epicondyle to the pronator teres and flexor carpi radialis muscles. Pain is increased with wrist flexion and forearm supination performed under resistance.
Elbow		Pronator Teres syndrome: Median nerve entrapment distal to the elbow		Hypertrophied pronator muscle distal to the antecubital fossa, often with a positive Tinel's sign.
Elbow		Biceps tendinosis		Anterior elbow pain in a patient who has engaged in activities involving repetitive elbow flexion and forearm supination leading to tenderness of the distal biceps tendon that increases with resisted flexion and supination.
Elbow		Ulnar nerve entrapment		Tenderness or a positive Tinel sign is present over the ulnar nerve within the groove of the medial epicondyle. Other possible physical findings include hypothenar atrophy and index pinch weakness.

(continued)

Table 4.3 (continued)

Joint	Test	Indication	Specificity and sensitivity	Technique
Elbow		Radial tunnel syndrome		Compression of the deep branch of the radial nerve at the radial tunnel causes pain that radiates into the dorsal forearm. The pain increases with activities involving repetitive pronation and supination. Night pain may be present.
Elbow		Olecranon impingement		Clicking or locking of the elbow with terminal extension. The elbow pain worsens with extension.
Hip	FABER test (flexion, abduction, external rotation): also called PATRICK TEST	Pathologies at the hip, lumbar and sacroiliac region.	Sensitivity 48% Specificity 99% [90]	Patient is supine and placed in a figure-4 position with hip flexed and abducted with the lateral ankle resting on the contralateral thigh proximal to the knee. The provider stabilizes the opposite side of the pelvis at the anterior superior iliac spine, an external rotation, abduction, and posterior force is then lightly applied to the ipsilateral knee until the end range of motion is achieved. A positive test reproduces the patient's pain or limits their range of movement.
Hip	FADIR test (flexion, adduction, internal rotation): also called impingement test		Sensitivity 96.5% Specificity 7% [91]	Patient is supine with affected hip fully flexed or 90° flexed. Adduct the hip with combined internal rotation of the hip. A positive test is production of pain in the groin.

(continued)

Table 4.3 (continued)

Joint	Test	Indication	Specificity and sensitivity	Technique
Hip	Log roll passive supine rotation): also called Freiberg test	Pathology within the joint		With the patient in a supine position, place one hand over the mid-thigh and passively externally and internally rotate the hip to the ends of its range of motion. Compare the range of motion on both sides.
Hip	Ober test	Passive adduction to determine tightness in tensor fascia Lata and Iliotibial band		The patient is side-lying affected hip side up. Examiner stands behind patient and firmly stabilize the pelvis/greater trochanter to prevent movement in any. Knee is bent at 90, examiner hold distal leg and extends and abduct the hip joint. Then the leg is slowly lowered and hip adducted until motion is restricted.
Knee	McMurray test	Assess medial meniscus	Sensitivity 79.7% Specificity 78.5% [85]	Patient is supine grasp the patient's heel with one hand and the joint line of the knee with the other hand. The knee is flexed maximally, with external tibial rotation (medial meniscus) or internal tibial rotation (lateral meniscus). The knee is brought to full extension while maintaining rotation. A positive test produces a pop or click.
Knee	Lachman test (anterior drawer test)	Assess anterior cruciate ligament	Sensitivity 77.7% Specificity 95% [92]	The patient is supine with knee flexed to 30° degrees. The physician stabilizes the distal femur with one hand, grasps the proximal tibia in the other hand, and then attempts to sublux the tibia anteriorly. ACL damage will show forward translation without firm end point.

(continued)

Table 4.3 (continued)

Joint	Test	Indication	Specificity and sensitivity	Technique
Knee	Posterior drawer test	Assess posterior cruciate ligament	Sensitivity 90% Specificity 99%	Patient is supine with flexion of hip and knees to 90°, feet flat on the table. Apply an anterior-posterior directed force through the proximal tibia. Note the degree of backward movement in the femur.
Knee	Valgus test	Assess medial collateral ligament		Place one hand at the lateral aspect of the knee joint and the other hand at the medial aspect of the distal tibia. Next, valgus stress is applied to the knee at both zero degrees (full extension) and 30° degrees of flexion.
Knee	Varus test	Assess lateral collateral ligament		Place one hand at the medial aspect of the patient's knee and the other hand at the lateral aspect of the distal fibula. Next, varus stress is applied to the knee, first at full extension (i.e., zero degrees), then with the knee flexed to 30°.
Knee	Noble test	Assess iliotibial band tendonitis	Unknown	Patient is supine, place a thumb over the lateral femoral epicondyle as the patient repeatedly flexes and extends the knee. Pain symptoms are most prominent with the knee at 30° of flexion.
Lumbar	Straight leg raise	Lumbar disc herniation	Sensitivity 83% specificity 36% [93]	Patient's legs are raised while remaining straight in supine position to test for provocation of pain.

(continued)

Table 4.3 (continued)

Joint	Test	Indication	Specificity and sensitivity	Technique
Lumbar	Slumped seat test	Neural tension test to test neural hypersensitivity	Sensitivity 84% Specificity 83% [94]	The patient is in sitting position and the examiner assist patients in successive motions—first to slump the thoracic and lumbar spine, then to flex the neck, and then extend the knee as much as possible.
Lumbar	Kerning test	Test for meningeal irritation		The elicitation of pain or resistance with extension of the knee past 135° degrees.
Lumbar	Kemp test or facet loading maneuver	Pain on the ipsilateral side in the back or above the knee is generally indicative of a facet etiology, with pain going below the knee indicating possible nerve root irritation	Sensitivity 50–70% [95] Lyle et al. Specificity 67.3% [96]	Patient is either sitting or standing. The examiner often braces the patient at the ilium and then guides the patient into lumbar flexion, rotation lateral flexion, and lastly extension; axial force can be added at any time.
SI joint	FABER	Sacroiliac dysfunction		Flexion, abduction, and external rotation of the contralateral hip; if pain is felt in the contralateral SI joint, the test is considered positive.
SI joint	Gaenslen test	May indicate SI joint pain, hip pathology, pubic symphysis instability, or L4 nerve root irritation.		With the patient in supine position, the painful leg is resting on the edge of the table; the examiner assists in sagittal flexing the asymptomatic leg while the knee is flexed. The examiner stabilizes the pelvis and applies passive pressure to the leg being tested to hold it in a hyperextended position with downward force applied to the lower leg.

(continued)

Table 4.3 (continued)

Joint	Test	Indication	Specificity and sensitivity	Technique
SI joint	Fortin finger test			In either sitting or standing, the patient is asked to identify with one finger the area of pain. Positive is pointing to the within 1 cm inferomedial to the PSIS at 2 distinct times

variables—in conjunction with adverse childhood experiences, socioeconomic and cultural factors, situational stressors, substance use patterns, and other contextual dynamics—also have the potential to impact response to treatment and are thus critical to assess [105, 106].

Additionally, PTSD continues to be a significant factor in the maintenance and development of chronic pain. Pain at the time of a trauma is related to PTSD symptoms in both adults and children. Elevated pain in the days and weeks after a traumatic injury was associated with greater posttraumatic stress symptoms at 6 months. Similarly, pain intensity at hospital discharge was significantly correlated with depressive and PTSD symptoms one year after a traumatic injury [106]. Research has well established the role of emotional distress in the pain experience, and research in the last three decades has shown that adverse childhood experiences (ACEs), defined as potentially traumatic events, are associated with higher rates of pain in adulthood, and adults with chronic pain are much more likely to report ACEs, even suggesting a cumulative effect. Research is looking into mechanisms, treatment options, and differentiating between types of ACEs and their impact on chronic pain. Given this, obtaining a history of ACEs should be considered part of the pain evaluation.

A psychiatric history should seek out previous diagnoses and treatment courses for said diagnosis. It should also inquire about the family history of psychopathology.

There are numerous surveying instruments used to assess patients. The tests that are typically used to assess these domains are listed in Table 4.4. There are several caveats to this, namely that the NIH has developed a standardized tool for assessing many of these measures. Known as PROMIS, these computer adaptive tests seek to minimize patient burden and are standardized to normative data with the goal of providing clinicians and researchers standardized tools and seek to replace the confusing multitude of tests that are currently used [107].

A large part of the evaluation is spent understanding the patient's coping style, meaning the behavioral and cognitive techniques to manage physical/emotional stress.

Table 4.4 Tests for the psychological examination

Psychological state	Test
Depression	Beck depression inventory
	Patient health questionnaire (PHQ-9)
Anxiety/fear	Generalized anxiety disorder scale
	State trait anxiety inventory
	Fear avoidance beliefs questionnaire
Post traumatic stress disorder	PTSD checklist for DSM-5 (PCL-5)
Sleep	Insomnia severity index
	Pittsburgh sleep quality index
Catastrophizing	Pain catastrophizing scale (PCS) (13 items)
Coping	Coping strategies questionnaire (6 items)
	Chronic pain coping inventory
Avoidance/Kinesiophobia	Tampa scale
	Fear avoidance beliefs questionnaire
Multidimensional	Multidimensional pain inventory (MPI) 56 items
Disability and pain related behaviors	Brief pain inventory
	Pain disability index
	Chronic disability index
	Oswestry low back disability questionnaire

1. Cognitive vs. behavioral
2. Active vs. passive coping
3. Problem focused vs. emotion focused
4. Avoidant/attentional
5. Adaptive vs. maladaptive

The provider will also seek to understand more fully the role of family and support groups in the patient's pain experience. Solicitous responses—associated with higher levels of reported pain, disability, pain behaviors, and negatively associated with pain acceptance. Punitive responses are often associated with poorer outcomes. Positive reinforcement/confidence—facilitative response to good behavior is associated with lower levels of pain behavior [106].

Assessment of Substance Use

The National Institute of Health (NIDA) modified ASSIST (NM-ASSIST) to is an enhancement of the World Health Organization (WHO) Alcohol, Smoking, and Substance Involvement Screening Test (ASSIST) Version (V) 3.0 for identifying substance use disorders. This tool guides clinicians through a series of questions to identify risky substance use in their adult patients. The accompanying resources assist clinicians in providing patient feedback and arranging for specialty care, where necessary, using the 5 As of intervention (ask, advise, assess, assist, and arrange) [108].

For adolescents, the Screening to Brief Intervention Tool is recommended to help understand risk as well as potential for interventions. This screening tool consists of frequency of use questions to categorize substance use by adolescent patients into different risk categories. The accompanying resources assist clinicians in providing patient feedback and resources for follow-up [109].

Opioid Risk of Abuse Assessment

For predicting prescription opioid misuse in chronic pain patients, the pain medication questionnaire (PMQ) and the screener and opioid assessment for patients with pain (SOAPP) have the best evidence according to a systematic review looking at all validated measurements [110]. The current opioid misuse measure (COMM) performed best screening for current misuse, developed and validated in three studies of acceptable quality [110]. Other screening tools include ORT, mORT, TAPS, SISAP, and DIRE. Features shared amongst various opioid assessment and risk prediction tools, and amongst state and national guidelines, include an assessment of an individual and family history of substance use disorder, history of comorbid psychiatric disease, and history of physical, emotional, or sexual abuse.

Appropriate tools to use when considering initiation of opioid therapy include the Opioid Risk Tool (ORT), the Brief Pain Questionnaire (BPQ) and the Pain Medication Questionnaire, which predicts the risk of future misuse. For ongoing monitoring COMM is frequently used.

Disability Assessment

Chronic pain is responsible for disability, inability to work, and need for long-term medical treatment. Pain specialists require an understanding of disability terminology to provide objective ongoing or independent assessment of pain patients with disabilities and impairments.

A variety of assessments have been developed to assess a patient's functional status. Referred to as a functional capacity evaluation (FCE), these assessments are a comprehensive and objective measurement of a patient's work ability [2]. The effect on a patient's ability to perform purposeful tasks is the focus of functional and/or work capacity evaluation (FCE/WCE) [111]. These evaluations are typically performed by a physical therapist or occupational therapist.

An independent medical evaluation (IME) is a comprehensive assessment of a patient performed by a trained physician who does not provide medical care and does not initiate a therapeutic relationship with the person undergoing the evaluation. An IME objectively assesses the impact of an injury and subsequent disability on the patients' ability to function in a variety of domains, including self-care, work duty, and leisure or recreational activity [112].

Studies in Pain Medicine

In addition to a thorough history and physical examination, a variety of imaging and diagnostic tools are available in the workup and treatment of painful conditions. Common imaging modalities include x-rays, magnetic resonance imaging (MRI), and computed tomography (CT). These are used to investigate spinal pain, especially in the contest of spondylosis or suspected radiculitis. Increasingly, ultrasound is also used to examine large joints to evaluate for effusion, vascularization, and ligamentous or tendinous injury. High-resolution ultrasound can also be used to evaluate peripheral neurosonology and can aid in the diagnosis of nerve entrapment, swelling, or even neuroma formation. In some cases, more specialized imaging may be utilized, including single photon emission computed tomography (SPECT) or triple-phase bone scans to evaluate low back pain or complex-regional pain syndrome patients, respectively. Nerve conduction studies are another diagnostic tool that can be very useful for the pain practitioner. They can identify the anatomic site of injury, the type of neurons or fibers involved, and the severity of the injury.

Imaging Studies in Pain

X-ray/radiographs: X-rays record differential attenuation of the x-ray beam by tissues based on their differential densities. In pain medicine, x-rays are used as a diagnostic tool for workup but also in the procedure space for procedural invention. Often underutilized, X-ray should be considered as an initial imaging modality in many pain conditions due to the wide availability and cost-effectiveness.

Common pain applications: assessing for scoliosis, facet arthritis, spinal instability secondary to spondylolisthesis, vertebral compression fractures, and hardware failure.

Computed Tomography (CT): As with conventional radiographs, CT imaging is based on differential attenuation of x-ray beams but can differentiate not only bone from soft tissue but also between different densities of bone and soft tissue structures. Although CT can be very useful in the evaluation of the pain patient, careful consideration should be given to the increased radiation exposure. Quantitative CT of the lumbar spine exposed a patient to an estimated effective dose of about 0.1 mSv with an estimated cancer risk of 1 in 200,000 compared to a typical chest radiograph estimated effective dose of 0.02 mSv, which gives a relative risk of causing cancer of about 1 in 1,000,000 [113].

Common pain applications: evaluation of the spine, brain, or extremities when MRI is contraindicated (implantable devices, claustrophobia, inability of patient to lie supine for prolonged period of time), assessment of spinal canal and neural foramina for stenosis or compression, rule out acute or red flag conditions including bleeding, infection, or mass (contrast frequently given in these situations.

Ultrasound: An ultrasound probe contains piezoelectric crystals that vibrate in response to an applied electric current. These sound waves create alternating areas of compression and rarefaction when propagating through body tissues. The ultrasound waves penetrate body tissues, each having a different acoustic impedance. Some sound waves are reflected back to the transducer (which are processed to generate an image), and some continue to penetrate deeper. Advantages of ultrasound include live, dynamic assessment of joints, muscle, tendon, blood vessels, and nerve with no exposure to ionizing radiation.

Common pain applications: assessment of large joints for effusion, tendinopathy, or ligamentous injury; visualization of vascularity in relation to potential interventional targets; evaluation of peripheral nerves for compression, swelling, or neuroma.

Magnetic Resonance Imaging (MRI): Uses magnetic fields and radiofrequency (RF) to generate a 3D image. Electricity passed through the magnet creates a permanent magnetic field whose strength is measured in tesla (T)—typically 1.5 to 3 T. MR provides good soft tissue definition and precise definition of extra-dural, intradural, extramedullary, and intramedullary pathology. Pulse sequences commonly used in MRI of the spine include sagittal and axial T1 and T2-weighted sequences as well as short tau inversion recovery (STIR) sequences [114].

§ T1 (longitudinal plane relaxation time)—weighted toward fat—excellent for imaging fat, blood, or proteinaceous fluid.

§ T2 (transverse plane relaxation time)—weighted towards water (bright on T2)— useful for contrasting normal and abnormal anatomy (most acute processes are hyperintense and associated with increased water content).

§ STIR—this sequence can increase conspicuity of osseous and ligamentous lesions, including compression fractures.

§ MR Neurography—enhanced MR visualization of the peripheral nerve and pathology by encompassing a combination of two-dimensional, three-dimensional, and diffusion imaging pulse sequences [115].

Common pain applications: Spinal, brain, and joint imaging. Evaluation of soft tissue structures, including muscle, tendon, and nerve.

fMRI—functional MRI—exploits the fact that an increase in blood flow is associated with neural activity in the brain. This results in a local reduction in deoxyhemoglobin (it is paramagnetic and alters T2 images) and functions as an endogenous contrast-enhancing agent for fMRI. In clinical settings, fMRI has been used to monitor disease progression and also to map the brain language centers for surgical planning for tumor resection; it is used primarily as a research tool [116].

Magnetic Resonance Spectroscopy (MRS)—is a measurement of brain chemistry used to monitor serial biochemical signals in patients with tumors, stroke, epilepsy, metabolic disorders, infections, and neurodegenerative diseases [116].

Positron Emission Tomography (PET)—A positron emission tomography scan is a nuclear medicine technique that utilizes a radioisotope tracer with the primary goal of examining the biochemical or metabolic function of your tissues or organs. While PET has lower resolution than fMRI, it is considered more hazardous. Clinically used in oncology, in pain limited to research, though there is interest in clinical use for inflammatory pathology (i.e., Baastrup's disease—close approximation of spinous processes results in inflammation of interspinous ligament and bursa) [117].

Non-imaging Modalities in Pain

Electroencephalogram (EEG)—EEG is recorded at the scalp by electrodes with direct contact with skin. The recordings show alpha, beta, delta, and theta waves, which are used most commonly to detect consciousness, seizures, and sleep [117].

Magnetoencephalography (MEG)—records magnetic activity of the brain by using an array of SQUIDs (super quantum induction devices) placed above the head. It carries the advantage of not needing to apply electrodes to the brain, but it is not very sensitive to brain currents, typically used for epilepsy and cortical mapping [117].

Electromyography (EMG)—is a recording of electrical activities generated by depolarization of muscle cells in an attempt to assess size, morphology, and firing characteristics of the electrical signal within skeletal muscles at rest and during contraction. At rest the muscle cell membrane is silent except at the neuromuscular junction where ACh vesicles are released spontaneously, causing endplate potentials. After inserting the needle into a resting muscle, a brief burst of electrical discharge from mechanical irritation occurs. This is known as insertional activity and can be pathologic in myopathic processes. The most common abnormal spontaneous activity: fibrillation and positive sharp waves. When a muscle is minimally contracted, muscle fiber action potentials (MFAPs) that belong to a single motor unit can be recorded with a needle. As strength of contraction is increased, motor units are recruited in sequence. The summated electrical signal is the motor unit potential (MUP), which helps differentiate neurogenic disease from myopathic in that the high amplitude, long duration, and greater number of phases are reflective of the remodeling of surviving motor units following the loss of a certain amount of motor neurons in neurogenic disease as opposed to the low amplitude, short duration MUP seen in myopathic disease. Motor response is composed of multiple muscle fiber action potentials—compound muscle action potential (CMAP). Amplitude is proportional to the number of motor axons stimulated. Latency represents three processes—(1) the nerve conduction time from stimulus to neuromuscular junction (2) time delay across the NMJ (3) depolarization time across muscle. Prolonged terminal latency—detect distal entrapment neuropathies or NMJ disorder. Motor nerve conduction velocity represents the distance/difference between terminal latencies—F response (or waves) or H reflexes are 2 types of late potentials that assess conduction in the more proximal segments (such as a plexus or roots). These provide info regarding radiculopathies, polyneuropathies, plexopathies, and proximal mononeuropathies Sensory nerve action potential (SNAP) is obtained by supramaximal electrical stimulation of sensory fibers and recording the nerve action potential a certain distance further along the same nerve [118].

Nerve conduction studies evaluate large myelinated nerves (sensory/motor) for speed of conduction and amplitude. This helps us determine fiber type specificity. In nerve conduction studies, one employs electrical stimulation proximal to the suspected lesion and with recording of electrical activity distal—allowing one to evaluate any event between the stimulator point and recording point. Nerve conductions studies are used for suspected diseases of peripheral nervous system and used to detect focal nerve damage to myelin (i.e., entrapment neuropathies) [118].

Peripheral Neuropathy

Axonal: If an injury occurs at the cell body or axon, axonal degeneration occurs, resulting in low-amplitude CMAPs/SNAPs throughout the nerve being studied.

Demyelinating: If an injury is directed against the myelin, demyelination ensues, resulting in slowed conduction velocity and prolonged latencies. Conduction blocks and temporal dispersions are also seen.

Quantitative Sensory Testing (QST)—formalized, standardized clinical sensitivity test using calibrated stimuli. This type of testing allows for detection of sensory positive and negative symptoms (hyperalgesia vs. hypoesthesia). Most often used for research studies, it is useful in neuropathic pain (polyneuropathies and small fiber neuropathies (cannot localize a lesion though) [119].

Somatosensory Evoked Potentials (SSEP)—SSEPs are produced by activation of large peripheral nerve fibers by mechanical or electrical stimuli. Following either mixed nerve or sensory nerve stimulation, SSEPs are recorded over proximal portions of peripheral/CNS and can help identify impaired conduction caused by axonal loss (reduced amplitude, loss) or demyelination (prolonged or absent wave form) and are often used for intraoperative monitoring during spinal procedures [120].

Laser Evoked Potentials (LEPs)—LEPs are specialized infrared lasers used to stimulate thermal nociceptors in the skin. They are used to monitor cortical responses and are similar to audio or visual evoked potentials, but these do not measure pain. Pain pathways can be studied using LEPs. There are 2 different lasers available—CO_2 and solid-state lasers (these penetrate deeper into skin with shorter wavelengths—reduce skin burns but vary penetration based on pigmentation). The patient may feel pricking and burning sensations due to laser activation of A-delta and C fibers [120].

Skin Punch Biopsy—Sural nerve biopsy has been used for histopathological diagnosis of peripheral neuropathies, but it is invasive and carries the risk of permanent nerve damage. Skin biopsy is a safer and inexpensive technique for the evaluation of small nerve fibers. Decreased nerve-fiber density is typically found in peripheral neuropathies. Innervation density is measured by intraepidermal nerve fiber density measurement via microscopy. Can quantify the disease severity in small-fiber neuropathy and monitor disease progression. Skin site heals within a week and can be performed multiple times. Note, you need to compare epidermal nerve fiber density to controls based on age, gender, and location of biopsy [121].

Autonomic testing—used in the evaluation of small fiber sensory neuropathy, autonomic neuropathy, or autonomic dysregulation. The composite autonomic scoring scale (CASS), which includes measurements of orthostatic blood pressure, the quantitative sudomotor axon reflex test, heart rate response to tilt, heart rate variability with deep breathing, and changes in blood pressure with the Valsalva maneuver, appears to provide a useful measure of autonomic function and can help support a diagnosis of small fiber sensory neuropathy The evaluation of intraepidermal sweat glands is a viable technique to evaluate sudomotor function [122].

Disclosures Dr. Anuj Aggarwal has nothing to disclose.
Dr. Meredith Barad has nothing to disclose.
Dr. Stephanie Jones has nothing to disclose.
Dr. Scott Pritzlaff: Consultant: SPR Therapeutics, EBT Medical, and Nalu Medical; Grant support: Medtronic, Abbott.
Dr. Alpana Gowda has nothing to disclose.
Dr. Ameet Nagpal—Consultant: Practicing Clinician Exchange; Avanos Pharmaceuticals.

References

1. IASP News. Classification of Chronic Pain, Second Edition (Revised). International Association for the Study of Pain (IASP). 2021. https://www.iasp-pain.org/publications/free-ebooks/classification-of-chronic-pain-second-edition-revised/
2. Raja SN, et al. The revised International Association for the Study of Pain definition of pain: concepts, challenges, and compromises. Pain. 2020;161:1976–82.
3. Treede R-D, et al. Chronic pain as a symptom or a disease: the IASP classification of chronic pain for the International Classification Of Diseases (ICD-11). Pain. 2019;160:19–27.
4. Malhotra A, Mackey S. Outcomes in pain medicine: a brief review. Pain Ther. 2012;1:5.
5. Price DD, McGrath PA, Rafii A, Buckingham B. The validation of visual analogue scales as ratio scale measures for chronic and experimental pain. Pain. 1983;17:45–56.
6. Younger J, McCue R, Mackey S. Pain outcomes: a brief review of instruments and techniques. Curr Pain Headache Rep. 2009;13:39–43.
7. Cleeland CS, Ryan KM. Pain assessment: global use of the brief pain inventory. Ann Acad Med Singap. 1994;23:129–38.
8. Melzack R. The short-form McGill pain questionnaire. Pain. 1987;30:191–7.
9. Kerns RD, Turk DC, Rudy TE. The West Haven-Yale Multidimensional Pain Inventory (WHYMPI). Pain. 1985;23:345–56.
10. Dworkin RH, et al. Interpreting the clinical importance of treatment outcomes in chronic pain clinical trials: IMMPACT recommendations. J Pain. 2008;9:105–21.
11. Hummel P, van Dijk M. Pain assessment: current status and challenges. Semin Fetal Neonatal Med. 2006;11:237–45.
12. Li D, Puntillo K, Miaskowski C. A review of objective pain measures for use with critical care adult patients unable to self-report. J Pain. 2008;9:2–10.
13. Gershon RC, Rothrock N, Hanrahan R, Bass M, Cella D. The use of PROMIS and assessment center to deliver patient-reported outcome measures in clinical research. J Appl Meas. 2010;11:304–14.

14. Amanzio M, Benedetti F. Neuropharmacological dissection of placebo analgesia: expectation-activated opioid systems versus conditioning-activated specific subsystems. J Neurosci. 1999;19:484–94.

15. Benedetti F. Placebo effects: from the neurobiological paradigm to translational implications. Neuron. 2014;84:623–37.

16. Oken BS. Placebo effects: clinical aspects and neurobiology. Brain. 2008;131:2812–23.

17. Frisaldi E, Shaibani A, Benedetti F. Understanding the mechanisms of placebo and nocebo effects. Swiss Med Wkly. 2020;150:w20340.

18. Cohen SP, Wallace M, Rauck RL, Stacey BR. Unique aspects of clinical trials of invasive therapies for chronic pain. Pain Rep. 2019;4:e687.

19. Arnold MH, Finniss DG, Kerridge I. Medicine's inconvenient truth: the placebo and nocebo effect. Intern Med J. 2014;44:398–405.

20. Mackey S. National Pain Strategy Task Force: the strategic plan for the IOM pain report. Pain Med. 2014;15:1070–1.

21. van Hecke O, Torrance N, Smith BH. Chronic pain epidemiology and its clinical relevance. Br J Anaesth. 2013;111:13–8.

22. Mackey S. Future directions for pain management: lessons from the Institute of Medicine Pain Report and the National Pain Strategy. Hand Clin. 2016;32:91–8.

23. Engel GL. The need for a new medical model: a challenge for biomedicine. Science. 1977;196:129–36.

24. Gatchel RJ. Comorbidity of chronic pain and mental health disorders: the biopsychosocial perspective. Am Psychol. 2004;59:795–805.

25. Gatchel RJ, Peng YB, Peters ML, Fuchs PN, Turk DC. The biopsychosocial approach to chronic pain: scientific advances and future directions. Psychol Bull. 2007;133:581–624.

26. Gatchel RJ, Turk DC. Criticisms of the biopsychosocial model in spine care: creating and then attacking a straw person. Spine. 2008;33:2831–6.

27. Taylor LEV, Stotts NA, Humphreys J, Treadwell MJ, Miaskowski C. A biopsychosocial-spiritual model of chronic pain in adults with sickle cell disease. Pain Manag Nurs. 2013;14:287–301.

28. Miaskowski C, et al. A biopsychosocial model of chronic pain for older adults. Pain Med. 2020;21:1793–805.

29. Baria AM, Pangarkar S, Abrams G, Miaskowski C. Adaption of the biopsychosocial model of chronic noncancer pain in veterans. Pain Med. 2019;20:14–27.

30. Novy DM, Aigner CJ. The biopsychosocial model in cancer pain. Curr Opin Support Palliat Care. 2014;8:117–23.

31. Najem C, et al. Religious beliefs and attitudes in relation to pain, pain-related beliefs, function, and coping in chronic musculoskeletal pain: a systematic review. Pain Physician. 2021;24:E1163–76.

32. Clark J, Robinson ME. The influence of patient race, sex, pain-related body postures, and anxiety status on pain management: a virtual human technology investigation. J Pain Res. 2019;12:2637–50.

33. Shavers VL, Bakos A, Sheppard VB. Race, ethnicity, and pain among the US adult population. J Health Care Poor Underserved. 2010;21:177–220.

34. Meghani SH, Byun E, Gallagher RM. Time to take stock: a meta-analysis and systematic review of analgesic treatment disparities for pain in the United States. Pain Med. 2012;13:150–74.

35. Green CR, et al. The unequal burden of pain: confronting racial and ethnic disparities in pain. Pain Med. 2003;4:277–94.

36. Shah AA, et al. Analgesic access for acute abdominal pain in the emergency department among racial/ethnic minority patients: a Nationwide examination. Med Care. 2015;53:1000–9.

37. Green CR, Baker TA, Sato Y, Washington TL, Smith EM. Race and chronic pain: a comparative study of young black and white Americans presenting for management. J Pain. 2003;4:176–83.

38. Burgess DJ, et al. Patient race and physicians' decisions to prescribe opioids for chronic low back pain. Soc Sci Med. 2008;67:1852–60.
39. Dovidio JF, Fiske ST. Under the radar: how unexamined biases in decision-making processes in clinical interactions can contribute to health care disparities. Am J Public Health. 2012;102:945–52.
40. Becker WC, et al. Racial differences in primary care opioid risk reduction strategies. Ann Fam Med. 2011;9:219–25.
41. Becker WC, Sullivan LE, Tetrault JM, Desai RA, Fiellin DA. Non-medical use, abuse and dependence on prescription opioids among U.S. adults: psychiatric, medical and substance use correlates. Drug Alcohol Depend. 2008;94:38–47.
42. Staton LJ, et al. When race matters: disagreement in pain perception between patients and their physicians in primary care. J Natl Med Assoc. 2007;99:532–8.
43. Bauchat J, Wong CA. Chapter 39 – Pain management during pregnancy and lactation. In: Benzon HT, Raja SN, Liu SS, Fishman SM, Cohen SP, editors. Essentials of pain medicine. 4th ed. Elsevier; 2018. p. 339–344.e1.
44. Turk DC, Fillingim RB, Ohrbach R, Patel KV. Assessment of psychosocial and functional impact of chronic pain. J Pain. 2016;17:T21–49.
45. Burke ALJ, Mathias JL, Denson LA. Psychological functioning of people living with chronic pain: a meta-analytic review. Br J Clin Psychol. 2015;54:345–60.
46. Howe CQ, Robinson JP, Sullivan MD. Psychiatric and psychological perspectives on chronic pain. Phys Med Rehabil Clin N Am. 2015;26:283–300.
47. Fillingim RB, et al. Psychological factors associated with development of TMD: the OPPERA prospective cohort study. J Pain. 2013;14:T75–90.
48. Diatchenko L, Fillingim RB, Smith SB, Maixner W. The phenotypic and genetic signatures of common musculoskeletal pain conditions. Nat Rev Rheumatol. 2013;9:340–50.
49. Huijnen IPJ, Rusu AC, Scholich S, Meloto CB, Diatchenko L. Subgrouping of low back pain patients for targeting treatments: evidence from genetic, psychological, and activity-related behavioral approaches. Clin J Pain. 2015;31:123–32.
50. Clauw DJ. Fibromyalgia and related conditions. Mayo Clin Proc. 2015;90:680–92.
51. Herr K, Titler M. Acute pain assessment and pharmacological management practices for the older adult with a hip fracture: review of ED trends. J Emerg Nurs. 2009;35:312–20.
52. Spilman SK, et al. Infrequent assessment of pain in elderly trauma patients. J Trauma Nurs. 2014;21:229–35; quiz 236–7.
53. Booker SQ, Herr KA. Assessment and measurement of pain in adults in later life. Clin Geriatr Med. 2016;32:677–92.
54. Rospand. AGS panel on persistent pain in older person. The management of persistent pain in older person. J Am Geriatr Soc. 2002;50:S205–24.
55. Herr KA, Mobily PR, Kohout FJ, Wagenaar D. Evaluation of the Faces pain scale for use with the elderly. Clin J Pain. 1998;14:29–38.
56. Perera S, et al. Gait speed predicts incident disability: a pooled analysis. J Gerontol A Biol Sci Med Sci. 2016;71:63–71.
57. Gender and health. https://www.who.int/health-topics/gender#tab=tab_1
58. Craft RM. Modulation of pain by estrogens. Pain. 2007;132(Suppl 1):S3–S12.
59. Craft RM, Mogil JS, Aloisi AM. Sex differences in pain and analgesia: the role of gonadal hormones. Eur J Pain. 2004;8:397–411.
60. Smith YR, et al. Pronociceptive and antinociceptive effects of estradiol through endogenous opioid neurotransmission in women. J Neurosci. 2006;26:5777–85.
61. Boerner KE, Birnie KA, Caes L, Schinkel M, Chambers CT. Sex differences in experimental pain among healthy children: a systematic review and meta-analysis. Pain. 2014;155:983–93.
62. Fillingim RB. Sex differences in analgesic responses: evidence from experimental pain models. Eur J Anaesthesiol Suppl. 2002;26:16–24.
63. Niesters M, et al. Do sex differences exist in opioid analgesia? A systematic review and meta-analysis of human experimental and clinical studies. Pain. 2010;151:61–8.

64. Keefe FJ, Brown GK, Wallston KA, Caldwell DS. Coping with rheumatoid arthritis pain: catastrophizing as a maladaptive strategy. Pain. 1989;37:51–6.
65. Jackson T, Iezzi T, Gunderson J, Nagasaka T, Fritch A. Sex Roles. 2002;47:561–8.
66. Fillingim RB. Sex, gender, and pain. International Assn for the Study of Pain; 2000.
67. Robinson ME, et al. Gender role expectations of pain: relationship to sex differences in pain. J Pain. 2001;2:251–7.
68. Sorge RE, Totsch SK. Sex differences in pain. J Neurosci Res. 2017;95:1271–81.
69. Meints SM, Cortes A, Morais CA, Edwards RR. Racial and ethnic differences in the experience and treatment of noncancer pain. Pain Manag. 2019;9:317–34.
70. Jensen MP, Moore MR, Bockow TB, Ehde DM, Engel JM. Psychosocial factors and adjustment to chronic pain in persons with physical disabilities: a systematic review. Arch Phys Med Rehabil. 2011;92:146–60.
71. Schreiber KL, et al. Persistent pain in postmastectomy patients: comparison of psychophysical, medical, surgical, and psychosocial characteristics between patients with and without pain. Pain. 2013;154:660–8.
72. Helmhout PH, Staal JB, Heymans MW, Harts CC, Hendriks EJ, de Bie RA. Prognostic factors for perceived recovery or functional improvement in non-specific low back pain: secondary analyses of three randomized clinical trials. Eur Spine J. 2009;19(4):650–9. (Epub ahead of print). *The Spine Journal* vol. 10 456–457 (2010)
73. Melloh M, et al. Who is likely to develop persistent low back pain? A longitudinal analysis of prognostic occupational factors. Work. 2013;46:297–311.
74. Melloh M, et al. Prognostic occupational factors for persistent low back pain in primary care. Int Arch Occup Environ Health. 2013;86:261–9.
75. Nijs J, et al. Sleep disturbances in chronic pain: neurobiology, assessment, and treatment in physical therapist practice. Phys Ther. 2018;98:325–35.
76. Bjørklund G, Dadar M, Chirumbolo S, Aaseth J. Fibromyalgia and nutrition: therapeutic possibilities? Biomed Pharmacother. 2018;103:531–8.
77. Scholten P, Chekka K, Benzon HT. Chapter 4 – Physical examination of the patient with pain. In: Benzon HT, Raja SN, Liu SS, Fishman SM, Cohen SP, editors. Essentials of pain medicine. 4th ed. Elsevier; 2018. p. 27–38.e1.
78. Hashim MM, Edgeworth DM, Saunders JA, Harmon DC. Patient's perceptions of physical examination in the setting of chronic pain. Ir J Med Sci. 2021;190:313–6.
79. Medical Research Council (Great Britain). Aids to the examination of the peripheral nervous system. H.M.S.O., 1976.
80. Dyck PJ, et al. History of standard scoring, notation, and summation of neuromuscular signs. A current survey and recommendation. J Peripher Nerv Syst. 2005;10:158–73.
81. Malanga GA, Mautner K. Musculoskeletal physical examination E-book: an evidence-based approach. Elsevier Health Sciences; 2016.
82. Wainner RS, et al. Reliability and diagnostic accuracy of the clinical examination and patient self-report measures for cervical radiculopathy. Spine. 2003;28:52–62.
83. Shah KC, Rajshekhar V. Reliability of diagnosis of soft cervical disc prolapse using Spurling's test. Br J Neurosurg. 2004;18:480–3.
84. Jain NB, et al. The diagnostic accuracy of special tests for rotator cuff tear: the ROW cohort study. Am J Phys Med Rehabil. 2017;96:176–83.
85. Rinonapoli G, Carraro A, Delcogliano A. The clinical diagnosis of meniscal tear is not easy. Reliability of two clinical meniscal tests and magnetic resonance imaging. Int J Immunopathol Pharmacol. 2011;24:39–44.
86. Hegedus EJ, et al. Which physical examination tests provide clinicians with the most value when examining the shoulder? Update of a systematic review with meta-analysis of individual tests. Br J Sports Med. 2012;46:964–78.
87. Miller CA, Forrester GA, Lewis JS. The validity of the lag signs in diagnosing full-thickness tears of the rotator cuff: a preliminary investigation. Arch Phys Med Rehabil. 2008;89:1162–8.
88. Holtby R, Razmjou H. Accuracy of the Speed's and Yergason's tests in detecting biceps pathology and SLAP lesions: comparison with arthroscopic findings. Arthroscopy. 2004;20:231–6.

89. Nakagawa S, et al. Forced shoulder abduction and elbow flexion test: a new simple clinical test to detect superior labral injury in the throwing shoulder. Arthroscopy. 2005;21:1290–5.

90. Albert H, Godskesen M, Westergaard J. Evaluation of clinical tests used in classification procedures in pregnancy-related pelvic joint pain. Eur Spine J. 2000;9:161–6.

91. Hoppe DJ, Truntzer JN, Shapiro LM, Abrams GD, Safran MR. Diagnostic accuracy of 3 physical examination tests in the assessment of hip microinstability. Orthop J Sports Med. 2017;5:2325967117740121.

92. Katz JW, Fingeroth RJ. The diagnostic accuracy of ruptures of the anterior cruciate ligament comparing the Lachman test, the anterior drawer sign, and the pivot shift test in acute and chronic knee injuries. Am J Sports Med. 1986;14:88–91.

93. Poiraudeau S, et al. Value of the bell test and the hyperextension test for diagnosis in sciatica associated with disc herniation: comparison with Lasègue's sign and the crossed Lasègue's sign. Rheumatology. 2001;40:460–6.

94. Majlesi J, Togay H, Unalan H, Toprak S. The sensitivity and specificity of the slump and the straight leg raising tests in patients with lumbar disc herniation. J Clin Rheumatol. 2008;14:87–91.

95. Lyle MA, Manes S, McGuinness M, Ziaei S, Iversen MD. Relationship of physical examination findings and self-reported symptom severity and physical function in patients with degenerative lumbar conditions. Phys Ther. 2005;85:120–33.

96. Manchikanti L, Pampati V, Fellows B, Baha AG. The inability of the clinical picture to characterize pain from facet joints. Pain Physician. 2000;3:158–66.

97. Calmbach WL, Hutchens M. Evaluation of patients presenting with knee pain: part I. History, physical examination, radiographs, and laboratory tests. Am Fam Physician. 2003;68:907–12.

98. Chamberlain R. Hip pain in adults: evaluation and differential diagnosis. Am Fam Physician. 2021;103:81–9.

99. Newman DP, Soto AT. Sacroiliac joint dysfunction: diagnosis and treatment. Am Fam Physician. 2022;105:239–45.

100. Physiopedia. physiopedia. https://www.physio-pedia.com/home/

101. Fishbain DA, Cutler RB, Rosomoff HL, Steele Rosomoff R. Is there a relationship between nonorganic physical findings (Waddell signs) and secondary gain/malingering? Clin J Pain. 2004;20:399–408.

102. Fishbain DA, et al. A structured evidence-based review on the meaning of nonorganic physical signs: Waddell signs. Pain Med. 2003;4:141–81.

103. Waddell Sign. StatPearls [Internet]. Waddell Sign [Updated 2021 Jul 18]. In: StatPearls [Internet]. Treasure Island: StatPearls Publishing; 2022 Jan-. Available from: https://www.ncbi.nlm.nih.gov/books/NBK519492/StatPearls

104. Main CJ, Waddell G. Behavioral responses to examination. A reappraisal of the interpretation of 'nonorganic signs'. Spine. 1998;23:2367–71.

105. Lerman SF, Haythornthwaite J. Chapter 6 – Psychological evaluation and testing. In: Benzon HT, Raja SN, Liu SS, Fishman SM, Cohen SP, editors. Essentials of pain medicine. 4th ed. Elsevier; 2018. p. 47–52.e2.

106. Darnall BD. The role of psychological factors in chronic pain. In: Psychological treatment for patients with chronic pain. American Psychological Association; 2019. p. 13–33. https://doi.org/10.1037/0000104-002.

107. PROMIS: Patient-Reported Outcomes Measurement Information System – Home Page. 2013. https://commonfund.nih.gov/promis/index

108. NIDA-Modified ASSIST (NM ASSIST): Clinician's Screening Tool for Drug Use in General Medical Settings. https://www.samhsa.gov/resource/ebp/nida-modified-assist-nm-assist-clinicians-screening-tool-drug-use-general-medical

109. Five Major Steps to Intervention (The '5 A's'). https://www.ahrq.gov/prevention/guidelines/tobacco/5steps.html

110. Lawrence R, Mogford D, Colvin L. Systematic review to determine which validated measurement tools can be used to assess risk of problematic analgesic use in patients with chronic pain. Br J Anaesth. 2017;119:1092–109.

111. Geisser ME, Robinson ME, Miller QL, Bade SM. Psychosocial factors and functional capacity evaluation among persons with chronic pain. J Occup Rehabil. 2003;13:259–76.
112. Quintero S, Manusov EG. The disability evaluation and low back pain. Prim Care. 2012;39:553–9.
113. Richards PJ, George J, Metelko M, Brown M. Spine computed tomography doses and cancer induction. Spine. 2010;35:430–3.
114. Ract I, et al. A review of the value of MRI signs in low back pain. Diagn Interv Imaging. 2015;96:239–49.
115. Chhabra A, Madhuranthakam AJ, Andreisek G. Magnetic resonance neurography: current perspectives and literature review. Eur Radiol. 2018;28:698–707.
116. Gevirtz. Review of clinical nerve function studies and imaging: part II. Top Pain Manag. 2011;26:1–7.
117. Chen AC. New perspectives in EEG/MEG brain mapping and PET/fMRI neuroimaging of human pain. Int J Psychophysiol. 2001;42:147–59.
118. Ginsberg MR, Morren JA, Levin K. Using and interpreting electrodiagnostic tests. Cleve Clin J Med. 2020;87:671–82.
119. Waldman SD, Waldman CW, Kidder KA. Evaluation and treatment of peripheral neuropathies. In: Pain Management; 2011. p. 260–7. https://doi.org/10.1016/b978-1-4377-0721-2.00028-3.
120. Waldman HJ. Evoked potential testing. In: Pain management; 2007. p. 192–6. https://doi.org/10.1016/b978-0-7216-0334-6.50021-2.
121. Lauria G, Cornblath DR, Johansson O, McArthur JC. FENS guidelines on the use of skin biopsy in the diagnosis of peripheral neuropathy. Eur J Neurol. 2005;12:747–58.
122. Novak P. Autonomic testing. J Clin Neurophysiol. 2021;38:251.

Non-procedural Interventions for Chronic Pain

5

Ashlyn Brown, Alexander Bautista, Dania Chastain, Charles DeMessa, Tina Doshi, Jason Friedrich, W. Michael Hooten, Mohammed Issa, Lori Urban, and Lynn Kohan

---

A. Brown (✉)
H. Ben Taub Department of Physical Medicine and Rehabilitation, Baylor College of Medicine, Houston, TX, USA
e-mail: Ashlyn.Brown@bcm.edu

A. Bautista
Department of Anesthesiology and Perioperative Medicine, University of Louisville, Louisville, KY, USA
e-mail: alexander.bautista@louisville.edu

D. Chastain · L. Urban · L. Kohan
Department of Anesthesiology, University of Virginia, Charlottesville, VA, USA
e-mail: DCC6W@uvahealth.org; LAU9C@uvahealth.org; LRK9G@uvahealth.org

C. DeMessa
Department of Anesthesia and Pain Medicine, University of California Davis Health, Sacramento, CA, USA
e-mail: Charles.DeMesa@hoag.org

T. Doshi
Department of Anesthesiology and Critical Care Medicine, Division of Pain Medicine, John Hopkins University, Baltimore, MD, USA
e-mail: tina.doshi@jhmi.edu

J. Friedrich
Department of Physical Medicine & Rehabilitation, University of Colorado School of Medicine, Aurora, CO, USA
e-mail: Jason.Friedrich@cuanschutz.edu

W. M. Hooten
Department of Anesthesiology and Perioperative Medicine, Mayo Clinic, Rochester, MN, USA
e-mail: hooten.william@mayo.edu

M. Issa
Department of Anesthesiology, Peri-operative and Pain Medicine, Brigham and Women's Hospital, Harvard Medical School, Boston, MA, USA
e-mail: missa1@bwh.harvard.edu

Abbreviations

AAPM	American Academy of Pain Medicine
ASRA	American Society of Regional Anesthesia and Pain Medicine
CAA	Controlled Substances Act
CBD	Cannabidiol
CBT	Cognitive-behavioral therapy
COMM	Current Opioid Misuse Measure
CYP	Cytochrome P450
DEA	Drug Enforcement Administration
DEI	Diversity, equity, and inclusion
EMG	Electromyography
FDA	Food and Drug Administration
GABA	Gamma-aminobutyric acid
GMI	Graded motor imagery
LILT	Low-intensity laser therapy
LLLT	Low-level laser therapy
MAOIs	Monoamine oxidase inhibitors
MME	Morphine milligram equivalent
MS	Multiple sclerosis
NCCIH	National Center for Complementary and Integrative Health
NMSK	Non-musculoskeletal
NSAIDs	Nonsteroidal anti-inflammatory drugs
OUD	Opioid use disorder
PAIN	Pain management (general use)
PNE	Pain neuroscience education
PRP	Platelet-rich plasma
PT	Physical therapy
PUFAs	Polyunsaturated fatty acids
S/L	Sublingual
SSRIs	Selective serotonin reuptake inhibitors
SUDs	Substance use disorders
TCAs	Tricyclic antidepressants
TEA	Trigger point dry needling
TENS	Transcutaneous electrical nerve stimulation
THC	Delta-9-tetrahydrocannabinol
VNS	Vagus nerve stimulation

Introduction

Non-procedural interventions for chronic pain are an integral part of multimodal treatment plans. These interventions encompass modalities that address pain without resorting to injections or surgery, incorporating both pharmacologic and non-pharmacologic management strategies. Pharmacologic therapies encompass a variety of drug classes, including nonsteroidal anti-inflammatory drugs (NSAIDs), acetaminophen, opioids, antidepressants, anticonvulsants, corticosteroids, muscle relaxants, benzodiazepines, topical agents, and cannabinoids. On the other hand, non-pharmacologic therapies embrace complementary and integrative health approaches, physical therapy, rehabilitation therapies, and psychosocial treatments. This section aims to provide an overview of these treatment options.

Introduction to the Biopsychosocial Pain Model

Traditionally, pharmacologic and procedural methods have dominated pain management paradigms, guided by a mind-body dualistic approach; however, the biopsychosocial model, introduced by Engel in 1977, revolutionized our understanding and treatment of pain [1]. This model proposes an integrated perspective that encompasses biological, psychological, and interpersonal/social dimensions. Recognizing the contextual factors surrounding medical conditions or illnesses is crucial, particularly in the realm of chronic pain [2]. The biological component pertains to the physical body, genetics, tissue damage, infection, and physical stressors. The psychological component encompasses cognitions, emotional responses, and behavioral patterns. Lastly, the interpersonal/social component delves into factors such as background, demographics, family dynamics, economic status, living conditions, and social interactions.

Integration of these components into treatment often leads to improved outcomes and enhanced quality of life. However, several barriers hinder the comprehensive adoption of the biopsychosocial approach, spanning three factorial levels [3]. Micro-level factors involve healthcare providers' attributes, knowledge base, misconceptions regarding clinical practice guidelines, perceptions of time constraints, and attitudes toward patient factors. Meso-level factors encompass the formulation of clinical practice guidelines, community dynamics, funding models, healthcare provision, resource allocation, and workforce training. Macro-level factors encompass health policy, organizational structures, and societal influences. Failure to address these barriers results in inadequate and unimodal pain treatment, posing a national challenge necessitating cultural transformation [4].

The incorporation of all facets of the biopsychosocial model in pain assessment and treatment is advocated as an ethical imperative and social responsibility [5]. A comprehensive diagnostic evaluation entails a clinical interview, physical examination, mental health and substance abuse screening, and diagnostic tests. Furthermore, a proposed treatment regimen based on the biopsychosocial paradigm includes psychological therapies (such as cognitive-behavioral therapy and acceptance and commitment therapy), pharmacotherapy, graded exercise or physical therapy, nutritional counseling, and social support [6]. Delivering cost-effective services with adequately trained healthcare providers specializing in pain management ultimately enhances patients' quality of life for those experiencing chronic pain. Achieving this necessitates ensuring access to services, educating providers, and acknowledging the heterogeneity of pain [7].

Yet, clinicians must now contextualize the biopsychosocial model within the realms of the opioid crisis and the COVID-19 pandemic. These dual challenges have reshaped the landscape of evaluating and treating both chronic and acute pain, exposing aspects of the biopsychosocial model that require careful consideration to optimize patient care.

In 2017, the US Department of Health and Human Services declared the opioid crisis a public health emergency [8]. According to the National Safety Council, opioid overdoses surpassed fatalities from car crashes, becoming the leading cause of unintentional deaths in the USA by 2018 [9, 10]. The National Institute on Drug Abuse reported approximately 92,000 deaths in the USA attributed to illicit and prescription opioids in 2020, with a further increase in deaths reported between December 2020 and December 2021 [10, 11]. Deaths associated with prescription opioids predominantly involve fentanyl and its analogs, with methamphetamine and cocaine combinations exacerbating the crisis [8, 11].

The opioid epidemic underscores the significance of addressing all components of the biopsychosocial model [8]. Failure to address psychosocial factors alongside medical issues contributes to ineffective patient care and exacerbates the crisis. Before integrating opioids into multifaceted treatment plans, prescribing providers must assess patients' ability to responsibly manage these medications, adhere to prescribed regimens, mitigate diversion risks, and ensure secure storage, particularly in environments with concerns about family members or environmental factors [10].

As the opioid crisis persists, the emergence of the COVID-19 virus further complicates the landscape of pain management. The pandemic disrupted access to medical care and support systems with social distancing and other mitigating practices, depriving high-risk individuals of essential treatments and interventions, such as 12-step meetings, routine medical and mental health appointments, and access to methadone or suboxone clinics [12]. Social distancing measures also led to increased instances of solitary drug use, reducing the availability of lifesaving naloxone for overdose situations. Healthcare providers were compelled to innovate and find alternative means of connecting with patients. The expansion of telehealth services, facilitated by relaxed regulations from insurance companies and government entities, proved to be beneficial and lifesaving. However, these challenges brought to light disparities in healthcare delivery that demand urgent attention.

While disparities in gender, race, ethnicity, cultural background, financial status, and access to pain management have long been documented, the convergence of the COVID-19 pandemic and the opioid crisis has reached a critical juncture. Disparities include undertreatment of pain among Black, Indigenous, and People of Color (BIPOC) patients, limited access to analgesic medications, including opioids, and inadequate diagnostic evaluations [13].

It is imperative for pain management providers to tailor recommendations to ensure accessibility for all patients. Considerations should include access to telehealth resources, transportation for physical therapy or clinic visits, pharmacy accessibility, participation in support groups, childcare arrangements, work commitments, and adequacy of health insurance coverage [13].

Healthcare professionals who use this model can improve the effectiveness of diagnosis and treatment [14]. Similarly, effective communication between the patient and the healthcare clinician can result in increased patient satisfaction and decreased conflicts [15].

Pharmacological Treatments

Chronic pain is multifactorial, and often associated with concurrent conditions such as depression, anxiety, mood disorders, and sleep disturbances. Treatment typically targets the underlying mechanism, whether neuropathic, nociceptive, or a combination thereof, yet is often influenced more by tradition and personal experience [16]. Pharmacotherapy remains a cornerstone in managing moderate to severe pain, offering potential benefits alongside risks and costs. However, effective treatment poses challenges due to barriers such as physician and patient misconceptions, development of drug tolerance, uncertain efficacy, and unfavorable side effects. Notably, there exists a significant disparity between the treatment goals perceived by physicians and those desired by patients. While physicians prioritize functionality improvement, enhanced quality of life, and avoidance of long-term opioid therapy, patients often seek symptom relief [17].

The principle underlying pharmacologic treatment is multifaceted, aiming to reduce sensitization, mitigate pain amplification, and restore normal pain thresholds [16]. Current treatment strategies increasingly favor multimodal and nonopioid therapies. Pharmacologic agents used in chronic pain management can be categorized into opioids, nonopioids, and adjuvants, the latter referring to medications with synergistic actions alongside other analgesics. Often, integrating one or more drug classes is necessary to manage moderate to severe pain effectively. Complementary and synergistic effects among drugs can provide sufficient pain relief with minimized adverse reactions.

Nonopioids

NSAIDs
Nonsteroidal anti-inflammatory drugs (NSAIDs) stand as the most widely used pain medications globally. Typically employed for mild to moderate pain accompanied by inflammation and swelling [18], NSAIDs serve as the first-line agents for conditions such as arthritis, muscle sprains, back and neck injuries, and menstrual cramps. NSAIDs exhibit three pharmacologic effects: anti-inflammatory, analgesic, and antipyretic. Their primary mechanism of action involves inhibiting prostaglandin synthesis via cyclooxygenase (COX) inhibition. While NSAIDs blocking Cox-1 enzymes may cause gastric upset and bleeding, Cox-2 inhibitors (e.g., celecoxib) act selectively on Cox-2 enzymes, offering gastric mucosal lining protection.

Various NSAIDs possess distinct molecular structures and chemical properties; for instance, diclofenac is a benzene acetic derivative, while ibuprofen and naproxen are propionic acid derivatives, celecoxib, and valdecoxib have a sulfonamide group, and etoricoxib and rofecoxib have a sulfonyl group [19]. Chronic NSAID use may lead to gastrointestinal, cardiovascular, and renal side effects, necessitating limited duration and dosage. Thromboembolic cardiovascular events associated with Cox-2 inhibitors arise from increased platelet activation and aggregation after selective blockade of prostacyclin formation, prooxidant activity, and reduction of endothelial factor expression [19]. The direct and indirect effect of NSAIDs in the kidneys via inhibition of prostaglandin synthesis leading to reduction of glomerular pressure and afferent arteriolar vasodilation has led to recommendations to avoid long-term use and avoidance in patients with borderline renal function. Nevertheless, recent evidence suggests oral NSAIDs can be judiciously used in selected individuals with chronic kidney disease [20].

Acetaminophen
Acetaminophen possesses both analgesic and antipyretic properties but lacks specific anti-inflammatory effects compared to NSAIDs. Although its mechanism remains unclear, acetaminophen likely blocks the Cox-3 enzyme, predominantly exerting a central nervous system effect on prostaglandin synthesis. Acetaminophen serves as a first-line option due to its favorable safety profile and cost-effectiveness. Recommended for mild to moderate musculoskeletal pain, acetaminophen usage should be capped at less than 3 g/day to avoid asymptomatic elevations in aminotransferases, with lower limits for frail patients and those who consume alcohol regularly [21].

Opioids

Opioid analgesics have been widely used in the treatment of severe acute pain and chronic pain related to cancer or at the end of life; however, their utility in treating non-cancer pain is always a subject of scrutiny and debate. Most opioids have a direct affinity to mu receptors to exert their analgesic effect. Opioids can be administered via different routes, including intravenous, intramuscular, intrathecal, transdermal, or oral. The oral and transdermal routes are the most common for the treatment of chronic pain. Opioids come in short-acting, long-acting, and abuse-deterrent formulations. Multiple pain societies comprising multidisciplinary groups of experts have issued guidelines regarding the tolerability, safety, and efficacy of opioids for persistent non-cancer pain [22, 23]. Initial risk assessments should be done before instituting medically directed opioid therapy with clearly defined goals, weighing potential benefits and risks. Sedation, gastrointestinal side effects, respiratory depression, hormonal alterations, tolerance, addiction, and opioid-induced hyperalgesia are known potential risks when used long term. Concurrent use of benzodiazepines and opioids should be avoided due to increased risk of overdose, respiratory depression, and

all-cause mortality. Concomitant use with alcohol, sedative-hypnotics, antide-
pressants, and anticonvulsants may potentiate the sedative effects of opioids.
Opioids may also interact with drugs that are either inhibitors or inducers of
CYP enzymes (CYP3A4 and CYP2D6). It is advisable to prescribe naloxone to
all patients receiving opioids, especially high-risk patients (patients with >50
MME and use of benzodiazepines) [22, 24].

Table 5.1 provides an overview of opioids.

Table 5.1 Opioids

Name	Mechanism	Route	Notes
Tramadol	Weak mu opioid Serotonin and norepinephrine reuptake inhibition	Oral Parenteral	Synthetic opioid Second-line agent for fibromyalgia Uncertain for chronic/neuropathic pain In combination with SSRI will increase the risk of seizure and serotonin syndrome
Tapentadol	Stronger affinity to mu compared to tramadol Noradrenergic reuptake inhibition	Oral	Synthetic opioid FDA indication for painful diabetic neuropathy In combination with SSRI will increase the risk of seizure and serotonin syndrome
Buprenorphine	Mu-receptor agonist Kappa-receptor antagonist	Oral Transdermal Parenteral Sublingual Buccal	Synthetic opioid Opioid use disorder Chronic pain Less physical dependence, opioid-induced hyperalgesia, respiratory depression
Codeine	Mu-opioid agonist	Oral	Natural opiates Mild to moderate pain Reduce chronic cough
Morphine	Primarily Mu-opioid agonist	Oral Parenteral	Natural opiates Has short-acting and long-acting formulations Moderate to severe pain Cancer pain
Hydromorphone	Mu-opioid agonist	Oral Rectal Parenteral Subcutaneous	Synthetic opioid Moderate to severe pain Cancer pain Has short and long-acting formulations (Exalgo)
Oxycodone	Highly selective mu agonist	Oral	Semi-synthetic opioid Short-acting and long-acting formulation Available in combination with paracetamol, aspirin, ibuprofen, naloxone, and naltrexone Moderate to severe acute or chronic pain

(continued)

Table 5.1 (continued)

Name	Mechanism	Route	Notes
Hydrocodone	Selective full mu agonist	Oral	Semi-synthetic opioid Short-acting and long-acting formulation (Hysingla ER) Available in combination with paracetamol, aspirin, ibuprofen Moderate to severe acute or chronic pain
Fentanyl	Binds to mu, delta, kappa receptors	Parenteral Transdermal Buccal	Synthetic opioids High lipid solubility, penetrates CNS easily Management of chronic and cancer pain When using a transdermal patch, advise to minimize external heat sources due to the release of too much medication
Methadone	Mu-receptor agonist NMDA antagonist	Oral Parenteral	Synthetic opioid Use of chronic pain, opioid dependence, OUD Has alpha metabolism (analgesia) and beta metabolism (detoxification/addiction)

SSRI Selective serotonin reuptake inhibitor, *FDA* Federal Drug Administration, *ER* Extended release, *CNS* Central nervous system, *OUD* Opioid use disorder [22]

Adjuvants

Adjuvant analgesics, medications primarily indicated for conditions other than pain, possess analgesic properties and are frequently employed as first-line agents in pain management. They encompass a diverse array of drugs utilized alone or alongside nonopioids or opioids to address chronic pain. Adjuvants aim to reduce opioid requirements, enhance pain relief synergistically, and manage pain inadequately responsive to other medications [25]. This category includes antidepressants, anticonvulsants, muscle relaxants, topical agents, and cannabinoids, each originally designed for distinct therapeutic purposes.

Antidepressants

Although traditionally used for clinical depression, antidepressants serve as adjuvants in treating neuropathic pain and chronic pain in patients with comorbid anxiety disorders and sleep disturbances. They demonstrate efficacy in conditions such as painful diabetic neuropathy, spinal cord injury, migraine headaches, and fibromyalgia [16]. Antidepressants function at the spinal level by inhibiting the reuptake of the neurotransmitters, namely, norepinephrine and serotonin. This leads to an increase in neurotransmitter concentration, which potentiates the inhibitory pathway in the dorsal horn of the spinal cord and at ectopic sites in the peripheral nerves by blocking Na channels, thereby producing analgesia. Tricyclic antidepressants (TCAs) like amitriptyline, desipramine, and imipramine, as well as serotonin-norepinephrine reuptake inhibitors such as duloxetine, venlafaxine, and milnacipran, have demonstrated efficacy across multiple pain conditions. However, TCAs may be limited by side effects such as sedation, confusion, and anticholinergic effects like dry mouth, blurry vision, and urinary retention. Additionally, they pose a risk of cardiotoxicity, for example, conduction disorders, arrhythmia, and heart failure, warranting caution in patients with cardiac history [26, 27]. Tricyclics are also contraindicated in patients with a known history of a narrow anterior chamber of the eye or prior attacks of acute glaucoma. Most antidepressants carry a black box warning due to an increased risk of suicidality [16]. Despite their favorable analgesic effects, antidepressants, when used in combination with other medications such as lithium, monoamine oxidase inhibitors (MAOIs), or drugs metabolized by CYP2D6, can lead to significant drug interactions. Polypharmacy, especially combining different types of antidepressants (TCAs, SSRIs, and selective norepinephrine reuptake inhibitors), should be avoided to prevent serotonin syndrome, which may include seizures [25].

Anticonvulsants

Originally developed for managing seizures, anticonvulsants are widely employed in treating neuropathic pain, migraine, fibromyalgia, and other headache disorders. These agents exert their analgesic effects by reducing ectopic neuronal discharges and stabilizing nerve membranes. Gabapentin and pregabalin, both believed to act as neuronal calcium channel $\alpha2-\delta$ ligands, mitigate hyperexcitability in excited neurons. Common side effects include sedation, dizziness, peripheral edema, and weight gain [18, 25].

Corticosteroids

Glucocorticoids, renowned for their anti-inflammatory effects, are utilized in various conditions associated with pain, including rheumatoid arthritis, neuropathic pain syndromes, and cancer pain. They exert their analgesic effects through inhibition of phospholipase, alteration of lymphocytes, cytokine expression inhibition, and membrane stabilization [25]. Prolonged steroid use may lead to adverse reactions such as fluid and electrolyte imbalance, osteoporosis, hyperglycemia, and psychiatric symptoms.

Muscle Relaxants

The true mechanism of muscle relaxants remains poorly understood. Most skeletal muscle relaxants are FDA-approved for either spasticity (such as baclofen, dantrolene, and tizanidine) or musculoskeletal conditions (including carisoprodol, chlorzoxazone, cyclobenzaprine, metaxalone, methocarbamol, and orphenadrine). Many of these muscle relaxants are associated with somnolence and sedation, making it somewhat challenging to determine whether their clinical effect is directly related to muscle action or primarily due to their sedative properties [28].

Benzodiazepines

Benzodiazepines enhance the action of gamma-aminobutyric acid (GABA) and are employed in conditions involving spasticity, such as spinal cord injury. Potential side effects include respiratory depression, somnolence, and dizziness, particularly when combined with opioid therapy. Caution is advised to minimize dose and long-term use [25, 28].

Topical Analgesics

Topical analgesic formulations (such as patches and creams) are utilized for localized pain, circumventing the systemic side effects of oral medications and potentially reducing drug-drug interactions [1]. These agents have demonstrated effectiveness in treating neuropathic pain syndromes and osteoarthritis. Their mechanism of action involves reducing peripheral pain processing from affected or injured nerves to the central processing in the brain. The FDA has approved Lidocaine 5% patches for post-herpetic neuralgia treatment. Capsaicin, an active ingredient in chili peppers, can be topically applied and leads to the defunctionalization of small afferent fibers through interaction with TRPV1 receptors, possibly resulting in decreased pain perception. While numerous topical anti-inflammatory formulations are available for musculoskeletal pain, their efficacy for neuropathic pain has yielded mixed results [16, 18].

Cannabinoids

The use of cannabinoids for the treatment of chronic pain has faced criticism due to the risks associated with long-term usage. The analgesic and anti-inflammatory effects of cannabinoids stem from the activation of different endocannabinoid systems in the CNS and PNS, immune, and hematologic systems. Among cannabinoids, delta-9-tetrahydrocannabinol (THC) and cannabidiol (CBD) have received the most research attention. THC inhibits glutamate and 5-hydroxytryptamine release while increasing dopamine secretion. On the other hand, CBD enhances adenosine receptor signaling, reduces reactive oxygen species, tumor necrosis factor, and T cell proliferation, all without the psychoactive effects of THC. Common side effects include cognitive impairment, drowsiness, and impaired attention span. However, the opioid-sparing effect of cannabinoids remains unclear, with clinical practice guidelines offering inconsistent recommendations [29].

Conclusion

The pharmacological management of chronic pain necessitates a comprehensive understanding of the pharmacokinetics and pharmacodynamics of medications. Treatment goals aim to reduce pain sensitization, pain amplification, and restore normal pain thresholds. Due to the potential side effects of high doses or combination therapy, it is essential to administer the lowest effective dose for the shortest duration possible to achieve symptom control.

Complementary and Integrative Health Approaches

The National Institutes of Health (NIH) National Center for Complementary and Integrative Health (NCCIH) delineates "complementary approaches" as non-mainstream healthcare approaches used alongside conventional medical care, while "alternative approaches" are those substituted for conventional medicine [30]. Integrative health entails the amalgamation of such practices with conventional medical care. According to the 2012 National Health Interview Survey, over 30% of US adults utilize complementary or alternative medicine (CAM) approaches [31]. In the same survey, 41.6% of adults with musculoskeletal pain disorders employ complementary health approaches, compared to 24.1% of those without musculoskeletal pain [31]. The Pain Management Best Practices Inter-Agency Task Force Report advocates for clinicians to contemplate integrative health approaches, including mind-body behavioral interventions, acupuncture, massage, osteopathic and chiropractic manipulation, meditative movement therapies (e.g., yoga, tai chi), and natural products [32]. CAM approaches can thus serve as a pivotal component of individualized, multimodal, multidisciplinary treatment for acute and chronic pain.

Dietary Approaches to Pain Management

The human diet encompasses essential macronutrients (fats, carbohydrates, proteins) and micronutrients (vitamins, minerals) and may incorporate non-vitamin, non-mineral dietary supplements. Diet and dietary supplements may influence pain through various mechanisms, including direct analgesic effects, modulation of analgesic drug pharmacokinetics or pharmacodynamics, and enhancement of nutritional status and overall fitness. Given nutrition's indispensable role in daily life, potential benefits of dietary approaches to pain management encompass heightened compliance and adherence, decreased cost compared to prescription medications, fewer potential side effects, and seamless integration into comprehensive pain treatment programs.

Dietary fat intake can influence pain pathways through various mechanisms, including neuropeptide and hormone synthesis, as well as neurotransmission involving serotonin, norepinephrine, and dopamine [33]. Notably, ω-3 and ω-6 polyunsaturated fats (PUFAs) serve as precursors in eicosanoid synthesis (e.g., prostaglandins, thromboxanes, and leukotrienes), which play crucial roles in inflammation and vasoactivity, thereby impacting cardiovascular health, neural development, and nociception [34]. While both ω-3 and ω-6 PUFAs contribute to pro- and anti-inflammatory compounds, ω-3 PUFAs are generally regarded as more anti-inflammatory [35]. Although most foods contain a mix of fat varieties, the typical North American diet is characterized by relatively high saturated fat (e.g., dairy, animal fats) and ω-6 PUFA (e.g., vegetable oils) content, with relatively low levels of ω-3 PUFAs (e.g., oily fish) [36].

A meta-analysis of 17 randomized, controlled trials focusing on inflammatory joint pain revealed that ω-3 PUFA supplementation significantly correlated with improvements in patient-reported joint pain, morning stiffness, and NSAID consumption [37]. Similarly, elevated ratios of ω-6 to ω-3 PUFAs have been linked to increased pain, reduced functioning, and heightened psychological distress in individuals with chronic knee pain [38]. Supplementation with PUFAs, such as fish oil, krill oil, or sourced from algae, is generally considered safe and well-tolerated [39]. However, the overall evidence for PUFA supplementation in chronic pain is limited by heterogeneity across studied pain conditions, as well as variations in type, dosage, and duration of supplementation [40].

Numerous micronutrients, such as glucosamine and chondroitin for osteoarthritis, vitamin B complex for peripheral neuropathy, vitamin D for chronic pain, magnesium for migraines, and curcuminoids, that is, turmeric extract for chronic pain, have been explored as potential analgesics [41–48]. While limited data suggest some potential benefits and minimal harm with such dietary supplements, high-quality evidence supporting their efficacy in chronic pain management for conditions including osteoarthritis, dysmenorrhea, cancer pain, and chronic musculoskeletal pain remains lacking [49–52]. The extensive diversity among clinical patients studied, variations in dosage and duration of interventions, utilization of combination treatments, and absence of randomization and/or controls hinder pain experts and professional societies from making definitive recommendations, emphasizing the necessity for ongoing research in this field.

Given the prevalence and assortment of dietary supplements, pain patients frequently seek recommendations from their pain physician. Practical advice for patients considering the use of dietary supplements for pain relief includes counseling regarding potential adverse effects, reviewing current medications and other supplements to prevent interactions, advising to obtain supplements from reputable sources, recommending checking for certification of good manufacturing practices by independent third parties (e.g., NSF International, U.S. Pharmacopeia, ConsumerLab.com), and starting at the lowest recommended dose, increasing gradually, and discontinuing use if adverse effects are observed.

Acupuncture

Acupuncture, originating from traditional Chinese medicine, is a procedural treatment aimed at restoring normal energy flow (qi) within the body [53]. Contemporary research, including sham-controlled trials, has highlighted the physiological effects of acupuncture on various pain pathways, involving modulation of endogenous opioids, neurotransmitters like serotonin and norepinephrine, and inflammatory cytokines. When administered by a well-trained, licensed practitioner using sterile techniques, acupuncture is generally considered low risk [32, 53]. While systematic reviews and meta-analyses suggest potential benefits for conditions such as osteoarthritis, migraine, low back pain, and neck pain, the quality of evidence is often questioned due to limitations in study design and execution, including small sample sizes, inadequate controls, and insufficient blinding [54–57]. Therefore, acupuncture for pain management should be approached within a patient-centered framework, considering factors such as the specific pain condition, associated benefits and risks, including cost implications, as well as the patient's preferences and expectations regarding treatment.

Mind-Body Therapies (Yoga and Tai Chi)/Impact of Exercise on Pain Management

Yoga, originating from ancient Indian practices, focuses on physical postures (asanas), breathing techniques (pranayama), and meditation (dyana) [30]. Tai chi, an ancient Chinese martial art, involves slow, gentle movements, postures, and controlled breathing within a meditative state [58]. These practices have become increasingly popular in Western culture as they offer low-impact exercises combined with spiritual and meditative elements. Yoga is generally regarded as safe, comparable to standard care and exercise [59], and has demonstrated efficacy similar to physical therapy in managing chronic low back pain [60, 61]. Additionally, systematic reviews suggest that yoga may provide modest benefits for neck pain, headaches, and osteoarthritis [62–64]. Tai chi research has shown potential benefits for conditions such as low back pain, osteoarthritis, rheumatoid arthritis, and fibromyalgia [65–69]. However, comprehensive reviews on both yoga and tai chi remain inconclusive, primarily due to the dominance of small, low-quality studies in the literature, with varying treatment protocols. Nonetheless, these modalities can be integrated into multimodal pain management strategies due to their potential for pain relief with minimal risk, cost-effectiveness (especially in group settings), and the ability to deliver sessions remotely via telehealth [32].

Physical Therapy Methods

Self-Efficacy

As Allied Health Professionals, physical therapists play a crucial role in treating patients with persistent pain while imparting education on prevention and health promotion strategies. They prioritize self-efficacy, which refers to an individual's belief in their capacity to achieve specific goals or desired outcomes, as a significant mediator between pain and disability. Physical therapists foster self-efficacy through techniques such as facilitating successful experiences, education, coaching, behavioral modeling, and exercise instruction. Physical activity and exercise are vital for individuals suffering from chronic pain as a sustainable long-term approach.

Addressing Pain-Related Fears

Pain-related avoidance behaviors, catastrophic beliefs, and fear of movement (kinesiophobia) can pose significant barriers to exercise adherence and progression [70, 71]. Physical therapists employ pain neuroscience education (PNE) to elucidate that "hurt does not always equal harm or damage" [70, 72–77]. By diminishing fear, patients become more accepting of discomfort and are more willing to engage in therapy programs and continue home exercise regimens.

Active Physical Therapy

Active treatments in physical therapy involve activities where the patient is actively engaged physically and/or cognitively as a participant. This includes learning and performing warm-up activities, stretching, strengthening exercises, and other prescribed physical therapy exercises. It is important to note that even self-application of passive modalities can be considered active because the patient takes responsibility. Active cognitive coping and self-management skills are recognized as significant mediators of positive outcomes in multidisciplinary pain rehabilitation programs [78–80]. Physical therapists employ various active strategies, including education, adaptations, facilitation, graded motor imagery (GMI), exercise-based interventions, and graded exposure techniques. Together, these active treatments aim to maintain long-term functionality in patients.

Passive Physical Therapy

Passive physical therapy involves treatments administered to a patient without their active participation, either by a practitioner or by a device. Examples include massage, electrical or thermal modalities, or manual joint manipulations. While these treatments can provide immediate pain relief, relying solely on passive interventions may compromise long-term outcomes if biopsychosocial factors are not fully considered due to the multidimensional complexity of persistent pain [78, 81].

Electrical Modalities

Electrical stimulation modalities aim to modulate all categories of pain mechanisms, including nociceptive, neuropathic, and central sensitization, to provide relief. Transcutaneous electrical nerve stimulation (TENS) is one such modality, delivering electrical stimulation through a portable device equipped with adhesive electrodes placed on the skin [82]. Clinical applications of TENS may involve various parameters such as low frequency (<10 Hz), high frequency (>50 Hz), sensory intensity level (tingling, tapping), motor level (muscle contraction), conventional TENS (high frequency applied at low intensity), and acupuncture-like TENS (low frequency applied at high intensity with motor contraction).

Thermal Modalities

Hot packs or heating pads provide pain relief through superficial heat application over the affected area for 15–30 minutes. They are commonly used for soft tissue pain, muscle spasms, sprains/strains, and osteoarthritis. Mechanisms of pain relief include increased blood flow, metabolism, and elasticity of connective tissues, that is, reduced tone [82].

Cold Packs and Ice Massage

Cold therapy, including ice packs and ice massage, reduces pain, blood flow, edema, inflammation, muscle spasms, and metabolic demand [82, 83]. Ice massage involves mechanical deformation forces aiding in fluid mobilization and reduction of edema and muscular relaxation. Treatment durations are typically 10–20 minutes for cold packs and 7–10 minutes for ice massage.

Low-Level Laser Therapy

Laser or light therapies, known as passively therapeutic modalities, include "3A or 3B" lasers, commonly referred to as low-level laser therapy (LLLT) and low-intensity laser therapy (LILT). These treatments involve administering non-thermal doses of light to painful tissues using devices that generate light with a wavelength between 600 and 1000 nm. The typical doses range from 820 to 830 nm, delivering 0.8–9.0 J per point, with an irradiation time of 15–180 s [84].

Several mechanisms of action are proposed for pain relief, including reduced inflammatory response (decrease in PGE2, mRNA Cox 2, IL-1β, TNFα), decreased neutrophil cell influx and oxidative stress, alteration of cell membrane and action potentials, prostaglandin reduction, inhibition of pain transmission at peripheral neuromuscular junctions, and selective inhibition of nerve conduction in Aδ and C fibers, which convey nociceptive stimulation [85–87].

Manual Therapy

Manual therapy encompasses techniques that mobilize or manipulate soft tissue and joints to modulate pain, reduce swelling and inflammation, induce relaxation, improve range of motion, and restore function [88, 89]. The evidence supporting the use of manual therapy varies depending on factors such as pain acuity, body region, and diagnosis. For patients with chronic musculoskeletal pain, manual therapy has been shown to produce slight improvements in temporal summation, an important characteristic of nociceptive processing associated with central sensitization [90]. Proposed mechanisms include biomechanical, neurophysiological, peripheral, spinal, and supraspinal effects [86, 87].

Impact of Exercise on Pain Management

Exercise Recommendations in Chronic Pain

Regular exercise is beneficial for most chronic medical conditions, including chronic low back pain, and significantly improves overall health [90–95]. Some patients benefit from specifically targeted exercise prescriptions. Patients with persistent pain engaging in movement and physical therapy programs may experience expected disruptive flare-up cycles. Using motivational interviews to modify behavioral change, address pain-related fear avoidance, and train patients in self-efficacy and self-treatment strategies, can be beneficial.

Adherence to a Movement Program

Exercise adherence is a significant challenge for individuals with persistent pain [95–98]. While no singular exercise (e.g., walking, swimming, biking) is superior to another, certain program characteristics predict higher adherence rates [95]. These include tailoring the program to the patient's goals and preferences, utilizing individualized supervised sessions when available, ensuring accessibility, and emphasizing self-efficacy [95, 99, 100]. Adherence to long-term behavioral strategies, such as positive reinforcement, exercise contracts, self-monitoring, and supervised follow-up sessions, enhances program effectiveness [95].

Low-Intensity Activity

Low-intensity activities like walking (land-based and aquatic), tai chi, yoga, Qi Gong, and gentle cycling have been shown to decrease pain and anxiety, reduce depression, improve balance and mobility, and are generally well-tolerated in chronic pain patients [34, 96]. Although low-intensity activity may not offer the same overall health benefits and functional improvements as moderate and vigorous exercise, it can serve as a starting point for patients unable to tolerate moderate-intensity activity, fostering self-efficacy [96, 99–101].

Aerobic Exercise

Aerobic exercise involves sustained movement of large muscle groups, increasing oxygen demand [96, 100–104]. Besides pain reduction, aerobic exercise benefits accessibility, as it involves simple movement patterns requiring minimal supervision or equipment, such as walking, jogging, cycling, dancing, and swimming [96, 97, 101–103]. Aerobic exercises can be modified to accommodate disabilities or other barriers.

Strength Training

Strength training offers clinical benefits for chronic pain patients, including increased muscle strength, pain relief, reduced disability, decreased depression, increased self-efficacy, and improved quality of life [96, 99, 100, 105, 107, 108]. These outcomes can be achieved with two training sessions per week [96–108]. Successful implementation strategies involve allowing patients to define volitional fatigue with each set of exercises, starting with simple exercises, and providing guidance for controlled exercise performance to avoid strain [97, 99, 107].

Flexibility

Flexibility exercises aimed at alleviating stiffness or tightness and improving joint range of motion modestly benefit pain and are more efficacious for anxiety, depression, and quality of life. Optimal outcomes are achieved when stretching is included as part of an overall fitness program [97, 105, 109].

Stimulation Produces Analgesia: Transcutaneous Electrical Nerve Stimulation (per ABA)

Transcutaneous electrical nerve stimulation (TENS) delivers electrical stimulation through the skin and is utilized for the treatment of acute and chronic pain. TENS is preferred over interferential current or other electrical stimulation for chronic pain treatment due to its cost-effectiveness and independent application [110]. TENS is often incorporated with exercise during physical therapy sessions [51, 111]. It does not necessarily require instruction by a skilled physical therapist, and these devices are readily available over the counter.

TENS is applied at varied frequencies, intensities, and pulse durations, working by muting central neuronal excitability and activating descending inhibitory pathways [110–116]. The efficacy of TENS remains equivocal, attributed to inconsistent methodology and heterogeneous subgrouping in clinical trials. Therefore, considerations for TENS use should encompass cost-effectiveness and its potential to support self-efficacy in patients with persistent pain [116–118].

Rehabilitation Techniques

Chronic pain rehabilitation programs integrate exercises aimed at increasing the patient's activity tolerance and range of motion. These exercises encompass stretching, conditioning, strengthening, and relaxation techniques. Combining exercise with other physical modalities proves more effective than employing any single modality. Rehabilitation techniques entail behavior modification to unlearn pain behaviors, coping strategies to promote better functioning, and assistance to family members in altering their responses to encourage improved outcomes [119]. Individualized education and psychosocial approaches serve to foster and reinforce the treatment regimen. Psychotherapy, whether in individual or group format, is an integral component. Stress management and other medical interventions, including medications, injections, stimulation, manual therapy, and physical modalities, constitute part of a multimodal approach for patients suffering from persistent pain.

Work Hardening Rehabilitation

Multidisciplinary rehabilitation encompasses a combination of physical, psychological, educational, and/or work-specific interventions, often delivered by a team of healthcare providers [120]. Within this framework, the pain physician must comprehend the concepts of physical conditioning programs. Physical conditioning programs are typically defined by the desired outcome. For injured workers with chronic pain, physical rehabilitation focuses on work-specific conditioning or functional training. The terms "work conditioning" or "work hardening" implies a structured program of exercises or tasks that are progressively graded to enhance physical and emotional tolerance for specific work tasks [121]. Work hardening emphasizes task-specific job deficits, often utilizing simulated or duplicated work tasks in a supervised environment, with daily sessions lasting several hours or even a full workday. A functional restoration program, a broader term emphasizing functional outcomes over pain, includes work conditioning and/or work hardening, intensive education, and psychology when the goal is to return to work [78].

Concerning outcomes in chronic spine pain, multidisciplinary biopsychosocial rehabilitation is recognized to decrease pain and disability beyond usual care and physical treatments, potentially improving work status compared to physical treatments alone [120–122]. It remains unclear which elements within the multidisciplinary rehab program provide benefit, nor is the optimal dose or intensity known for a given outcome. Physical conditioning programs alone have little effect on return-to-work rates in acute low back pain but confer a slight positive effect at 1 year for reducing sick leave use in patients with chronic low back pain [121]. To achieve this positive result, patients with chronic low back pain likely need more than five 1- or 2-hour sessions, ranging up to 8-hour sessions for at least 2 weeks. There is insufficient evidence that work hardening or work conditioning is superior to an active therapeutic exercise program or guideline-based physical therapy [123]. Given the low to moderate quality evidence, further research is likely to have a high impact on our understanding and utilization of structured physical conditioning programs for return to work. Physical conditioning programs should be considered as part of a multidisciplinary approach for those with chronic pain impeding their return to work.

Psychological Approaches to Treat Chronic Pain

Psychological treatments, whether alone or within an interdisciplinary program, boast the greatest empirical evidence for success. There exists an overwhelming body of research supporting the effectiveness of various psychological approaches, especially cognitive-behavioral therapy. It is therefore prudent to consider the use of psychological treatment in conjunction with traditional medical interventions.

Psychological interventions include the following:
Cognitive-behavioral therapy
Behavioral approaches
Motivational interviewing
Biofeedback
Meditation
Guided imagery
Hypnosis

Cognitive-Behavioral Therapy

The CBT approach combines cognitive and behavioral techniques, including assertiveness, stress management, relaxation training, goal setting, guided imagery, and pacing of activities [124, 125]. Biofeedback, meditation, and hypnosis can all be incorporated within the framework of CBT. The focus is to provide patients with more adaptive ways of thinking, feeling, and behaving so they can better respond to pain.

Patients should actively collaborate in changing their thoughts, feelings, and behaviors.

Components of CBT (Four):

- Education: Help the patient become more aware of their negative thoughts and emotions, and their role in maintaining stress and physical symptoms. Steps include identifying maladaptive thoughts during problematic situations such as pain exacerbations, introducing and practicing coping thoughts, shifting from self-defeating to coping thoughts, introducing and practicing positive or reinforcing thoughts, and finally practicing at home and follow-up [126–129].
- Skills acquisition.
- Consolidation: Goal of skills acquisition and consolidation is to help patients learn new skills for pain management behavior and stress reduction, including training in relaxation, distraction, problem-solving, activity pacing, and communication.
- Generalization and maintenance are aimed at solidifying those skills and preventing relapse.

CBT helps restore function and mood, as well as reduce pain and disability-related behavior. Its efficacy has been demonstrated in many studies of chronic pain disorders. Despite CBT being undoubtedly the most common intervention used in chronic pain, it may not work for everyone, and other interventions may be considered.

Behavioral Approaches

Classical (respondent) conditioning involves the repeated pairing of a neutral stimulus with a nociceptive stimulus, leading the neutral stimulus to elicit a pain response over time [73, 130]. Treatment typically consists of exposing the patient to feared or avoided activities that result in less pain than anticipated, and providing corrective feedback in the process.

Operant conditioning, on the other hand, focuses on extinguishing pain behavior by withdrawing positive attention from such behavior and reinforcing good behavior [131]. This approach aims to modify behavior through a process of reinforcement and punishment, encouraging patients to engage in more adaptive behaviors and discouraging maladaptive responses to pain.

Motivational Interviewing

Motivational interviewing, originally developed for substance use disorders (SUDs), has seen increasing use in chronic pain management. It operates on the framework of the stages of readiness to change, which include precontemplation, contemplation, preparation, action, and maintenance.

- Precontemplation stage: Patients still view their pain as purely somatic and have adopted a passive role as they wait for their provider to identify and provide appropriate treatment. The clinician educates the patient about the risks and problems resulting from inactivity, such as increased pain and deconditioning.
- Contemplation stage: The goal is to encourage the patient to conclude that the risks associated with inactivity outweigh the perceived benefits.
- Preparation stage: The clinician helps outline appropriate structured physical activities in which the patient is willing to participate.
- Action stage: The clinician helps the patient increase activity levels.
- Maintenance: Geared toward the individual's ongoing motivation and commitment.

Throughout these stages, clinicians encourage patients to transition by providing motivational statements, listening with empathy, asking open-ended questions, providing feedback and affirmation, and handling resistance. Since motivational interviewing has been applied to chronic pain only recently, its efficacy has not yet been well documented [132, 133].

Biofeedback

Biofeedback is a self-regulation technique that assists individuals in exerting control over their physiological processes. During biofeedback sessions, the patient is connected to equipment via electrodes, which record physiological responses such as skin conductance, respiration, heart rate, skin temperature, and muscle tension.

These readings are then translated into visual or auditory signals displayed on a monitor that the patient can observe. Consequently, the patient can manipulate these auditory or visual signals to alter their physiological responses. With practice, most individuals can learn to voluntarily control crucial physiological functions associated directly with pain and stress, thereby inducing a state of general relaxation. Patients are instructed to practice the methods that have successfully altered their physiological parameters.

Forms of biofeedback may include EMG biofeedback, commonly used for tension headaches, thermal biofeedback as seen with migraine headaches, and biofeedback associated with heart variability as seen in those complaining of pain.

Biofeedback empowers patients with a general sense of control over their bodies, a critical aspect given the high levels of helplessness observed in individuals with chronic pain problems [134–136].

Meditation

Meditation involves a systematic inner focus on particular aspects of inner and outer experience. Unlike many approaches in behavioral medicine, meditation was developed in a spiritual context. However, as a healthcare intervention, it has been effective regardless of the patient's cultural or religious background [134, 137, 138]. There are two common forms of meditation: Transcendental meditation and Zen or Mindfulness meditation. Transcendental meditation involves focusing on one of the senses, like a zoom lens focusing on a specific object. For example, the individual repeats a silent word (mantra) with the goal of transcending the ordinary stream of mental discourse.

On the other hand, Zen or Mindfulness meditation aims for awareness of the whole perceptual field, akin to a wide-angle lens. It incorporates focused attention and whole-field awareness in the present moment. Mindfulness meditation reframes the experience of discomfort such that physical pain, malaise, or suffering becomes the object of meditation. Rather than being avoided, which is the most common reaction, they are investigated, experienced, and explored. Mindfulness-based interventions have been found to decrease pain, increase healing, reduce stress, and improve mood.

Guided Imagery

Guided imagery entails using visualization or imagination to evoke specific pleasant images. These images can be sensory or affective, with the most successful ones involving all five senses (vision, sound, touch, smell, taste). Guided imagery has been shown to reduce presurgical anxiety, postsurgical pain, and accelerate healing [139].

Hypnosis

Hypnosis is defined as a natural state of aroused attentive focal concentration coupled with a relative suspension of peripheral awareness [140–143]. It consists of three key components: absorption, dissociation, and suggestibility. Absorption refers to the intense involvement in the central object of concentration, while dissociation involves experiences that would commonly be felt consciously occurring outside of conscious awareness. Suggestibility, the third component, indicates that individuals are more likely to accept outside input without cognitive censorship or criticism. Hypnosis has been proven beneficial in relieving pain among patients suffering from various conditions such as headaches, arthritis, burn injuries, cancer, and chronic back pain.

Substance Use Disorders and Pain

Substance use disorders are highly prevalent in patients with chronic pain (15–28%) [144]. Lifetime rates range from 23% to 41%. Substance use disorders are more common in males than females. The most commonly abused substances in chronic pain patients are alcohol (current and lifetime) and narcotics (current). Substance use disorders often precede the onset of chronic pain [144]. The incidence of addiction in patients on chronic opioid therapy varies widely and is greatest in individuals with a prior history of substance use disorder and/or a history of abuse [145–148]. Chronic pain patients with comorbid substance diagnoses have higher rates of depression, anxiety, and personality disorders than patients with no substance diagnosis [149–151].

Identifying substance use disorders in chronic pain patients may be difficult, secondary to fears that pain-relieving medications will be reduced or discontinued, that they will not be considered good candidates for pain rehabilitation programs, and/or that this information will work against them in potential future worker's compensation litigation.

Evaluation of Opioid Risk

The prevalence of opioid misuse in chronic non-cancer pain patients treated with opioids is around 20%. Misuse is defined as the use of medications other than as directed, whether willfully or unintentionally, and whether harm results or not. The prevalence of opioid use disorder is much lower (around 2–5%).

Prescription Opioid Use Disorder is defined as a primary, chronic, neurobiological disease that is characterized by behaviors that include one or more of the following (4 C's) [152]: Loss of Control over the drug, Compulsive drug use, Cravings (strong urges to use), and Continued use despite harm.

Screening tools for substance abuse [such as Pain Medicine Questionnaire, Current Opioid Misuse Measure (COMM), and Screener and Opioid Assessment for Patients with Pain—Revised (SOAPP-R)] may be beneficial in assessing the risk of addiction to opioids before initiation and during maintenance with opioid therapy. The utilization of prescription drug monitoring programs is another complementary tool that helps identify patients who "doctor shop." Urine toxicology screens are the most widely used and possibly the gold standard for detecting illicit substance use in chronic pain patients treated with opioids [153].

Opioid therapy agreements, signed by both patient and clinician, may be an appealing tool for managing many of the potential difficulties related to chronic non-cancer opioid therapy [154]. Screening for the risk of opioid abuse/misuse is directed toward identifying aberrant drug behaviors resulting from the 4 C's. A history of personal and/or family history of addiction significantly increases the risk of opioid misuse. It is also important to assess for any implications on work, interpersonal, or social function with opioid use. Additionally, comorbid mood problems, anxiety, and emotional distress significantly increase the risk of misusing prescribed opioids if not appropriately treated.

Buprenorphine

Sublingual (S/L) buprenorphine is FDA approved only for the treatment of opioid use disorder (opioid detoxification and maintenance). Buprenorphine in the patch and buccal forms is approved only for analgesia. However, buprenorphine is present at a significantly lower dose in the patch and buccal forms compared to the S/L forms (Table 5.2).

Mechanism of Action

Buprenorphine acts as a partial agonist at the μ-opioid receptor with unusually high affinity [155]. It has a weak partial antagonist effect on the κ-opioid receptor (with anti-depressant effects) and a ceiling effect on respiration and CNS depression, providing a considerable margin of safety in a high-risk population. Several side effects have been described with the use of buprenorphine (Table 5.3).

Table 5.2 Common buprenorphine formulations

Generic dose	Brand name	Starting
Buprenorphine patch	Butrans	5–10 mcg/h
Buprenorphine buccal film	Belbucca	75–150 mcg/twice daily
Buprenorphine/Naloxone Sublingual	Suboxone	4–8/1–2 mg

Note: Adapted from Suboxone product information. Retrieved from http://www.suboxone.com

Table 5.3 Side effects of buprenorphine

Common	Rare
Sedation	Weight gain
Headache	Hepatotoxicity
Constipation	Oral hypoesthesia (film)
Nausea	Glossodynia (film)

Note: Adapted from Suboxone product information. Retrieved from http://www.suboxone.com

Drug Interactions and Clinical Indications

Buprenorphine is metabolized by CYP 450 3A4, leading to fluctuations in blood levels if co-administered with medications that induce or inhibit the CYP 450 3A4 enzyme, such as several anticonvulsants and protease inhibitors. The most common clinical indications for buprenorphine formulations are the treatment of chronic pain and opioid addiction [156, 157].

Initiation

Sublingual (S/L) buprenorphine, used for addiction treatment, should only be initiated when the patient is experiencing mild to moderate withdrawals (W/Ds) to prevent precipitated W/Ds. The typical starting dose for S/L buprenorphine is 4 mg, titrating up every 1/2 to 1 hour in 2–4 mg increments until W/D symptoms improve. The dose can be increased every week by 4–8 mg increments to alleviate cravings and/or improve pain until reaching a maximum recommended daily dose of 24 mg daily (however, doses higher than 24 mg daily have been reported with improved analgesia).

Butrans should be initiated at 5 mcg/h in opioid-naïve patients and titrated up by 5 mcg every week to a maximum dose of 20 mcg/h (possible QT prolongation with doses >20 mcg/h). If the patient is opioid-tolerant with an oral morphine equivalent of 30–80 mg/day, the starting patch dose is 10 mcg/h. Similarly, Belbuca should commence at 75 mcg films twice daily in opioid-naïve patients, and 150 mcg twice daily in opioid-tolerant patients. Dose adjustments can be made every 1–2 weeks to achieve effective analgesia, up to a maximum dose of 900 mcg twice daily.

Of note, abrupt discontinuation can lead to opioid withdrawal symptoms; however, these symptoms are usually milder compared to full agonist opioids. However, buprenorphine may precipitate withdrawal symptoms in patients currently on opioid therapy.

Clinical Pearls

An amendment to the Controlled Substances Act (CAA) has exempted certain Schedule III, IV, and V narcotic drugs from X-Waiver requirements. Buprenorphine, classified as a Schedule III narcotic, can now be prescribed for opioid use disorder (OUD) treatment by any DEA-registered prescriber with Schedule III authority, without patient caps.

However, the CAA introduced a new training mandate for all DEA registrants prescribing controlled substances. Effective June 21, 2023, prescribers must complete an 8-hour training program before obtaining or renewing their DEA registration [158].

Sublingual buprenorphine can effectively treat both addiction and pain in high-risk patients. It is essential to conduct liver function tests before and during Suboxone treatment. In cases where patients on Suboxone develop acute pain, several options are available:

- Divide the buprenorphine dose to every 6 hours
- Gradually increase the buprenorphine dose to achieve analgesia

- Stop buprenorphine and start a full opioid agonist
- Continue buprenorphine and add a full opioid agonist

For options 3 and 4 above, naloxone should be readily available at the bedside as patients may easily develop respiratory/CNS depression.

Summary

This chapter underscores the significance of exercise in managing chronic pain, detailing specific exercise recommendations and various rehabilitation techniques. In concluding our exploration into chronic pain management, several pivotal insights emerge, offering valuable guidance for clinicians and researchers alike.

Foremost among these insights is the indispensable role of exercise as a foundational component of effective pain management. Through targeted exercise prescriptions and tailored physical therapy programs, patients can achieve substantial improvements not only in pain levels but also in overall health and well-being. The significance of regular exercise cannot be overstated in the context of chronic pain management.

However, the challenge of exercise adherence looms large, underscoring the importance of personalized programs aligned with individual patient goals and preferences. Incorporating behavioral modification techniques such as motivational interviewing can empower patients to overcome barriers to adherence, fostering long-term engagement with exercise regimens.

Moreover, our exploration into multidisciplinary rehabilitation underscores the holistic nature of effective pain management. By integrating exercise, behavioral modification, and psychosocial interventions, clinicians can address the intricate interplay of physical and emotional factors inherent in chronic pain. The superiority of comprehensive treatment approaches over traditional physical interventions alone is evident.

In parallel, the pivotal role of psychological interventions, particularly cognitive-behavioral therapy (CBT), emerges as a cornerstone of chronic pain management. By guiding patients in identifying and challenging maladaptive thoughts and behaviors, CBT equips them with invaluable coping skills essential for navigating the complexities of chronic pain.

Additionally, the value of complementary interventions such as biofeedback, meditation, and guided imagery cannot be understated. These techniques offer supplementary avenues for pain management, promoting self-regulation, relaxation, and mindfulness, thus augmenting the efficacy of traditional medical interventions.

Amidst our discussions on treatment modalities, the complex issue of substance use disorders in chronic pain patients warrants careful consideration. Thoughtful evaluation and management, supported by screening tools and individualized treatment plans, are essential for addressing substance misuse effectively.

Finally, our examination of buprenorphine as a therapeutic option underscores the importance of understanding its mechanisms, clinical indications, and dosing considerations. By leveraging this medication judiciously, clinicians can provide safe and efficacious pain management solutions for high-risk patients.

In summary, our journey through chronic pain management has illuminated the multifaceted nature of this condition and underscored the imperative for a personalized, patient-centered approach. By integrating exercise, behavioral modification, psychological interventions, and substance use disorder management strategies, clinicians can navigate the complexities of chronic pain effectively, empowering patients to reclaim their quality of life.

Multiple-Choice Questions

Pharmacology

Question 1. In patients with known painful diabetic neuropathy, which of the following opioids have been FDA-approved for its use?
A. Morphine
B. Hydromorphone
C. Tapentadol
D. Oxydocone
Answer: C. Currently, there are few medications with FDA approval for use in painful diabetic peripheral neuropathy. These include pregabalin, duloxetine, and tapentadol. Morphine, hydromorphone, and oxycodone are opioids used for chronic pain but long-term chronic use of these patients even in neuropathic pain is controversial.

Question 2. A patient is diagnosed with CRPS type 1 and has benign prostatic hypertrophy. He is intolerant to gabapentinoids and NSAIDs. Which of the following medications is *MOST* appropriate for use to treat his pain?
A. Amitriptyline
B. Selegiline
C. Desipramine
D. Venlafaxine
Answer: C. The tricyclics block muscarinic acetylcholine receptors and cause anticholinergic effects such as blurred vision, constipation, dry mouth (which may lead to dental caries), and urinary retention. In addition, these anticholinergic effects can cause tachycardia, ocular crisis in patients with narrow-angle glaucoma, and confusion and delirium. Among the choices, desipramine has the least anticholinergic effect and can be safely used in patients with benign prostatic hypertrophy. Amitriptyline, selegiline, and venlafaxine have significant anticholinergic effects.

Question 3. An elderly male with a known history of rheumatoid arthritis presents with increased swelling and pain in the interphalangeal joints of his hand. Which of the following medications would *LEAST* likely provide therapeutic benefit?
A. Naproxen

B. Meloxicam
C. Indomethacin
D. Acetaminophen

Answer: D. NSAIDs have been found to have profound analgesic, antipyretic, and anti-inflammatory effects. The reduction of prostaglandin synthesis through the inhibition of cyclooxygenase enzyme is responsible for its mechanism of action. Even though it is an effective analgesic, Acetaminophen has a weaker anti-inflammatory effect and would not be very effective in treating acute arthritic pain.

Alternative Therapy

Question 4. Which of the following is true about the relationship between dietary fats and pain?
A. Ω-3 polyunsaturated fatty acids (PUFAs) are essential for the production of anti-inflammatory prostaglandins, while ω-6 PUFAs are essential for the production of pro-inflammatory prostaglandins.
B. Chronic pain patients should be counseled to minimize dietary fat intake as much as possible.
C. Increased dietary intake of saturated fats (e.g., animal fats, dairy) and ω-3 polyunsaturated fatty acids (PUFAs) (e.g., fish oil) is associated with increased inflammation compared to diets rich in ω-6 PUFAs (e.g., vegetable oils).
D. Dietary fats may affect pain through a variety of mechanisms, including modulation of inflammatory pathways, neuropeptide and hormone synthesis, and neurotransmission.

Answer: D. Synthesis of eicosanoids (e.g., prostaglandins, thromboxanes, leukotrienes) is a major role of PUFAs in the body, but fats can also influence pain through other physiological pathways. Both types of PUFAs play a role in the synthesis of both pro- and anti-inflammatory eicosanoids. Fats are an essential part of the human diet, and some fats may have beneficial properties for pain, inflammation, and general health. High intake of saturated fats and ω-6 PUFAs, with low intake of ω-3 PUFAs, is associated with increased inflammation and pain symptoms.

Question 5. Which of the following experimental observations would be *MOST* consistent with the putative mechanism of action of acupuncture?
A. Patients with chronic neck pain reported significant improvements in pain relief and function after an 8-week course of acupuncture performed by a licensed acupuncturist.
B. In chronic pain patients with depression, acupuncture treatment combined with duloxetine provided better pain relief than duloxetine alone.
C. Administration of naloxone blocks the analgesic effect of acupuncture in migraine.
D. A 4-week course of acupuncture provides greater pain relief for pain in fibromyalgia compared to sham acupuncture or no treatment.

Answer: C. Acupuncture exerts some analgesic effects through modulation of the endogenous opioid system. There is no control arm, and this information does not provide any information to suggest the mechanism of action of acupuncture. Although acupuncture may exert some analgesic effects via serotonin and norepinephrine pathways, this observation does not mean that acupuncture acts through the same mechanism as duloxetine. Although this observation suggests that acupuncture analgesia is separate from placebo response, it does not provide any information to suggest the mechanism of action.

Question 6. You refer a patient with low back pain for physical therapy. She asks if she can do yoga instead. In counseling your patient, which of the following statements is true?

A. Overall, the evidence in favor of yoga for chronic pain is limited by low-quality studies, small sample sizes, and high variability in treatment regimens.
B. To be effective for pain relief, yoga instruction must be delivered in person, in a group class setting.
C. Yoga is not as effective as physical therapy for low back pain.
D. Yoga is more risky than physical therapy because it is not performed under the guidance of a licensed physical therapist.

Answer: A. Although there is some evidence of benefit, most published studies of yoga in chronic pain are small, often with substantial heterogeneity and a high risk of bias. One benefit of yoga is that it can easily be delivered via telemedicine. Studies have found yoga to be comparable in efficacy to physical therapy for low back pain. Studies have demonstrated yoga to be as safe as usual care and exercise, with overall low risk of harm.

Physical Therapy Methods

Question 7. Which of the following physical therapy modalities is *MOST* likely to improve in chronic musculoskeletal pain by decreasing temporal summation?

A. Manual therapy
B. Therapeutic exercise
C. High-frequency transcutaneous electrical nerve stimulation (TENS)

Answer: A. Manual therapy techniques, neural mobilization exercises, and high-velocity mobilizations have been shown to produce significant changes in mechanical temporal summation (TS) which is an important nociceptive processing characteristic of central sensitization. Patients with chronic musculoskeletal pain have alterations in the processing of the central nervous system with central sensitization (CS). This generalized hypersensitivity of the somatosensory system can be measured quantitatively by two measures: one which is pronociceptive and a second which is antinociceptive. TS measures the state of hyperactivity in the dorsal horn of the pain facilitation pathways, while conditioned pain modulation (CPM) measures the disturbance of the descending pain inhibitory system, respectively. A Systematic Review and Meta-analysis had reported the Efficacy of Physical Therapy on

Nociceptive Pain Processing Alterations in Patients with Chronic Musculoskeletal Pain with one of the key findings serving the clinical relevance of this question. The effect of therapeutic exercise (answer choice b) on TS is mixed and acupuncture (choice c) has not demonstrated changes in TS [159].

Question 8. A 53-year-old woman with fibromyalgia complains of worsening bilateral shoulder pain. X-rays excluded fracture, subluxation, or osteoarthritis. There is no evidence of rotator cuff tears or cervical radiculopathy. She was referred to physical therapy (PT). Which of the following PT interventions is *MOST* effective in the long-term management of this patient?

A. The therapist educates the patient on thermal modalities before applying a heating pad on the shoulder and the patient performs a mental distraction technique.
B. The therapist applies an active massage treatment to the soft tissues of the deltoid and the patient remains supine.
C. The therapist provides technical instruction on the use of a shoulder pulley apparatus and the patient performs passive range-of-motion exercises.

Answer: B. Active treatments in physical therapy are activities in which the patient is physically and/or cognitively engaged. They tend to provide a long-term, sustainable approach to managing pain. Passive treatments in physical therapy involve activities that are performed on the patient. For example, massage, the use of heating pads, and cold packs are passive treatments [122].

Impact of Exercise on Pain Management

Question 9. Which of the following interventions is *MOST* likely to reduce pain and disability in patients with chronic low back pain?

A. Education
B. Electrotherapy
C. Exercise

Answer: C. Exercise may reduce pain and improve disability compared to common treatments such as electrotherapy or education. In a 2021 Cochrane Review by Hayden et al., chronic low back pain was defined as pain, muscle tension, or stiffness lasting longer than 12 weeks *or* recurrent low back pain with two episodes in a year, lasting more than 24 hours, with more than 30 days pain-free between. These persistent back pain populations were categorized as "chronic." Examples of exercise treatment included general physical fitness programs prescribed by health professionals delivered in a group setting, aerobic exercise in the form of walking programs, and focused muscle strengthening and core stability exercises. The systematic review evaluated the impact of exercise treatment on pain and functional limitations in adults with chronic non-specific low back pain compared to no treatment, usual care, placebo, and other conservative treatments. Exercise was determined to reduce pain and improve disability in comparison to electrotherapy or education [92].

Stimulation Produces Analgesia: TENS (per ABA)

Question 10. A 63-year-old male presents with chronic neuropathic and nociceptive pain affecting his right posterolateral hip. Which of the following *BEST* describes the utility of a trial of transcutaneous electrical nerve stimulation (TENS) therapy in his case?
  A. Utility is low because it is costly and requires physical therapy assistance to apply it correctly.
  B. Utility is equivocal because it may reduce neuropathic pain but not nociceptive pain.
  C. Utility is high because of low-risk and promotion of self-reliance for managing pain.
Answer: C. TENS therapy can reduce pain in some patients and is a low-cost, low-risk therapy that can be administered by the patient independently. Conventional TENS therapy utilizes high-frequency, low-intensity stimulation through adhesive pads on the skin and can be used to treat acute or chronic neuropathic, nociceptive, or nociplastic (i.e., central sensitization) pain. Its mechanism of action may include the activation of large-diameter afferent fibers leading to the facilitation of descending inhibitory systems. TENS therapy will not be effective for all patients. However, despite its equivocal efficacy in systematic reviews, TENS therapy is relatively inexpensive, requires little instruction, and can be delivered independently by the patient, thereby promoting patient self-efficacy. TENS is also safe but should be avoided in patients with implanted electronic devices, and TENS adhesive pads should not be placed over damaged skin, hematoma, or possible thrombosis, and should not be used on the head or throat [111, 118].

Rehabilitation Techniques

Question 11. Which of the following strategies is *MOST* likely to promote adherence to an exercise program in patients with chronic widespread musculoskeletal pain?
  A. Engaging in psychodynamic therapy
  B. Promoting self-efficacy
  C. Incorporating passive treatments from licensed physical therapists
Answer: B. Emphasizing self-efficacy is a recommended approach to help patients with chronic widespread pain or fibromyalgia adhere to an exercise program. Several psychological techniques including cognitive restructuring and relaxation may be applied to achieve goals of reducing pain and disability in patients with chronic widespread pain, persistent pain, or fibromyalgia. Approaches may involve adaptation, pain coping skills, and self-management to reduce disability associated with pain symptoms. The perspective is to decrease reliance on passive, reactive, and dependent circumstances to active and self-directed approaches in coping with symptoms and improving quality of life.

Strategies to achieve improved outcomes include but are not limited to (1) tailoring the program to the patient's own goals and preferences, (2) using individualized supervised sessions when available, (3) ensuring accessibility, and (4) emphasizing self-efficacy [101, 119, 160].

Work Hardening Rehabilitation

Question 12. A 44-year-old male delivery driver presents with lower back pain for the last 4 months. He has been off work due to pain for the last 8 weeks. He has had 10 visits with physical therapy including stretches, dry needling, and e-stim. He has taken meloxicam 15 mg daily and completed a 2-week trial of cyclobenzaprine. He still reports moderate-severe daily lower back pain worse with bending and lifting. No red flags. His neurological exam is normal and imaging shows age-appropriate mild spondylosis. Which of the following would be the *BEST* option to facilitate return to work?
A. Refer for a 4-week functional restoration program.
B. Refer to a pain psychologist for a 10-week cognitive-behavioral therapy program.
C. Extend his current physical therapy prescription for another 4 weeks and encourage a daily home stretching program.
Answer: A. Multidisciplinary biopsychosocial rehabilitation and active (rather than passive) treatment approaches can improve the work status of patients with chronic low back pain. Concerning outcomes in chronic spine pain, multidisciplinary biopsychosocial rehabilitation is known to decrease pain and disability beyond usual care and can improve work status. Extended prescriptions for passive PT approaches or referral for passive chiropractic care are unlikely to reduce disability in chronic low back pain. Medications and injections are also passive treatments. Cognitive-behavioral therapy (CBT) is an active therapy and may assist in reducing pain catastrophizing and fear avoidance, but CBT will not prepare the spine for manual labor. When return to work is the goal, functional restoration programs should include work conditioning and/or work hardening, in addition to education and psychology [120–122].

Psychological Treatments

Question 13. A 34-year-old man presents with anxiety and chronic generalized abdominal pain. His diagnostic work-up was unremarkable. He was diagnosed with functional abdominal pain, and referred for cognitive-behavioral therapy (CBT). Which of the following is the *MAIN* component of cognitive-behavioral therapy intervention for chronic pain?
A. Accept and modify negative (maladaptive) thoughts related to pain
B. Employ relaxation strategies to decrease pain
C. Use distraction techniques to reduce pain

Answer: A. CBT involves relaxation and distraction, but at its core, it focuses on maladaptive thoughts.

Question 14. Which of the following brain regions do exogenous opioids affect to reinforce addictive behavior as part of the "dopamine reward pathway"?

A. Globus pallidus

B. Frontal cortex

C. Ventral tegmental area

Answer: C. The key brain regions constituting the brain networks for addiction are found within the mesocorticolimbic dopamine systems, which start in the ventral tegmental area and connect to the amygdala, prefrontal cortex, and nucleus accumbens. This pathway has been called the "dopamine reward pathway," and all addictive drugs ultimately act through different mechanisms to potentiate euphoria or other positive reward symptoms that subsequently reinforce behavior for ongoing use of the drug. Opioids, in particular, work by inducing the release of dopamine in the ventral tegmental area and by binding to receptors in the nucleus accumbens.

Question 15. A 73-year-old man with multiple medical problems, including hypertension, hyperlipidemia, benign prostatic hypertrophy, and a remote history of bilateral pulmonary emboli, was brought to the emergency room after reporting suicidal ideations to his primary care physician. An initial assessment revealed a 4-week history of increasingly depressed mood in the context of worsening lower abdominal pain. A chart review revealed seven medical admissions in the past year for work-up of this gastrointestinal pain, which was largely unremarkable. Which of the following is *MOST* characteristic for diagnosis of somatic symptom disorder in this patient?

A. Presence of four different pain symptoms.

B. Pain is not required to be continuously present.

C. Absence of a medical condition explaining the somatic symptom.

Answer: B. Somatic symptom disorder (SSD) is characterized by preoccupation with one or more distressing physical symptoms, resulting in disruption of daily life. According to the Diagnostic and Statistical Manual Fifth Edition (DSM-5), a known medical condition explaining the somatic symptom does not preclude the diagnosis of SSD. Rather, considering the medical diagnosis, the patient's distress and dysfunction are more than what would be expected. SSD is a new disorder defined in the DSM-5, replacing somatoform and related disorders from the DSM-4-Text Revision (TR). For example, the criteria for somatization disorder required the patient's constellation of somatic symptoms to include four different pain symptoms, two gastrointestinal symptoms, one sexual symptom, and one pseudoneurological symptom. In contrast, diagnosis of SSD requires the presence of just a single somatic symptom. Further, any one somatic symptom is not required to be continuously present, but rather the state of being symptomatic, with any variation of symptoms, is required for the diagnosis of SSD.

Question 16. A 23-year-old woman with a history of depression and post-traumatic stress disorder presents with generalized body pain and aches that have progressively worsened over the past year. She is wheelchair-bound. On examination, she was extremely sensitive to touch all over her body. Neurologic examination was intact and brain/spine imaging was unremarkable. Which of the following tools is *BEST* to assess catastrophizing behaviors in this patient?

A. The Profile of Mood States (POMS)
B. Fear Avoidance and Beliefs Questionnaire (FABQI)
C. Coping Strategies Questionnaire (CSQ)

Answer: C. Pain catastrophizing is defined as an exaggerated negative orientation toward actual or anticipated pain experiences. It is a cognitive and emotional process that involves the magnification of pain-related stimuli, feelings of helplessness, and a negative orientation to pain and life circumstances. Several self-report measures of catastrophizing have been developed and shown to have good psychometric properties—the most significant of which are the Coping Strategies Questionnaire [CSQ] and the Pain Catastrophizing Scale [PCS]. These measures have been used in both clinical research and contexts and have shown to have predictive validity for disability and response to various treatments.

Question 17. A 40-year-old policeman comes to the primary care clinic with complaints of intermittent episodes of low back pain, for the past year, that has been progressively worsening. No precipitating factors could be identified except that his workload as a police traffic officer has increased. Physical examination and diagnostic testing were unremarkable. Which of the following resilience factors is considered the *MOST* important in determining his adjustment to chronic pain?

A. Anxiety sensitivity
B. Optimism
C. Neuroticism

Answer: B. Three potential resilience factors are particularly relevant in chronic pain: optimism, hope, and psychological flexibility. Optimism may be one of the most important personality traits concerning adjustment to chronic pain. Dispositional optimism is defined as "the tendency to believe that one will generally experience good outcomes in life." Optimism was found to be associated with better general health, adaptation to chronic disease, and recovery after various surgical procedures.

References[1]

1. Engel GL. The need for a new medical model: a challenge for biomedicine. Science. 1977;196(4286):129–36.
2. Gatchel RJ, Peng YB, Peters ML, Fuchs PN, Turk DC. The biopsychosocial approach to chronic pain: scientific advances and future directions. Psychol Bull. 2007;133(4):581–624.
3. Ng W, Slater H, Starcevich C, Wright A, Mitchell T, Beales D. Barriers and enablers influencing healthcare professionals' adoption of a biopsychosocial approach to musculoskeletal pain: a systematic review and qualitative evidence synthesis. Pain. 2021 Aug;162(8):2154–85.

[1](*) denotes essential references for additional reading.

4. Living well with chronic illness: a call for public health action [Internet]. Washington, DC: National Academies Press; 2012 [cited 2024 Aug 18]. Available from: http://www.nap.edu/catalog/13272.
5. Darnall BD, Carr DB, Schatman ME. Pain psychology and the biopsychosocial model of pain treatment: ethical imperatives and social responsibility. Pain Med. 2016;18:pnw166.
6. Cheatle MD. Biopsychosocial approach to assessing and managing patients with chronic pain. Med Clin North Am. 2016;100(1):43–53.
7. Darnall BD. Psychological treatment for chronic pain: improving access and integration. Psychol Sci Public Interest. 2021;22(2):45–51.
8. Montiel Ishino FA, McNab PR, Gilreath T, Salmeron B, Williams F. A comprehensive multi-variate model of biopsychosocial factors associated with opioid misuse and use disorder in a 2017–2018 United States national survey. BMC Public Health. 2020;20(1):1740.
9. Harmon ZS, Welch EN, Ruby CL. Conceptualizing drug addiction and chronic pain through a biopsychosocial framework to improve therapeutic strategies. In: Meil WM, Mills JA, editors. Addictions – diagnosis and treatment [Internet]. IntechOpen; 2021. [cited 2024 Aug 18]. Available from: https://www.intechopen.com/books/addictions-diagnosis-and-treatment/conceptualizing-drug-addiction-and-chronic-pain-through-a-biopsychosocial-framework-to-improve-thera.
10. Overdose Death Rates [Internet]. 2022. Available from: Nida.nih.gov.
11. Issue brief: Nation's drug-related over-dose and death epidemic continues to worsen. [Internet]. 2022. Available from: Ama-assn.org.
12. Bao Y, Williams AR, Schackman BR. COVID-19 could change the way we respond to the opioid crisis—for the better. Psychiatr Serv. 2020;71(12):1214–5.
13. Ghoshal M. Special report: race, pain management, and the system. Pract Pain Manag. 2020;20(5).
14. Makivić I, Kersnik J, Klemenc-Ketiš Z. The role of the psychosocial dimension in the improvement of quality of care: a systematic review. Slov J Public Health. 2016;55(1):86–95.
15. Xiao X, Song H, Sang T, Wu Z, Xie Y, Yang Q. Analysis of real-world implementation of the biopsychosocial approach to healthcare: evidence from a combination of qualitative and quantitative methods. Front Psych. 2021;12:725596.
16. *Varrassi G, Müller-Schwefe G, Pergolizzi J, Orónska A, Morlion B, Mavrocordatos P, et al. Pharmacological treatment of chronic pain – the need for CHANGE. Curr Med Res Opin. 2010;26(5):1231–45.
17. Henry SG, Bell RA, Fenton JJ, Kravitz RL. Goals of chronic pain management: do patients and primary care physicians agree and does it matter? Clin J Pain. 2017;33(11):955–61.
18. Park HJ, Moon DE. Pharmacologic management of chronic pain. Korean J Pain. 2010;23(2):99–108.
19. Ho KY, Gwee KA, Cheng YK, Yoon KH, Hee HT, Omar AR. Nonsteroidal anti-inflammatory drugs in chronic pain: implications of new data for clinical practice. J Pain Res. 2018;11:1937–48.
20. Barreto EF, Feely MA. Can NSAIDs be used safely for analgesia in patients with CKD?: PRO. Kidney360. 2020;1(11):1184–8.
21. American Geriatrics Society Panel on the Pharmacological Management of Persistent Pain in Older Persons. Pharmacological management of persistent pain in older persons. J Am Geriatr Soc. 2009;57(8):1331–46.
22. *Dowell D, Ragan KR, Jones CM, Baldwin GT, Chou R. CDC clinical practice guideline for prescribing opioids for pain — United States, 2022. MMWR Recomm Rep. 2022;71(3):1–95.
23. Petzke F, Bock F, Hüppe M, Nothacker M, Norda H, Radbruch L, et al. Long-term opioid therapy for chronic noncancer pain: second update of the German guidelines. Pain Rep. 2020;5(5):e840.
24. *Finnerup NB, Attal N, Haroutounian S, McNicol E, Baron R, Dworkin RH, et al. Pharmacotherapy for neuropathic pain in adults: a systematic review and meta-analysis. Lancet Neurol. 2015;14(2):162–73.

25. *Lussier D, Huskey AG, Portenoy RK. Adjuvant analgesics in cancer pain management. Oncologist. 2004;9(5):571–91.
26. Marano G, Traversi G, Romagnoli E, Catalano V, Lotrionte M, Abbate A, et al. Cardiologic side effects of psychotropic drugs. J Geriatr Cardiol JGC. 2011;8(4):243–53.
27. Hopkins T, Kominek C. Medication management of chronic pain in patients with comorbid cardiovascular disease. 7th ed. Pract Pain Manag. 2019;19.
28. Fine PG. Treatment guidelines for the pharmacological management of pain in older persons. Pain Med Malden Mass. 2012;13(Suppl 2):S57–66.
29. Busse JW, Vankrunkelsven P, Zeng L, Heen AF, Merglen A, Campbell F, et al. Medical cannabis or cannabinoids for chronic pain: a clinical practice guideline. BMJ. 2021:n2040.
30. National Center for Complementary and Integrative Health (NCCIH). Yoga: what you need to know. n.d. Retrieved May 20, 2022, from https://www.nccih.nih.gov/health/yoga-what-you-need-to-know.
31. Clarke TC, Black LI, Stussman BJ, Barnes PM, Nahin RL. Trends in the use of complementary health approaches among adults: United States, 2002–2012. Natl Health Stat Rep. 2015;79:1–16.
32. U.S. Department of Health and Human Services. Pain management best practices interagency task force report. 2020. Retrieved from https://www.hhs.gov/sites/default/files/pmtf-final-report-2019-05-23.pdf.
33. Yehuda S, Rabinovitz S, Carasso RL, Mostofsky DI. Fatty acids and brain peptides. Peptides. 1998;19(2):407–19.
34. Neitzel JJ. Fatty acid molecules: a role in cell signaling. Nat Educ. 2010;3(9):57. Retrieved from https://www.nature.com/scitable/topicpage/fatty-acid-molecules-a-role-in-cell-14231940/.
35. Bagga D, Wang L, Farias-Eisner R, Glaspy JA, Reddy ST. Differential effects of prostaglandin derived from ω-6 and ω-3 polyunsaturated fatty acids on COX-2 expression and IL-6 secretion. Proc Natl Acad Sci. 2003;100(4):1751–6.
36. Tick H. Nutrition and pain. Phys Med Rehabil Clin N Am. 2015;26(2):309–20.
37. Goldberg RJ, Katz J. A meta-analysis of the analgesic effects of omega-3 polyunsaturated fatty acid supplementation for inflammatory joint pain. Pain. 2007;129(1):210–23.
38. Sibille KT, King C, Garrett TJ, Glover TL, Zhang H, Chen H, et al. Omega-6: omega-3 PUFA ratio, pain, functioning, and distress in adults with knee pain. Clin J Pain. 2018;34(2):182–9.
39. National Institutes of Health Office of Dietary Supplements. Omega-3 fatty acids – health professional fact sheet. n.d. Retrieved May 20, 2022, from https://ods.od.nih.gov/factsheets/Omega3FattyAcids-HealthProfessional/.
40. Takkouche B. Polyunsaturated fatty acids and chronic pain: a systematic review and meta-analysis. Pain Physician. 2016;19(8):521–35.
41. Wandel S, Juni P, Tendal B, Nuesch E, Villiger PM, Welton NJ, et al. Effects of glucosamine, chondroitin, or placebo in patients with osteoarthritis of hip or knee: network meta-analysis. BMJ. 2010;341:c4675.
42. Ang CD, Alviar MJM, Dans AL, Bautista-Velez GGP, Villaruz-Sulit MVC, Tan JJ, et al. Vitamin B for treating peripheral neuropathy. Cochrane Neuromuscular Group, editor. Cochrane Database Syst Rev [Internet]. 2008 [cited 2024 Aug 18]. Available from: https://doi.wiley.com/10.1002/14651858.CD004573.pub3.
43. Yong WC, Sanguankeo A, Upala S. Effect of vitamin D supplementation in chronic widespread pain: a systematic review and meta-analysis. Clin Rheumatol. 2017;36(12):2825–33.
44. Pramono A, Jocken JWE, Blaak EE, Van Baak MA. The effect of vitamin D supplementation on insulin sensitivity: a systematic review and meta-analysis. Diabetes Care. 2020;43(7):1659–69.
45. Straube S, Derry S, Straube C, Moore RA. Vitamin D for the treatment of chronic painful conditions in adults. Cochrane Pain, Palliative and Supportive Care Group, editor. Cochrane Database Syst Rev [Internet]. 2015 [cited 2024 Aug 18]. Available from: https://doi.wiley.com/10.1002/14651858.CD007771.pub3.

46. Banerjee S, Jones S. Magnesium as an alternative or adjunct to opioids for migraine and chronic pain: a review of the clinical effectiveness and guidelines. CADTH rapid response reports. 2017. Retrieved from https://www.ncbi.nlm.nih.gov/books/NBK475794/.

47. Park R, Ho AMH, Pickering G, Arendt-Nielsen L, Mohiuddin M, Gilron I. Efficacy and safety of magnesium for the management of chronic pain in adults: a systematic review. Anesth Analg. 2020;131(3):764–75.

48. Sahebkar A, Henrotin Y. Analgesic efficacy and safety of curcuminoids in clinical practice: a systematic review and meta-analysis of randomized controlled trials. Pain Med. 2015;17:pnv024.

49. Liu X, Machado GC, Eyles JP, Ravi V, Hunter DJ. Dietary supplements for treating osteoarthritis: a systematic review and meta-analysis. Br J Sports Med. 2018;52(3):167–75.

50. Pattanittum P, Kunyanone N, Brown J, Sangkomkamhang US, Barnes J, Seyfoddin V, et al. Dietary supplements for dysmenorrhoea. Cochrane Gynaecology and Fertility Group, editor. Cochrane Database Syst Rev [Internet]. 2016 [cited 2024 Aug 18];2016(3). Available from: http://doi.wiley.com/10.1002/14651858.CD002124.pub2.

51. Yilmaz ST, Elma Ö, Deliens T, Coppieters I, Clarys P, Nijs J, Malfliet A. Nutrition/dietary supplements and chronic pain in patients with cancer and survivors of cancer: a systematic review and research agenda. Pain Physician. 2021;24:335–44.

52. Crawford C, Boyd C, Paat CF, Meissner K, Lentino C, Teo L, et al. Dietary ingredients as an alternative approach for mitigating chronic musculoskeletal pain: evidence-based recommendations for practice and research in the military. Pain Med. 2019;20(6):1236–47.

53. Kelly RB, Willis J. Acupuncture for pain. Am Fam Physician. 2019;100(2):89–96.

54. Hempel S, Taylor SL, Solloway MR, Miake-Lye IM, Beroes JM, Shanman R, et al. Evidence map of acupuncture [Internet]. Washington, DC: Department of Veterans Affairs (US); 2014 [cited 2024 Aug 18]. (VA Evidence-based Synthesis Program Reports). Available from: http://www.ncbi.nlm.nih.gov/books/NBK185072/.

55. Trinh K, Graham N, Irnich D, Cameron ID, Forget M. Acupuncture for neck disorders. In: The Cochrane Collaboration, editor. Cochrane database of systematic reviews [Internet]. Chichester: Wiley; 2016 [cited 2024 Aug 18]. p. CD004870.pub4. Available from: https://doi.wiley.com/10.1002/14651858.CD004870.pub4.

56. Witt CM, Vertosick EA, Foster NE, Lewith G, Linde K, MacPherson H, et al. The effect of patient characteristics on acupuncture treatment outcomes: an individual patient data meta-analysis of 20,827 chronic pain patients in randomized controlled trials. Clin J Pain. 2019;35(5):428–34.

57. MacPherson H, Vertosick EA, Foster NE, Lewith G, Linde K, Sherman KJ, et al. The persistence of the effects of acupuncture after a course of treatment: a meta-analysis of patients with chronic pain. Pain. 2017;158(5):784–93.

58. National Center for Complementary and Integrative Health (NCCIH). Tai Chi: what you need to know. n.d. Retrieved May 20, 2022, from https://www.nccih.nih.gov/health/tai-chi-what-you-need-to-know.

59. Cramer H, Ward L, Saper R, Fishbein D, Dobos G, Lauche R. The safety of yoga: a systematic review and meta-analysis of randomized controlled trials. Am J Epidemiol. 2015;182(4):281–93.

60. Wieland LS, Skoetz N, Pilkington K, Vempati R, D'Adamo CR, Berman BM. Yoga treatment for chronic non-specific low back pain. Cochrane Back and Neck Group, editor. Cochrane Database Syst Rev [Internet]. 2017 [cited 2024 Aug 18];2017(1). Available from: http://doi.wiley.com/10.1002/14651858.CD010671.pub2.

61. Saper RB, Lemaster C, Delitto A, Sherman KJ, Herman PM, Sadikova E, et al. Yoga, physical therapy, or education for chronic low back pain: a randomized noninferiority trial. Ann Intern Med. 2017;167(2):85.

62. Li Y, Li S, Jiang J, Yuan S. Effects of yoga on patients with chronic nonspecific neck pain: a PRISMA systematic review and meta-analysis. Medicine (Baltimore). 2019;98(8):e14649.

63. Anheyer D, Klose P, Lauche R, Saha FJ, Cramer H. Yoga for treating headaches: a systematic review and meta-analysis. J Gen Intern Med. 2020;35(3):846–54.

64. Kolasinski SL, Neogi T, Hochberg MC, Oatis C, Guyatt G, Block J, et al. 2019 American College of Rheumatology/Arthritis Foundation guideline for the management of osteoarthritis of the hand, hip, and knee. Arthritis Rheumatol. 2020;72(2):220–33.

65. Qin J, Zhang Y, Wu L, He Z, Huang J, Tao J, et al. Effect of Tai Chi alone or as additional therapy on low back pain: systematic review and meta-analysis of randomized controlled trials. Medicine (Baltimore). 2019;98(37):e17099.

66. Mudano AS, Tugwell P, Wells GA, Singh JA. Tai Chi for rheumatoid arthritis. Cochrane Musculoskeletal Group, editor. Cochrane Database Syst Rev [Internet]. 2019 [cited 2024 Aug 18]. Available from: https://doi.wiley.com/10.1002/14651858.CD004849.pub2.

67. Hu L, Wang Y, Liu X, Ji X, Ma Y, Man S, et al. Tai Chi exercise can ameliorate physical and mental health of patients with knee osteoarthritis: systematic review and meta-analysis. Clin Rehabil. 2021;35(1):64–79.

68. Cheng CA, Chiu YW, Wu D, Kuan YC, Chen SN, Tam KW. Effectiveness of Tai Chi on fibromyalgia patients: a meta-analysis of randomized controlled trials. Complement Ther Med. 2019;46:1–8.

69. Kong LJ, Lauche R, Klose P, Bu JH, Yang XC, Guo CQ, et al. Tai Chi for chronic pain conditions: a systematic review and meta-analysis of randomized controlled trials. Sci Rep. 2016;6(1):25325.

70. Brox JI, Storheim K, Grotle M, Tveito TH, Indahl A, Eriksen HR. Systematic review of back schools, brief education, and fear-avoidance training for chronic low back pain. Spine J. 2008;8(6):948–58.

71. Vlaeyen JWS, Crombez G. Fear of movement/(re)injury, avoidance and pain disability in chronic low back pain patients. Man Ther. 1999;4(4):187–95.

72. Louw A, Diener I, Butler DS, Puentedura EJ. The effect of neuroscience education on pain, disability, anxiety, and stress in chronic musculoskeletal pain. Arch Phys Med Rehabil. 2011;92(12):2041–56.

73. Vlaeyen JWS, Linton SJ. Fear-avoidance and its consequences in chronic musculoskeletal pain: a state of the art. Pain. 2000;85(3):317–32.

74. Moseley GL. Evidence for a direct relationship between cognitive and physical change during an education intervention in people with chronic low back pain. Eur J Pain. 2004;8(1):39–45.

75. Ryan CG, Gray HG, Newton M, Granat MH. Pain biology education and exercise classes compared to pain biology education alone for individuals with chronic low back pain: a pilot randomised controlled trial. Man Ther. 2010;15(4):382–7.

76. Zimney K, Louw A, Puentedura EJ. Use of Therapeutic Neuroscience Education to address psychosocial factors associated with acute low back pain: a case report. Physiother Theory Pract. 2014;30(3):202–9.

77. Dolphens M, Nijs J, Cagnie B, Meeus M, Roussel N, Kregel J, et al. Efficacy of a modern neuroscience approach versus usual care evidence-based physiotherapy on pain, disability and brain characteristics in chronic spinal pain patients: protocol of a randomized clinical trial. BMC Musculoskelet Disord. 2014;15(1):149.

78. Edwards RR, Dworkin RH, Sullivan MD, Turk DC, Wasan AD. The role of psychosocial processes in the development and maintenance of chronic pain. J Pain. 2016;17(9):T70–92.

79. Rooij A, Boer M, Leeden M, Roorda L, Steultjens M, Dekker J. Cognitive mechanisms of change in multidisciplinary treatment of patients with chronic widespread pain: a prospective cohort study. J Rehabil Med. 2014;46(2):173–80.

80. Burns JW, Nielson WR, Jensen MP, Heapy A, Czlapinski R, Kerns RD. Specific and general therapeutic mechanisms in cognitive behavioral treatment of chronic pain. J Consult Clin Psychol. 2015;83(1):1–11.

81. Gaskin DJ, Richard P. The economic costs of pain in the United States. J Pain. 2012;13(8):715–24.

82. Frontera WR, DeLisa JA, Gans BM, Walsh NE, Robinson LR, editors. Physical medicine and rehabilitation: principles and practice. 5th ed. Philadelphia: Lippincott Williams & Wilkins Health; 2018.

83. Malanga GA, Yan N, Stark J. Mechanisms and efficacy of heat and cold therapies for muscu-loskeletal injury. Postgrad Med. 2015;127(1):57–65.
84. Chow RT, Johnson MI, Lopes-Martins RA, Bjordal JM. Efficacy of low-level laser therapy in the management of neck pain: a systematic review and meta-analysis of randomised placebo or active-treatment controlled trials. Lancet. 2009;374(9705):1897–908.
85. Karu T. Low intensity laser light action upon fibroblasts and lymphocytes. In: Progress in laser therapy: selected papers from the October 1990 ILTA Congress; 1991. p. 175–9.
86. Tsuchiya K, Kawatani M, Takeshige C, Matsumoto I. Laser irradiation abates neuronal responses to nociceptive stimulation of rat-paw skin. Brain Res Bull. 1994;34(4):369–74.
87. Watson T. Chapter 11. In: Electrotherapy: evidence-based practice. Churchill Livingstone; 2008.
88. Seffinger M, editor. Foundations of osteopathic medicine. 4th ed. Lippincott Williams and Wilkins; 2018.
89. Bialosky JE, Bishop MD, Price DD, Robinson ME, George SZ. The mechanisms of man-ual therapy in the treatment of musculoskeletal pain: a comprehensive model. Man Ther. 2009;14(5):531–8.
90. Kujala UM. Evidence on the effects of exercise therapy in the treatment of chronic disease. Br J Sports Med. 2009;43(8):550–5.
91. Hoffmann TC, Maher CG, Briffa T, Sherrington C, Bennell K, Alison J, et al. Prescribing exer-cise interventions for patients with chronic conditions. Can Med Assoc J. 2016;188(7):510–8.
92. Hayden JA, Ellis J, Ogilvie R, Malmivaara A, Van Tulder MW. Exercise therapy for chronic low back pain. Cochrane Back and Neck Group, editor. Cochrane Database Syst Rev [Internet]. 2021 [cited 2024 Aug 18];9(9):CD009790. Available from: http://doi.wiley.com/10.1002/14651858.CD009790.pub2. PMID: 34580864; PMCID: PMC8477273.
93. Centers for Disease Control and Prevention. Measuring physical activity. n.d.. Retrieved from https://www.cdc.gov/physicalactivity/basics/measuring/.
94. Hordern MD, Dunstan DW, Prins JB, Baker MK, Singh MAF, Coombes JS. Exercise prescrip-tion for patients with type 2 diabetes and pre-diabetes: a position statement from Exercise and Sport Science Australia. J Sci Med Sport. 2012;15(1):25–31.
95. *Jordan JL, Holden MA, Mason EE, Foster NE. Interventions to improve adherence to exer-cise for chronic musculoskeletal pain in adults. Cochrane Musculoskeletal Group, editor. Cochrane Database Syst Rev [Internet]. 2010 [cited 2024 Aug 18]. Available from: https://doi.wiley.com/10.1002/14651858.CD005956.pub2.
96. Ambrose KR, Golightly YM. Physical exercise as non-pharmacological treatment of chronic pain: why and when. Best Pract Res Clin Rheumatol. 2015;29(1):120–30.
97. Jones KD, Adams D, Winters-Stone K, Burckhardt CS. A comprehensive review of 46 exercise treatment studies in fibromyalgia (1988–2005). Health Qual Life Outcomes. 2006;4(1):67.
98. Giannotti E, Koutsikos K, Pigatto M, Rampudda ME, Doria A, Masiero S. Medium-/long-term effects of a specific exercise protocol combined with patient education on spine mobil-ity, chronic fatigue, pain, aerobic fitness and level of disability in fibromyalgia. Biomed Res Int. 2014;2014:1–9.
99. *Brosseau L, Wells GA, Tugwell P, Egan M, Wilson KG, Dubouloz CJ, et al. Ottawa panel evidence-based clinical practice guidelines for strengthening exercises in the management of fibromyalgia: part 2. Phys Ther. 2008;88(7):873–86.
100. Jones KD, Burckhardt CS, Clark SR, Bennett RM, Potempa KM. A randomized controlled trial of muscle strengthening versus flexibility training in fibromyalgia. J Rheumatol. 2002;29(5):1041–8.
101. Busch AJ, Webber SC, Brachaniec M, Bidonde J, Bello-Haas VD, Danyliw AD, et al. Exercise therapy for fibromyalgia. Curr Pain Headache Rep. 2011;15(5):358–67. https://doi.org/10.1007/s11916-011-0214-2.
102. U.S. Department of Health and Human Services. 2008 Physical activity guidelines for Americans. 2008. Retrieved from www.health.gov/paguidelines.
103. Haskell WL, Lee IM, Pate RR, Powell KE, Blair SN, Franklin BA, Macera CA, Heath GW, Thompson PD, Bauman A. Physical activity and public health: updated recommendation for

adults from the American College of Sports Medicine and the American Heart Association. Circulation. 2007;116(9):1081–93.

104. Dimeo FC. Effects of exercise on cancer-related fatigue. Cancer. 2001;92(S6):1689–93.

105. Sañudo B, Carrasco L, De Hoyo M, McVeigh JG. Effects of exercise training and detraining in patients with fibromyalgia syndrome: a 3-yr longitudinal study. Am J Phys Med Rehabil. 2012;91(7):561–73.

106. Häkkinen A, Häkkinen K, Hannonen P, Alen M. Strength training induced adaptations in neuromuscular function of premenopausal women with fibromyalgia: comparison with healthy women. Ann Rheum Dis. 2001;60(1):21–6.

107. Valkeinen H, Häkkinen K, Pakarinen A, Hannonen P, Häkkinen A, Airaksinen O, et al. Muscle hypertrophy, strength development, and serum hormones during strength training in elderly women with fibromyalgia. Scand J Rheumatol. 2005;34(4):309–14.

108. Valkeinen H, Alén M, Häkkinen A, Hannonen P, Kukkonen-Harjula K, Häkkinen K. Effects of concurrent strength and endurance training on physical fitness and symptoms in postmenopausal women with fibromyalgia: a randomized controlled trial. Arch Phys Med Rehabil. 2008;89(9):1660–6.

109. Gavi MBRO, Vassalo DV, Amaral FT, Macedo DCF, Gava PL, Dantas EM, et al. Strengthening exercises improve symptoms and quality of life but do not change autonomic modulation in fibromyalgia: a randomized clinical trial. Cordero MD, editor. PLoS One. 2014;9(3):e90767.

110. Sluka KA, Walsh D. Transcutaneous electrical nerve stimulation: basic science mechanisms and clinical effectiveness. J Pain. 2003;4(3):109–21.

111. Vance CG, Dailey DL, Rakel BA, Sluka KA. Using tens for pain control: the state of the evidence. Pain Manag. 2014;4(3):197–209. https://doi.org/10.2217/pmt.14.13.

112. Kalra A, Urban MO, Sluka KA. Blockade of opioid receptors in rostral ventral medulla prevents antihyperalgesia produced by transcutaneous electrical nerve stimulation (TENS). J Pharmacol Exp Ther. 2001;298(1):257–63.

113. Sluka KA, Lisi TL, Westlund KN. Increased release of serotonin in the spinal cord during low, but not high, frequency transcutaneous electric nerve stimulation in rats with joint inflammation. Arch Phys Med Rehabil. 2006;87(8):1137–40.

114. Ma YT, Sluka KA. Reduction in inflammation-induced sensitization of dorsal horn neurons by transcutaneous electrical nerve stimulation in anesthetized rats. Exp Brain Res. 2001;137(1):94–102.

115. Sluka KA, Deacon M, Stibal A, Strissel S, Terpstra A. Spinal blockade of opioid receptors prevents the analgesia produced by TENS in arthritic rats. J Pharmacol Exp Ther. 1999;289(2):840–6.

116. Sluka KA, Vance CGT, Lisi TL. High-frequency, but not low-frequency, transcutaneous electrical nerve stimulation reduces aspartate and glutamate release in the spinal cord dorsal horn. J Neurochem. 2005;95(6):1794–801.

117. Rutjes AW, Nüesch E, Sterchi R, Kalichman L, Hendriks E, Osiri M, et al. Transcutaneous electrostimulation for osteoarthritis of the knee. Cochrane Musculoskeletal Group, editor. Cochrane Database Syst Rev [Internet]. 2009 [cited 2024 Aug 18]. Available from: https://doi.wiley.com/10.1002/14651858.CD002823.pub2.

118. Bennett MI, Hughes N, Johnson MI. Methodological quality in randomised controlled trials of transcutaneous electric nerve stimulation for pain: LOW fidelity may explain negative findings. Pain. 2011;152(6):1226–32. https://doi.org/10.1016/j.pain.2010.12.009.

119. Institute of Medicine (US) Committee on Pain, Disability, and Chronic Illness Behavior. Pain and disability: clinical, behavioral, and public policy perspectives. Washington, DC: National Academies Press (US); 1987. PMID: 25032476.

120. Kamper SJ, Apeldoorn AT, Chiarotto A, Smeets RJEM, Ostelo RWJG, Guzman J, et al. Multidisciplinary biopsychosocial rehabilitation for chronic low back pain: cochrane systematic review and meta-analysis. BMJ. 2015;350:h444. PMID: 25694111; PMCID: PMC4353283.

121. Schaafsma FG, Whelan K, Van Der Beek AJ, Van Der Es-Lambeek LC, Ojajärvi A, Verbeek JH. Physical conditioning as part of a return to work strategy to reduce sickness absence

for workers with back pain. Cochrane Back and Neck Group, editor. Cochrane Database Syst Rev [Internet]. 2013 [cited 2024 Aug 18];2013(8):CD001822. Available from: http://doi. wiley.com/10.1002/14651858.CD001822.pub3. PMID: 23990391; PMCID: PMC7074637.

122. Roche-Leboucher G, Petit-Lemanac'h A, Bontoux L, Dubus-Bausière V, Parot-Shinkel E, Fanello S, et al. Multidisciplinary intensive functional restoration versus outpatient active physiotherapy in chronic low back pain: a randomized controlled trial. Spine (Phila Pa 1976). 2011;36(26):2235–42. https://doi.org/10.1097/BRS.0b013e3182191e13. PMID: 21415807.

123. Kreiner DS, Matz P, Bono CM, Cho CH, Easa JE, Ghiselli G, et al. Guideline summary review: an evidence-based clinical guideline for the diagnosis and treatment of low back pain. Spine J. 2020;20(7):998–1024.

124. Otis J. Managing chronic pain: a cognitive-behavioral therapy approach. Oxford, UK: Oxford University Press; 2007.

125. Murphy JL, Cordova MJ, Dedert EA. Cognitive behavioral therapy for chronic pain in veterans: evidence for clinical effectiveness in a model program. Psychol Serv. 2022;19(1):95–102.

126. Stanos S. Focused review of interdisciplinary pain rehabilitation programs for chronic pain management. Curr Pain Headache Rep. 2012;16(2):147–52.

127. Ektor-Andersen J, Ingvarsson E, Kullendorff M, Orbaek P. High cost-benefit of early team-based biomedical and cognitive-behaviour intervention for long-term pain-related sickness absence. J Rehabil Med. 2008;40(1):1–8.

128. Patrick LE, Altmaier EM, Found EM. Long-term outcomes in multidisciplinary treatment of chronic low back pain: results of a 13-year follow-up. Spine. 2004;29(8):850–5.

129. Lambeek LC, Anema JR, van Royen BJ, Buijs PC, Wuisman PI, van Tulder MW, et al. Multidisciplinary outpatient care program for patients with chronic low back pain: design of a randomized controlled trial and cost-effectiveness study [ISRCTN28478651]. BMC Public Health. 2007;7:254.

130. Dolce JJ, Crocker MF, Moletteire C, Doleys DM. Exercise quotas, anticipatory concern and self-efficacy expectancies in chronic pain: a preliminary report. Pain. 1986;24(3):365–72.

131. Fordyce WE. Behavioral methods in chronic pain and illness. St. Louis: Mosby; 1976.

132. Thieme K, Gromnica-Ihle E, Flor H. Operant behavioral treatment of fibromyalgia: a controlled study. Arthritis Care Res. 2003;49(3):314–20.

133. Jensen MP, Nielson WR, Kerns RD. Toward the development of a motivational model of pain self-management. J Pain. 2003;4(9):477–92.

134. Astin JA, Shapiro SL, Eisenberg DM, Forys KL. Mind-body medicine: state of the science, implications for practice. J Am Board Fam Pract. 2003;16(2):131–47.

135. Seers K, Carroll D. Relaxation techniques for acute pain management: a systematic review. J Adv Nurs. 1998;27(3):466–75.

136. Benson H, Goodale IL. The relaxation response: your inborn capacity to counteract the harmful effects of stress. J Fla Med Assoc. 1981;68(4):265–7.

137. Goleman DJ, Schwartz GE. Meditation as an intervention in stress reactivity. J Consult Clin Psychol. 1976;44(3):456–66.

138. Schmidt S, Grossman P, Schwarzer B, Jena S, Naumann J, Walach H. Treating fibromyalgia with mindfulness-based stress reduction: results from a 3-armed randomized controlled trial. Pain. 2011;152(2):361–9.

139. Halpin LS, Speir AM, CapoBianco P, Barnett SD. Guided imagery in cardiac surgery. Outcomes Manag. 2002;6(3):132–7.

140. Spiegel D, Moore R. Imagery and hypnosis in the treatment of cancer patients. Oncol Williston Park N. 1997;11(8):1179–89; discussion 1189–1195.

141. Patterson DR, Jensen MP. Hypnosis and clinical pain. Psychol Bull. 2003;129(4):495–521.

142. Jensen M, Patterson DR. Hypnotic treatment of chronic pain. J Behav Med. 2006;29(1):95–124.

143. Montgomery GH, DuHamel KN, Redd WH. A meta-analysis of hypnotically induced analgesia: how effective is hypnosis? Int J Clin Exp Hypn. 2000;48(2):138–53.

144. Cicero TJ, Lynskey M, Todorov A, Inciardi JA, Surratt HL. Co-morbid pain and psychopathology in males and females admitted to treatment for opioid analgesic abuse. Pain. 2008;139(1):127–35.

145. Polatin PB, Kinney RK, Gatchel RJ, Lillo E, Mayer TG. Psychiatric illness and chronic low-back pain. The mind and the spine--which goes first? Spine. 1993;18(1):66–71.
146. Katon W, Egan K, Miller D. Chronic pain: lifetime psychiatric diagnoses and family history. Am J Psychiatry. 1985;142(10):1156–60.
147. Fishbain DA, Goldberg M, Meagher RB, Steele R, Rosomoff H. Male and female chronic pain patients categorized by DSM-III psychiatric diagnostic criteria. Pain. 1986;26(2):181–97.
148. Dersh J, Polatin PB, Gatchel RJ. Chronic pain and psychopathology: research findings and theoretical considerations. Psychosom Med. 2002;64(5):773–86.
149. Wasan AD, Butler SF, Budman SH, Benoit C, Fernandez K, Jamison RN. Psychiatric history and psychologic adjustment as risk factors for aberrant drug-related behavior among patients with chronic pain. Clin J Pain. 2007;23(4):307–15.
150. Jamison RN. Introduction to special edition. Clin J Pain. 2002;18(suppl):S1–2.
151. Nedeljkovic SS, Wasan A, Jamison RN. Assessment of efficacy of long-term opioid therapy in pain patients with substance abuse potential. Clin J Pain. 2002;18(4 Suppl):S39–51.
152. Savage SR, Joranson DE, Covington EC, Schnoll SH, Heit HA, Gilson AM. Definitions related to the medical use of opioids: evolution towards universal agreement. J Pain Symptom Manag. 2003;26(1):655–67.
153. Katz N, Fanciullo GJ. Role of urine toxicology testing in the management of chronic opioid therapy. Clin J Pain. 2002;18(4 Suppl):S76–82.
154. Burchman SL, Pagel PS. Implementation of a formal treatment agreement for outpatient management of chronic nonmalignant pain with opioid analgesics. J Pain Symptom Manag. 1995;10(7):556–63.
155. Suboxone product information. Retrieved from http://www.suboxone.com.
156. Davis MP. Twelve reasons for considering buprenorphine as a frontline analgesic in the management of pain. J Support Oncol. 2012;10(6):209–19.
157. Daitch J, Frey ME, Silver D, Mitnick C, Daitch D, Pergolizzi J. Conversion of chronic pain patients from full-opioid agonists to sublingual buprenorphine. Pain Physician. 2012;15(3 Suppl):ES59–66.
158. Substance Abuse and Mental Health Services Administration (SAMHSA). Waiver Elimination (MAT Act). Available at https://www.samhsa.gov/medications-substance-use-disorders/waiver-elimination-mat-act. Accessed 25 Apr 2024.
159. Arribas-Romano A, Fernández-Carnero J, Molina-Rueda F, Angulo-Diaz-Parreño S, Navarro-Santana MJ. Efficacy of physical therapy on nociceptive pain processing alterations in patients with chronic musculoskeletal pain: a systematic review and meta-analysis. Pain Med. 2020;21(10):2502–17. https://doi.org/10.1093/pm/pnz366. PMID: 32100027.
160. Scheidt CE, Waller E, Endorf K, Schmidt S, König R, Zeeck A, Joos A, Lacour M. Is brief psychodynamic psychotherapy in primary fibromyalgia syndrome with concurrent depression an effective treatment? A randomized controlled trial. Gen Hosp Psychiatry. 2013;35(2):160–7. https://doi.org/10.1016/j.genhosppsych.2012.10.013. Epub 2012 Dec 4. Erratum in: Gen Hosp Psychiatry. 2014;36(1):124. PMID: 23218844.

Use of Opioids in Chronic Pain Management

6

Ameet Nagpal, Tyler Kalajian, Brian Boies, Hussein Musa, Rani Chovatiya, and Gina Votta-Velis

Abbreviations

ADE	Adverse drug effects
APS	American Pain Society
cAMP	Cyclic adenosine monophosphate
CDC	Center for Disease Control and Prevention
CNS	Central nervous system
DEA	Drug Enforcement Administration
DENk	Dual opioid peptides enkephalinase
DOP	Delta opioid peptide receptor
EDDP	Ethylideine-1,5-dimethyl-3,3-dipyhenylpyrrolidine
GC-MS	Gas chromatography mass spectrometry

A. Nagpal (✉)
Department of Orthopaedics and Physical Medicine & Rehabilitation, Medical University of South Carolina, Charleston, SC, USA
e-mail: nagpal@musc.edu

T. Kalajian
Department of Anesthesiology, Medical University of South Carolina College of Medicine, Charleston, SC, USA
e-mail: kalajian@musc.edu

B. Boies
Cone Health, Greensboro, NC, USA
e-mail: brian.boies@conehealth.com

H. Musa
Department of Anesthesiology, UT Health San Antonio School of Medicine, San Antonio, TX, USA

R. Chovatiya · G. Votta-Velis
Department of Anesthesiology, University of Illinois at Chicago College of Medicine, Chicago, IL, USA
e-mail: rchova1@uic.edu

© The Author(s), under exclusive license to Springer Nature Switzerland AG 2025
M. Anitescu (ed.), *Multidisciplinary Pain Medicine Fellowship*,
https://doi.org/10.1007/978-3-031-88357-6_6

GI   Gastro-intestinal
GPCR   G protein-coupled receptor
GWAS   Genome wide association study
HSV   Herpes simplex virus
IL   Interleukine
KOP   Kappa opioid peptide receptor
MAT   Medication assisted treatment
MME   Morphine miligram equivalents
MOP   Mu opioid peptide receptor
NMDA   N-methyl-D aspartate
NOP   Nociceptin opioid peptide receptor
ORL   Opioid receptor like
OUD   Opioid use disorder
PAG   Peri aqueductal gray
PCP   Phencyclidine
PDMP   Prescription drug monitoring program
PNS   Peripheral nervous system
RVM   Rostro-ventral medulla
SNP   Single nucleotide polymorphism
TNF   Tumor necrosis factor

Introduction

The utilization of opioids as a form of analgesia dates back to 3400 BC when the opium poppy was cultivated in lower Mesopotamia. Since then, its popularity has gained global traction for its application in both acute and chronic pain management. The global opioid market was valued at USD 22.8 billion in 2022 with an anticipated growth rate of 1.4% from 2023 to 2030. The growth of this market is sought to be due to new opioid derivatives in the management of chronic pain. In this chapter we aim to explore the pharmacology of opioids, their clinical applications, and methods for combatting addiction.

Pharmacology of Opioid Medication

Opioids exert their effects on a variety of receptors in multiple areas of the body, with the CNS being the most relevant for analgesia. Opioid receptors themselves are G protein-coupled receptors (GPCRs), and specifically are coupled to Go/Gi inhibitory proteins [1]. Classical opioid agonism leads to inhibition of cyclic adenosine monophosphate (cAMP) within the cell, hyperpolarizing the cell via its downstream effects by increasing potassium conductance while conversely inhibiting calcium conductance [2]. Historically, the primary opioid receptors were considered to be the Mu (μ) opioid peptide receptor (MOP), Kappa (κ) opioid peptide receptor

(KOP), and Delta (δ) opioid peptide receptor (DOP), which are primarily differentiated from a structural perspective by the extracellular components of the GPCR [1].

The nociceptin opioid peptide receptor (NOP), also known as the opioid receptor-like 1 receptor (ORL1), is structurally similar to the above but is considered to be a non-opioid branch of the opioid receptor family [2, 3] and has little affinity for traditional opioid substances such as morphine [4]. Uniquely, it does not bind naloxone and many traditional opioids [5]. Sigma (σ) receptors were once believed to be in the opioid class of receptors, but these are structurally distinct from opioids receptors and produce psychomimetic effects from substances including phencyclidine (PCP) and its analogs [6]. Zeta (ζ) receptors regulate developmental events related to embryonic development and cancer cell proliferation [7, 8].

Clinical Effects of Classic Opioid Receptors

The opioid receptors noted above have a wide range of effects on the body, with varying levels of individual receptor subtype activation based upon the opioid used. Below is a brief outline of some of the more pertinent effects [6, 7].

MOP receptors are found in the CNS, GI system, and peripheral nervous system (PNS). It has several subtypes, with $\mu1$ and $\mu2$ being the most clinically relevant. $\mu1$ is associated with analgesia and physical dependence, with $\mu2$ having many of the "unwanted" effects of opioids, such as euphoria, respiratory depression, miosis, reduced GI motility, and physical dependence.

KOP receptors are found in the CNS and PNS, and their activation provides analgesia, sedation, dysphoria, diuresis, and respiratory depression, along with hallucinogenic/psychomimetic effects due to its action in the limbic system.

DOP receptors are primarily located in the brain and PNS, with analgesia and constipation being some of the primary effects.

NOP receptors are primarily in the CNS and may regulate both analgesia and hyperalgesia, along with emotional behaviors. They may have potential uses as non-addictive analgesics [9].

Mechanisms of Pain Relief

While a full description of the pain pathways associated with opioid therapy is outside of the scope of this review, the spinal and supraspinal mechanisms are briefly outlined below. For further information on these mechanisms, we recommend review of Bonica Chapter 79 or Wall and Melzack Chapter 30.

Spinal analgesia is elicited at a segmental level in predominantly Rexed lamina I and II (marginal zone and substantial gelatinosa) in the dorsal horn via the opioid receptors noted above [10]; specifically, the estimated total opiate binding in the spinal cord is predominantly via the μ receptor, contributing 70%, with δ and κ contributing 23% and 7%, respectively [1, 10]. Greater than 70% of these receptors exist on the presynaptic terminals of Aδ and C fibers, which are the nociceptive fiber types, and are absent on large-diameter A fibers such as Aβ fibers, which are associated with proprioception and fine touch. Activation of these receptors decreased the release of excitatory neurotransmitters, thus reducing the transmission of pain signals further into the CNS.

From a supraspinal perspective, opioids act at several sites, including the thalamus, amygdala, and sensory cortex [1]. Most importantly are structures in the midbrain and brainstem, such as the periaqueductal gray (PAG) the rostroventral medulla (RVM). Binding of these receptors causes an activation of a descending inhibitory pathway projecting to the spinal cord, thus exerting an overall antinociceptive effect.

Classification of Opioids

Opioid compounds can be classified in several ways, from chemical structure and receptor agonism to the Drug Enforcement Agency (DEA) schedule of controlled drugs.

There are four chemical classes of opioids: phenanthrenes, benzomorphans, phenylpiperidines, and diphenylheptanes [6, 11]. Phenanthrenes refer to opioids derived from the opium plant itself and typically have multiple fused rings. These include morphine, hydromorphone, oxymorphone, codeine, and hydrocodone, to name a few. Benzomorphans only have pentazocine as a member of the class. Phenylpiperidines have a high utility in pain management and include synthetic opioids such as fentanyl, alfentanil, sufentanil, and meperidine. Diphenylheptanes include propoxyphene and methadone.

Another important classification method is based on activity at the opioid receptors. Most commonly used opioids are considered agonists, directly activating different opioid receptor types at various degrees of activity and efficacy [6]. However, other agents exist to include partial agonists, agonists-antagonists, and antagonists. Partial agonists (such as buprenorphine) have a partial effect when binding opioid receptors; these tend to have an analgesic ceiling effect, with potential safety with regards to respiratory depression, and can precipitate withdrawal if given to those taking traditional opioid agonists. Agonists-antagonists (such as nalbuphine and butorphanol) have an antagonist effect at the MOP with agonism at other receptor types, having a constellation of effects based on their relative activity. Finally, antagonists, as expected, do not have any opioid activity and therefore are competitive antagonists for other opioids; these include naloxone and naltrexone.

Finally, several opioids have mechanisms of action beyond simple opioid receptor binding. These include methadone (NMDA antagonism), tramadol (serotonin/norepinephrine reuptake inhibition), and tapentadol (norepinephrine reuptake inhibition), which may contribute to their analgesic effects in ways distinct from pure opioid agonism.

Pharmacogenetics and Opioid Medications

Opioid therapy is commonly used as an analgesic in treating pain of varying types; this includes acute pain, chronic pain, and chronic cancer pain associated with palliative care [12]. Several evidence-based guidelines and tools exist to assist providers in proper prescribing and dosing of opioids. However, challenges arise in the form of adverse effects, opioid use disorder, and overdose. Such issues have contributed to the current public health dilemma facing the U.S. and the declaration of national epidemic by the Centers for Disease Control [13].

Efficacy of opioid medications, as well as associated side effects and dependence risk, has been shown to vary based on genetic factors [14]. Numerous studies have reported genes can significantly affect pain sensitivity, perception, and predisposition to chronic pain. This is the foundation for pharmacogenetics, which is the study of how genes affect an individual's response to medications—in this case, opioids. Evidence supports that genes contribute to inter-individual differences in analgesic requirements [15]. This is further compounded by individual differences that exist in pain reporting and management. The progress in identifying genetic variants and their correlation to personalized pain management has been shown in genome-wide association studies (GWAS), single nucleotide polymorphisms (SNPs), and epigenetic studies in modulation of pain [16]. SNPs are the most common cause of genetic variation and further understanding offers promise for improving disease detection and treatments. The aim of this narrative is to highlight the role of genetics in hopes of optimizing individual opioid therapy, minimizing associated side effects, in addition to the risk of opioid dependence.

Genetic Polymorphism Related to Opioid Analgesia

Pharmacokinetics involves the process of how the body acts on the medication; this involves the processes of drug absorption, distribution, metabolism, and excretion. Pharmacodynamics, on the other hand, concerns the effect of the drug on the body. Knowledge of these processes, in addition to drug receptor types, nociceptive pathways, and antinociceptive pathways, can further enhance understanding of the differential response to opioids in patients [15]. Genetic polymorphisms in opioid metabolism, enzymes, and opioid receptors have been shown to contribute to variability in analgesic doses and associated side effects. Opioids are metabolized by the cytochrome P450 (CYP 450) enzymes in the liver. SNP polymorphisms in the genes encoding CYP 450 enzymes are linked to variations in the pharmacogenetics of various opioids. There are individuals that may be categorized as ultra-rapid, normal, intermediate, or poor metabolizers based on the level of enzymatic activity during drug metabolism.

More than 20 genes have been identified as important biological features relevant to opioid analgesia and involved in the metabolism of opioids. Several pharmacokinetic-related candidate genes (CYP2D6, CYP3A4/A5, UGT2B7, ABCB1, ABCC3, SLC22A1) and pharmacodynamic-related candidate genes

(OPRM1, COMT, KCNJ6) are presently under investigation and hold promise for clinical use in the future. CYP2D6 is responsible for the metabolism of commonly prescribed opioid medications, including codeine, tramadol, hydrocodone, oxycodone, and methadone. This enzyme has been shown to be highly polymorphic and displays significant variability across race and ethnicity [17]. As such, this has been associated with varying clinical effects in different patient populations. In addition to CYP2D6, the genotypes OPRM1 and COMT have been identified as having an impact on opioid analgesia and adverse events. Sufficient data supports that CYP2D6 genotype test results can be used to provide therapeutic recommendations specific to codeine and tramadol. However, there is limited data to support its clinical application for the following opioid medications: hydrocodone, oxycodone, and methadone, as well as for OPRM1 and COMT [18].

Multiple SNPs in genes are involved in catecholamine metabolism [19]. COMT is a key regulator of catecholamine concentrations in the pain perception pathway. As such, it also regulates pain perception and has been evaluated for its influence on the response of opioid medications in the body. Polymorphism of this enzyme has been shown to modulate opioidergic activity [20]. Inhibition of COMT enzymatic activity has been shown to increase pain sensitivity [21]. The implications of this can be especially helpful in providing guidance in managing opioid therapies amongst different patient populations.

OPRM1 is highly polymorphic and has been studied for its role in opioid responsiveness and addictive properties. There is a known association between increased OPRM1 activity and substance use disorders. Mu opioid receptors (MORs) are encoded by the OPRM1, and the high concentration dopaminergic neurons in the brain in the presence of MORs correlates directly with the development of dependence [23]. OPRM1 activity and MORs have also been associated with alcohol and nicotine abuse, heroin dependence, and oxycodone sensitivity [22, 24, 25]. Understanding OPRM1 activity and genetic variation may offer guidance in identifying patients at higher risk for dependency, and more research on how SNPs may promote dependence liability in certain populations is necessary.

Variability in Responsiveness/Genetic Influences

Clearly, genetic polymorphism in select opioid receptors, enzymatic activity, and metabolic pathways influence pain perception and analgesia in individuals. Clinical factors such as age, gender, and ethnicity have been shown to contribute to differences in opioid response. Though the effect of age and gender on the opioid response is inconclusive at this time [26, 27], the role of ethnicity has been shown to be correlative [28]. Different genetic variations can contribute to altered enzymatic activity and protein function, which in turn affects a patient's response to different analgesics—in this case, opioids.

With further understanding of a patient's genetic makeup, providers can potentially determine which opioid medications can provide optimal (or suboptimal) analgesic response in said patient. Several opioid medications that are commonly prescribed are under investigation for their effect on various patient populations. These include codeine, tramadol, hydrocodone, oxycodone, and methadone.

Therapeutic Applications

Codeine
Codeine is not nearly as potent as morphine since it is a pro-drug that undergoes O-demethylation by CYP2D6 to form the active metabolite of morphine. As such, codeine should not be prescribed to individuals that are considered CYP2D6 ultrarapid metabolizers, where higher levels of morphine would accumulate, contributing to higher toxicity risk. In contrast, codeine should also be avoided in CYP2D6 poor metabolizers where greatly reduced morphine formation leads to diminished analgesia. By understanding the phenotypic variation of CYP2D6 across different ethnicities, codeine therapy guidelines may be modified accordingly.

Tramadol
Tramadol is metabolized by CYP2D6 to form the active metabolite O-desmethyltramadol. In CYP2D6 ultrarapid metabolizers, higher levels of O-desmethyltramadol would accumulate, leading to increased toxicity risk. In contrast, CYP2D6 poor metabolizers would have diminished levels of the active metabolite and lead to diminished analgesia. In both these patient groups, a non-codeine opioid would be better suited for adequate and safer analgesia.

Hydrocodone
Hydrocodone undergoes metabolism via CYP3A4 and CYP2D6, the former producing the inactive metabolite norhydrocodone [29] and the latter producing its active metabolite of hydromorphone. Hydromorphone has significantly higher affinity toward mu-opioid receptors in comparison to hydrocodone [30]. Insufficient evidence is currently available to offer guidelines on managing hydrocodone in patients who may be CYP2D6 ultrarapid metabolizers or poor metabolizers.

Oxycodone
Oxycodone undergoes metabolism to water-soluble compounds via CYP3A-mediated N-demethylation and CYP2D6 O-demethylation; the former produces noroxycodone and the latter produces oxymorphone. Oxymorphone is responsible for the majority of oxycodone's analgesic effects [18, 31] as well as euphoria, sedation, and cough suppression [32]. However, due to its poor bioavailability at less than 10%, it is only 3 times more active than oral morphine.

Methadone
Methadone is metabolized by CYP3A4 to largely form the inactive metabolite ethylideine-1,5-dimethyl-3,3,-dipyhenylpyrrolidine (EDDP). It is also metabolized by CYP2D6 to lesser extent. This genotype does not significantly alter methadone adverse effects, opioid dose requirements, or analgesia.

Chronic pain is multifactorial and can vary across multiple dimensions. It is important to take into consideration social, demographic, clinical, psychological, biological, and lifestyle variations that vary between individuals. Pharmacogenetics has the potential to improve prescribing practices and optimize pain control in select patient populations. CYP2D6, OPRM1, and COMT are only a few of the many important genes that have been identified as influencing opioid analgesia and associated adverse events. Targeting these genes has the potential to yield promising results, but there is currently insufficient knowledge and understanding of their precise role in the pain pathway and opioid responsiveness. As more research and studies are conducted, the potential of pharmacogenetic testing may be better realized and contribute to the development of individualized guidelines for patients and personalized medicine [19, 28].

New Opioid Targets

Opioids continue to remain one of the most potent analgesics used for the management of severe pain conditions. However, there have been growing concerns in recent years as opioid use has escalated in the general population, contributing to opioid use disorders. Additionally, more evidence has indicated questionable long-term effectiveness of opioids in treating intractable pain. There is uncertainty about the frequency at which opioids should be prescribed and the associated severity of multiple poorly characterized adverse drug events (ADEs). There is a more urgent need for the development of safer opioid medications with less side effects. New approaches are being explored for development of safer prescription practices. These approaches include targeting specific opioid receptors in the periphery, biased ligand agonism, development of heteromers or multiligand receptor splice variants, degradation and synthesis of endogenous opioid peptides, and gene therapy.

As previously mentioned, the μ opioid receptor (MOR) is considered a key therapeutic target for clinically used opioids, including fentanyl, oxycodone, morphine, and methadone. Activation of MOR can substantially relieve severe pain in patients; however, there are also dose-limiting ADEs such as abuse liability, respiratory depression, constipation, itching, and physical dependence to take into consideration [33, 34]. These ADEs frequently compromise the therapeutic effects of opioids and in turn contribute to the development of opioid use disorders. Opioid use disorder and overdoses are considered an epidemic in North America. It is vital to develop novel and safe opioid medications that may produce potent analgesia in patients with serious medical conditions and simultaneously minimize unwanted ADEs. The aim of this narrative is to discuss novel opioid targets that may offer optimal therapeutic treatment of pain and reduce dependence/abuse.

Opioid Receptors

Several opioid receptors are responsible for physiologic responses when stimulated. They belong to the family of G protein-coupled receptors (GPCRs) and include the following subtypes: μ-opioid receptors (MORs), k-opioid receptor (KORs), and δ-opioid receptor (DORs). The MORs gather the most attention relatively, as their activation is responsible for both the therapeutic effects of opioids and the unwanted, adverse effects. But all of these opioid receptors are widely expressed in the central nervous system (CNS) and peripheral nervous system (PNS)—in addition to non-neuronal tissues—which also play a role in the mechanism of analgesia and propagation of side effects [35].

Activation of MORs is associated with respiratory depression, sedation, constipation, nausea, vomiting, analgesic tolerance, euphoria, depression, and withdrawal. Activation of KORs is associated with sedation, analgesic tolerance, diuresis, and central psychomimetic effects. Activation of DORs is associated with analgesic tolerance, aversion, dysphoria, and convulsions [35]. Activation of the nociceptin/orphanin FQ opioid peptide receptor (NOP) modulates the actions of the MORs associated with analgesia, tolerance, and reward.

Peripheral opioid agonists selectively activate opioid receptors outside of the CNS, thus avoiding all centrally mediated unwanted effects. They selectively target opioid peptide-containing cells that are prevalent at sites of inflammation or injury. The augmentation of opioid synthesis may also be possible via gene transfer. Such novel approaches have the ability to provide personalized pain treatment in patients [36].

Kappa opioid agonists can target receptors in the CNS and PNS. When peripheral KORs are targeted on visceral and somatic afferent nerves, lower abuse potential and less risk for physical dependence have been observed in addition to increased analgesia and antihyperalgesia. Unwanted centrally mediated KOR effects frequently mimic the effects of psychotomimetics. Peripherally restricted KOR agonists have been developed to target KORs located on visceral and somatic nerves to treat inflammatory visceral pain and chronic neuropathic pain. However, only a few pharmacologic agents are available that target KORs predominantly [37].

Biased Ligands

Opioid receptors are GPCRs that when activated, undergo conformational changes at the extracellular ligand-binding site to the intracellular end of the receptor, which leads to the coupling of intracellular G family proteins. The activated opioid receptors are phosphorylated by GPCR kinases, followed by the recruitment of multifunctional proteins referred to as β-arrestin (β-arr). Some ligands equally activate G protein and β-arr pathways, which can be referred to as "balanced" agonists. Other ligands preferentially activate more G protein or β-arr pathways—these ligands are considered "functionally selective" or "biased" agonists. These ligands can more precisely regulate biological functions of GPCRs, which has the potential to lead to further development of drugs with superior efficacy but reduced side effects. By stabilizing receptors in various active states, biased agonists can trigger preferred pathways via G protein-mediated or β-arr pathways. Designing biased ligands that elicit G protein activation without (or with minimal) β-arrestin-2 recruitment has the potential to provide efficient analgesia and avoid unwanted side effects such as respiratory depression, sedation, physical dependence, addiction, and tolerance [35, 38].

Current evidence supports that biased agonism exists for all three opioid receptors [38]. Oliceridine (TRV 130) is a G protein-biased μ-receptor agonist that was approved by the FDA in 2020, which simultaneously disfavors β-arrestin-2 signaling and is associated with less respiratory depression compared to nonbiased opioids (such as morphine) [39].

Heteromers, Bivalent, and Multifunctional Ligands

Heteromers, bivalent, and multifunctional ligands are composed of at least two functional receptor units and demonstrate different properties than the individual units. They may be non-selective and bind at two different targets. The goal of such compounds would be to promote profound analgesia with minimal to no side effects. For example, combined MOR agonist/DOR antagonist compounds specifically targeting said receptors would provide increased antinociception, reduced tolerance, decreased physical dependence, reduced respiratory depression, and decreased gastrointestinal inhibition [40].

Development of Dual Opioid Peptides Enkephalinase (DENk) Inhibitors

Dual enkephalinase (DENk) inhibitors have been shown to improve inflammatory-mediated, neuropathic-mediated, cancer-mediated, and postoperative pain. At higher doses, DENk inhibitors have been shown to have less side effects when compared to morphine (which include tolerance, withdrawal, reward, respiratory depression, and constipation). More data has yet to become available as clinical trials are currently underway [35].

Gene Therapy

Consideration should also be given to gene therapy and splicing as a mechanism to promote opioid targeting and further personalize pain treatment amongst patients. Introduction of DNA or mRNA encoding into a protein receptor could allow for manipulation of and long-term expression in the tissue. Alternative splicing of MOR coding exons is being evaluated and is leading to the discovery of multiple splice variants in humans. MOR splice variants may help explain the clinical variability of MOR agonist medications across a diverse patient population and provide further insight on the importance of individualizing pain therapies. The herpes simplex virus (HSV) has been explored and investigated as a vector in altering the endogenous genomes of nociceptors for genes of interest in neurons; they were shown to selectively and successfully knock down several proteins involved in various pain states [41]. Proinflammatory cytokines have been shown to play a role in the underlying mechanism of neuropathic pain and chronic opioid tolerance/withdrawal. Gene therapy strategies to enhance the expression of anti-inflammatory markers (such as IL-4, IL-10, or TNF) could be employed to reduce neuropathic pain and opioid tolerance/withdrawal [42].

Uncovering mechanisms that may enhance the availability of endogenous opioids within injured tissue, augment signal transduction of peripheral opioid receptors, and improve biased ligand agonism has the potential of opening exciting possibilities for pain therapy. Understanding these concepts further can contribute to the formulation of novel opioid drugs that are functionally selective between CNS and PNS. Identification of genetic differences in addition to genetic splicing also play a role in further individualizing pain therapy among patients. Going forward, a more detailed understanding of these concepts through clinical trials involving in vivo studies will be of crucial importance.

Prescribing Opioids Practices in Chronic Pain

Opioid use for pain has changed dramatically over the past several decades. While the pain-relieving properties of opium and its derivatives have been well described for millennia, the addictive potential has also been well established. Physicians trained during the 1970s and 1980s were commonly taught to avoid these medications for chronic non-cancer pain if possible and to use the lowest doses needed when required.

In 1995, Dr. James Campbell presented, in his presidential address to the American Pain Society (APS), the idea that pain should be evaluated as a vital sign. This, along with a misinterpreted "Letter to the Editor" in 1980 in the New England Journal of Medicine by Jane Porter and Dr. Hershel Jick allowed pharmaceutical companies to push the idea that pain should be aggressively treated and that development of addiction was rare in patients without a history of addiction [43]. The increased prescription patterns ushered in the opioid epidemic, which led to increased governmental regulation and guideline publications.

To battle addiction and the opioid epidemic, the Centers for Disease Control and Prevention (CDC) released guidelines for the prescription of opioids in 2016, updated in 2022 [44]. These updated guidelines recommend treating acute pain with 3 days or less of opioids, stating that rarely more than 7 days of treatment are necessary. From a chronic pain perspective, it also noted that nonpharmacologic and nonopioid pharmacologic therapy are preferred for chronic pain, and should opioids be necessary for chronic pain, short-acting agents are the preferred initial treatment as compared to long acting. A study by Shah et al. in 2017 noted that opioid-naïve and cancer-free patients, the highest probabilities of continued opioid use at 1 and 3 years, were those who were started on long-acting opioids, with those who were started on tramadol having the second highest probability [45]. It also found that the risk of chronic opioid use increases with each additional day of medication after the second day, and that the risk of chronic use doubles after a second prescription is given.

The CDC also recommends the use of prescription drug monitoring programs and drug testing for patients undergoing long-term opioid therapy [44]. The goal is for evaluation of other prescription medications that may interact with opioids, such as benzodiazepines and barbiturates, and also monitoring for potential divergence of opioids and concurrent use of illicit substances. While screening immunoassays are inexpensive, they tend to have low sensitivities and specificities, leading to inaccuracies [46, 47]. More accurate definitive tests are available (typically consisting of gas or liquid chromatography and mass spectroscopy), but are typically more costly [46]. Lack of the prescribed opioid in the urine may be an indicator that diversion has occurred, but discussion with the testing laboratory should occur for verification; the entire picture, including an individual's risk factors (such as history of substance abuse), should be evaluated in cases of abnormal results [46, 48].

However, there has been opposition to the CDC recommendations as well, with some arguing that there are unintended consequences of limiting or reducing opioids in many situations for patients who are already on chronic opioid therapy [49]. For example, dramatically reducing the amount of prescription opioids could precipitate withdrawal or worsen pain; this, in turn, may encourage patients to seek out other means of obtaining opioids, either legally from other providers or illegally obtaining either prescription or recreational opioids.

There also remains the overall question of effectiveness as a chronic long-term therapy; as implied by the CDC guidelines, opioids avoid much of the risk of tolerance and addiction if taken primarily for acute pain. The effectiveness of long-term opioid use for chronic non-cancer pain has not been well described. A study by Veiga et al. found in a 2-year prospective study that opioid users reported no improvement in pain symptoms, physical function, emotional function, or social disability, though there was patient-reported satisfaction with outcomes [50]. If opioids are prescribed to an individual, some organizations, such as the American Academy of Physical Medicine and Rehabilitation, suggest that the goal be weighted towards functional improvement over that of numerical pain relief, include multimodal pharmacotherapy, and utilize the lowest opioid dosage to achieve that goal [51].

For cancer pain, opioids are still commonly used as a primary therapy. Cancer pain itself is challenging to treat, with pain being significant in 75–90% of patients with advanced or terminal cancer [52]. The benefit of opioids from an analgesic perspective typically is seen to outweigh the risks of respiratory depression, addiction, tolerance, etc., for terminally ill patients with their shortened life expectancy. However, this treatment is not benign, and many patients expire due to the side effects of aggressive pain treatment during hospice and palliative care—an ethical principle known as the doctrine of double effect where treatment of pain is the primary motive rather than the death of a patient [53]. There is also the concern that opioids may increase tumor growth and angiogenesis and modulate the immune system, hastening the demise of a cancer patient [54]. While this concern should be explained to a patient, patient comfort often outweighs the impact on life expectancy in many cases.

Opioid Use Monitoring Techniques

The safe usage of opioid medications in chronic pain patients requires multiple forms of surveillance and monitoring. Pain medicine physicians will often treat patients with incurable conditions that may be managed with long-term opioid therapy. In the past few years, the most influential guideline regarding the use of opioids in the treatment of chronic pain patients was published by the Centers for Disease Control and Prevention (CDC) in 2016 and was updated in 2022 [44]. This document also provided specific recommendations for opioid use monitoring in patients.

Multiple clinically published guidelines recommend checking prescription drug monitoring programs (PDMPs) prior to initiation and during the treatment of patients with opioid therapy [55]. The 2016 CDC guidelines also advise that "clinicians should review the patient's history of controlled substance prescriptions using state prescription drug monitoring program (PDMP) data to determine whether the patient is receiving opioid dosages or dangerous combinations that put him or her at high risk for overdose [44]. Most patients treated for chronic pain will often have a complex medical history and typically have a medical care team that consists of various medical specialties. In our current environment of siloed health care in which physicians do not always communicate, the use of the PDMP is essential. The pain medicine physician will often be the prescriber of opioid medications and should have some form of a pain contract or an informed consent for opioid therapy with their patients. The pain medicine physician often plays a critical role in the early recognition and prevention of dangerous prescription drug combinations. In accordance with the CDC guidelines, "clinicians should review PDMP data when starting opioid therapy for chronic pain and periodically during opioid therapy for chronic pain, ranging from every prescription to every 3 months" [44].

The use of drug screens for monitoring opioid use in chronic pain patients is an important tool for clinicians. Drug screens should be used in the initial evaluation of patients for possible opioid treatment, continued monitoring of compliance, and documentation of possible aberrant drug behaviors. This task is usually completed using urine drug screens, but oral fluids may be screened also [56]. Immunoassays are the most common method for initial urine drug screening because of their low cost and quick results. These tests, however, can have cross-reactivity with other prescribed medications, causing false positives for illicit substances. False negatives may also occur if the concentration of the drug in the sample is below the assay's cutoff or if the sample is diluted or adulterated [57]. It is considered best practice to obtain a confirmatory test on any questionable sample using a more specific test such as gas chromatography mass spectrometry (GC-MS) or liquid chromatography [57].

The importance of the relationship between the pain medicine physician and the patient is often overlooked as a valuable component of opioid use monitoring in patients. Patients should be told why they are undergoing drug screening with opioid therapy to help improve compliance. A good physician-patient relationship can help navigate difficult scenarios, such as when a patient may have an abnormal drug screen result. A good relationship can encourage productive communication instead of immediate termination of an opioid treatment plan. Erroneous or premature discontinuation of an opioid treatment plan can increase a patient's risk of use of illicit opioids, leading to significant harm and possible development of opioid use disorder.

The CDC 2016 guidelines noted that "clinicians prescribing opioids to chronic pain patients should include strategies to mitigate risk, including considering offering naloxone when factors that increase risk for opioid overdose, such as history of overdose, history of substance use disorder, higher opioid dosages ($\geq$50 MME/day), or concurrent benzodiazepine use, are present" [44]. There can be significant overlap between patients with chronic pain and opioid use disorder. In addition to PDMP checks, drug screens, and pain contracts, some high-risk patients may benefit from periodic pill counts of their prescribed opioid medication.

Risk of Addiction in Chronic Opioid Therapy

Pain medicine physicians are justifiably concerned about the risk of their patients becoming addicted to opioid medications. First, it is important to differentiate physical dependence from opioid addiction. Physical dependence can be simply defined as the development of tolerance to a drug and the experience of a withdrawal syndrome in the absence of the drug [58]. The most useful definition of addiction in relation to opioid usage is provided by the DSM-V, which stratifies the severity of opioid use disorder (OUD) by symptoms. Opioid use disorder is defined by the number of symptoms in the categories of impaired control, social impairment, and risky use, in addition to having physical dependence. Unfortunately, the majority of patients who are treated with chronic opioid therapy will develop some level of physical dependence. A patient's physical dependence on an opioid medication alone is not sufficient for the diagnosis of opioid use disorder.

The most commonly associated risk factors for the development of OUD in patients treated for chronic pain include young age, smoking, poor social support, personal history of substance abuse, psychological stress, psychological trauma, psychological disease, psychotropic substance use, focus on opioids, preadolescent sexual abuse, history of legal problems, history of substance abuse treatment, craving for prescription drugs, mood swings, and childhood adversity [59, 60].

Prior to the initiation of chronic opioid therapy, it is important to identify patients most at risk for the development of OUD [28]. It is suggested that the highest risk of development of OUD is greatest when risk factors in the categories of psychosocial factors, drug-related factors, and genetic factors occur in the same patient. In the absence of psychosocial comorbidities and genetic predisposition, patients with chronic pain on a stable regimen of opioid medication in a monitored environment are not likely to develop OUD. It is known, however, that patients with a personal or family history of substance use disorder and psychosocial comorbidity are at higher risk of developing OUD, especially when not treated in a structured care setting [61].

Most patients treated for chronic pain have a complex medical history. It can be very challenging for a pain medicine physician to obtain a complete biopsychosocial history to screen for risk factors for addiction in a normal appointment time frame. The majority of pain medicine physicians will spend their allotted time with patients obtaining a focused history and physical to determine the etiology of their pain and to develop a multimodal treatment plan. It can be tremendously beneficial to use a validated screening tool to help with the risk assessment of patients being considered for opioid therapy in a limited amount of time.

There are several validated risk assessment tools that have been published to determine the probability that certain patients will develop non-adherence behaviors with prescribed opioid medication that could indicate possible OUD [62]. Prescreening tools that were developed to assess risk in patients being evaluated for the initiation of opioid therapy include the Opioid Risk Tool [60], Screener and Opioid Assessment for Patients with Pain [62], and the Diagnosis, Intractability, Risk, Efficacy [63, 64]. A common assessment tool designed to check for active signs of OUD in patients currently prescribed opioids is the Current Opioid Misuse Measure [65].

No single assessment tool will allow for complete accuracy in identifying patients who will develop opioid use disorder when prescribed opioid medications for chronic pain [66].

It is important for the pain medicine physician to evaluate the risks and benefits of opioid therapy in each patient using their best clinical judgment given their patient's unique clinical condition, along with currently accepted validated screening tools.

Addiction Treatments in Patients Suffering from Chronic Pain

Chronic pain patients with comorbid opioid use disorder (OUD) provide a unique challenge for pain medicine physicians. It is likely that treatment for opioid addiction can exclude these patients from obtaining opioids to manage their pain. It is important to maximize the usage of nonopioid medications and interventional pain medicine options in this patient population. There are currently three medications in the US approved for medication-assisted treatment (MAT) of OUD [67]. These medications are methadone, buprenorphine, and naltrexone.

Methadone

Methadone is considered the gold standard for treatment of OUD. Methadone is a full mu receptor opioid agonist that produces dose-dependent sedation, analgesia, and risk of respiratory depression that can lead to overdose. Methadone has a long yet variable half-life ranging from 13 to 30 hours. Methadone is known to prolong the QT interval in a dose-dependent fashion and can rarely lead to ventricular tachycardia torsades de point [68]. The risk of immediate patient harm with continued opioid addiction typically far outweighs the risk of side effects with methadone so that most patients start MAT for OUD without obtaining a baseline EKG. Methadone prevents withdrawal symptoms and reduces cravings in people addicted to opioids. It does not cause a euphoric feeling once patients become tolerant to its effects. It is important for the pain medicine physician to note that methadone can only be prescribed in specially regulated clinics when treating patients primarily for OUD. Most patients start with a single daily dose of 30 mg of methadone, which adequately prevents opioid withdrawal for 24 hours [67]. The dose of methadone is gradually increased by 5–10 mg increments over several days until a patient reaches a stable dose in which cravings and withdrawal symptoms are completely resolved. Most patients will require a dose of 60–100 mg of methadone to reach a stable dose that reduces the risk of relapse and promotes adherence to treatment [69]. Patients with chronic pain who have developed OUD without history of heroin use will often require a lower dose of methadone to reach a stable dose.

Buprenorphine

Buprenorphine is widely used to treat OUD in MAT treatment centers and in outpatient physician offices. Buprenorphine is a partial agonist at the mu opioid receptor with a high binding affinity [70]. Buprenorphine blocks the effects of other opioids, reduces or eliminates withdrawal symptoms, and reduces cravings. This medication is typically combined with naloxone for abuse deterrence. Buprenorphine also has the potential to prolong the QT interval, but EKGs are not routinely obtained in MAT treatment centers prior to initiation of therapy. Most patients start with an initial dose of 8 mg, which can prevent opioid withdrawal symptoms for opioid-dependent patients for 24 hours [71]. The dose of buprenorphine is gradually increased by 2–4 mg increments over several days until a stable dose that prevents withdrawals and cravings is reached. Chronic pain patients with OUD without history of heroin use will typically reach a stable dose at around 16 mg of buprenorphine daily [71]. Buprenorphine at higher doses is still far less effective than methadone at treating OUD patients with illicit heroin usage [67]. Buprenorphine is an excellent option to treat OUD patients without illicit heroin usage in the office setting and may allow for more comprehensive treatment of their pain.

Naltrexone

Naltrexone is less frequently used than both buprenorphine and methadone to treat OUD. Naltrexone is a mu-opioid receptor antagonist and blocks the effects of other opioids, preventing the feeling of euphoria. It is available from office-based providers in pill form or as a monthly injection. It can precipitate withdrawal if given to patients actively dependent on opioids. The initial dose of naltrexone is 25 mg orally once daily and is increased to 50 mg daily maintenance dose once the 25 mg dose is tolerated. It is difficult to induct patients on naltrexone because an abstinence period is required prior to starting treatment. This leads to poor compliance. Intramuscular naloxone is dosed at 380 mg once a month. Naltrexone is most effective clinically as an aid to sustaining abstinence and reducing risk of relapse in patients with OUD [72].

Pain medicine physicians will undoubtedly see chronic pain patients who develop OUD, and early referral to treatment programs or initiation of office-based MAT can be critical to saving a patient's life.

Summary

The use of opioids has incredible implications in both the chronic and acute pain settings, as highlighted in this chapter. It is imperative that attention be paid to the prescribing practices of opioids as this has enormous repercussions in the progression of addictive behaviors and opioid use disorders. Opioid care plans and monitoring should always be implemented in any long-term practice.

References[1]

1. McMahon S, Koltzenburg M. Preface. In: Wall and Melzack's textbook of pain. Published online 2014. p. 1184. https://doi.org/10.1016/b0-443-07287-6/50004-7.
2. *Pathan H, Williams J. Basic opioid pharmacology: an update. Br J Pain. 2012;6(1):11–6. https://doi.org/10.1177/2049463712438493.
3. Dhawan B, Cesselin F, Raghubir R, et al. International Union of Pharmacology. XII. Classification of opioid receptors. Pharmacol Rev. 1996;48(4).
4. Butour JL, Moisand C, Mazarguil H, Mollereau C, Meunier JC. Recognition and activation of the opioid receptor-like ORL1 receptor by nociceptin, nociceptin analogs and opioids. Eur J Pharmacol. 1997;321(1):97–103. https://doi.org/10.1016/S0014-2999(96)00919-3.
5. Calo' G, Guerrini R, Rizzi A, Salvadori S, Regoli D. Pharmacology of nociceptin and its receptor: a novel therapeutic target. Br J Pharmacol. 2000;129(7):1261–83. https://doi.org/10.1038/sj.bjp.0703219.
6. *Trescot AM. Opioid pharmacology and pharmacokinetics. In: Controlled substance management in chronic pain. Published online 2016. p. 45–62. https://doi.org/10.1007/978-3-319-30964-4_4.
7. Dhaliwal A, Gupta M. Physiology, opioid receptor. In: StatPearls. StatPearls Publishing; 2023. http://www.ncbi.nlm.nih.gov/books/NBK546642/. Accessed 12 Jan 2024.
8. Toubia T, Khalife T. The endogenous opioid system: role and dysfunction caused by opioid therapy. Clin Obstet Gynecol. 2019;62(1):3–10. https://doi.org/10.1097/GRF.0000000000000409.
9. *Zhou J, Ma R, Jin Y, et al. Molecular mechanisms of opioid tolerance: from opioid receptors to inflammatory mediators (Review). Exp Ther Med. 2021;22(3):1004. https://doi.org/10.3892/etm.2021.10437.
10. Besse D, Lombard MC, Zajac JM, Roques BP, Besson JM. Pre- and postsynaptic distribution of μ, δ and κ opioid receptors in the superficial layers of the cervical dorsal horn of the rat spinal cord. Brain Res. 1990;521(1–2):15–22. https://doi.org/10.1016/0006-8993(90)91519-m.

---

[1] (*) denotes essential references for additional reading.

11. Edinoff AN, Kaplan LA, Khan S, et al. Full opioid agonists and tramadol: pharmacological and clinical considerations. Anesth Pain Med. 2021;11(4):e119156. https://doi.org/10.5812/aapm.119156.

12. Rosenblum A, Marsch LA, Joseph H, Portenoy RK. Opioids and the treatment of chronic pain: controversies, current status, and future directions. Exp Clin Psychopharmacol. 2008;16(5):405–16. https://doi.org/10.1037/a0013628.

13. CDC grand rounds: prescription drug overdoses — a U.S. epidemic. https://www.cdc.gov/mmwr/preview/mmwrhtml/mm6101a3.htm. Accessed 28 Jan 2024.

14. Angst MS, Lazzeroni LC, Phillips NG, et al. Aversive and reinforcing opioid effects: a pharmacogenomic twin study. Anesthesiology. 2012;117(1):22–37. https://doi.org/10.1097/ALN.0b013e31825a2a4e.

15. Smith H. Variations in opioid responsiveness. Pain Phys. 2008;11(2):237–48. https://doi.org/10.36076/ppj.2008/11/237.

16. Singh A, Zai C, Mohiuddin AG, Kennedy JL. The pharmacogenetics of opioid treatment for pain management. J Psychopharmacol. 2020;34(11):1200–9. https://doi.org/10.1177/0269881120944162.

17. Trescot AM. Genetics and implications in perioperative analgesia. Best Pract Res Clin Anaesthesiol. 2014;28(2):153–66. https://doi.org/10.1016/j.bpa.2014.03.004.

18. Crews KR, Monte AA, Huddart R, Caudle KE, Kharasch ED, Gaedigk A, Dunnenberger HM, Leeder JS, Callaghan JT, Samer CF, Klein TE. Clinical pharmacogenetics implementation consortium guideline for CYP2D6, OPRM1, and COMT genotypes and select opioid therapy. Clin Pharmacol Ther. 2021;110(4):888–96.

19. Diatchenko L, Slade GD, Nackley AG, et al. Genetic basis for individual variations in pain perception and the development of a chronic pain condition. Hum Mol Genet. 2005;14(1):135–43. https://doi.org/10.1093/hmg/ddi013.

20. Zubieta JK, Smith YR, Bueller JA, et al. Regional mu opioid receptor regulation of sensory and affective dimensions of pain. Science. 2001;293(5528):311–5. https://doi.org/10.1126/science.1060952.

21. Nackley AG, Tan KS, Fecho K, Flood P, Diatchenko L, Maixner W. Catechol-O-methyltransferase inhibition increases pain sensitivity through activation of both beta2- and beta3-adrenergic receptors. Pain. 2007;128(3):199–208. https://doi.org/10.1016/j.pain.2006.09.022.

22. Reyes-Gibby CC, Shete S, Rakvåg T, et al. Exploring joint effects of genes and the clinical efficacy of morphine for cancer pain: OPRM1 and COMT gene. Pain. 2007;130(1–2):25–30. https://doi.org/10.1016/j.pain.2006.10.023.

23. Kreek MJ, Levran O, Reed B, Schlussman SD, Zhou Y, Butelman ER. Opiate addiction and cocaine addiction: underlying molecular neurobiology and genetics. J Clin Invest. 2012;122(10):3387–93. https://doi.org/10.1172/JCI60390.

24. Chen YT, Tsou HH, Kuo HW, et al. OPRM1 genetic polymorphisms are associated with the plasma nicotine metabolite cotinine concentration in methadone maintenance patients: a cross sectional study. J Hum Genet. 2013;58(2):84–90. https://doi.org/10.1038/jhg.2012.139.

25. Kreek MJ. Methadone-related opioid agonist pharmacotherapy for heroin addiction. History, recent molecular and neurochemical research and future in mainstream medicine. Ann N Y Acad Sci. 2000;909:186–216. https://doi.org/10.1111/j.1749-6632.2000.tb06683.x.

26. Kanbayashi Y, Hosokawa T, Okamoto K, et al. Factors predicting requirement of high-dose transdermal fentanyl in opioid switching from oral morphine or oxycodone in patients with cancer pain. Clin J Pain. 2011;27(8):664–7. https://doi.org/10.1097/AJP.0b013e3182168fed.

27. Li MH, Yeh ET, Huang SC, Wang HM, Su WR, Lai YL. Clinical experience with strong opioids in pain control of terminally ill cancer patients in palliative care settings in Taiwan. J Exp Clin Med. 2010;2(6):292–6. https://doi.org/10.1016/j.jecm.2010.10.004.

28. Kaye AD, Garcia AJ, Hall OM, et al. Update on the pharmacogenomics of pain management. Pharmgenomics Pers Med. 2019;12:125–43. https://doi.org/10.2147/PGPM.S179152.

29. Hutchinson MR, Menelaou A, Foster DJR, Coller JK, Somogyi AA. CYP2D6 and CYP3A4 involvement in the primary oxidative metabolism of hydrocodone by human liver microsomes. Br J Clin Pharmacol. 2004;57(3):287–97. https://doi.org/10.1046/j.1365-2125.2003.02002.x.
30. Smith HS. Opioid metabolism. Mayo Clin Proc. 2009;84(7):613–24.
31. Trescot AM, Datta S, Lee M, Hansen H. Opioid pharmacology. Pain Physician. 2008;11(2 Suppl):S133–53.
32. Kapur BM, Lala PK, Shaw JLV. Pharmacogenetics of chronic pain management. Clin Biochem. 2014;47(13–14):1169–87. https://doi.org/10.1016/j.clinbiochem.2014.05.065.
33. Ferrari A, Coccia CPR, Bertolini A, Sternieri E. Methadone – metabolism, pharmacokinetics and interactions. Pharmacol Res. 2004;50(6):551–9. https://doi.org/10.1016/j.phrs.2004.05.002.
34. Günther T, Dasgupta P, Mann A, et al. Targeting multiple opioid receptors – improved analgesics with reduced side effects? Br J Pharmacol. 2018;175(14):2857–68. https://doi.org/10.1111/bph.13809.
35. Machelska H, Celik MÖ. Advances in achieving opioid analgesia without side effects. Front Pharmacol. 2018;9:1388. https://doi.org/10.3389/fphar.2018.01388.
36. Arendt-Nielsen L, Olesen AE, Staahl C, et al. Analgesic efficacy of peripheral kappa-opioid receptor agonist CR665 compared to oxycodone in a multi-modal, multi-tissue experimental human pain model: selective effect on visceral pain. Anesthesiology. 2009;111(3):616–24. https://doi.org/10.1097/ALN.0b013e3181af6356.
37. Vanderah TW. Delta and kappa opioid receptors as suitable drug targets for pain. Clin J Pain. 2010;26(Suppl 10):S10–5. https://doi.org/10.1097/AJP.0b013e3181c49e3a.
38. Mafi A, Kim SK, Goddard WA 3rd. Mechanism of β-arrestin recruitment by the μ-opioid G protein-coupled receptor. Proc Natl Acad Sci USA. 2020;117(28):16346–55.
39. Simons P, van der Schrier R, van Lemmen M, et al. Respiratory effects of biased ligand oliceridine in older volunteers: a pharmacokinetic-pharmacodynamic comparison with morphine. Anesthesiology. 2023;138(3):249–63. https://doi.org/10.1097/ALN.0000000000004473.
40. Azzam AAH, McDonald J, Lambert DG. Hot topics in opioid pharmacology: mixed and biased opioids. Br J Anaesth. 2019;122(6):e136–45. https://doi.org/10.1016/j.bja.2019.03.006.
41. Goswami R, Subramanian G, Silayeva L, et al. Gene therapy leaves a vicious cycle. Front Oncol. 2019;9:297. https://doi.org/10.3389/fonc.2019.00297.
42. Guedon JMG, Wu S, Zheng X, et al. Current gene therapy using viral vectors for chronic pain. Mol Pain. 2015;11:27. https://doi.org/10.1186/s12990-015-0018-1.
43. Porter J, Jick H. Addiction rare in patients treated with narcotics. N Engl J Med. 1980;302(2):123. https://doi.org/10.1056/nejm198001103020221.
44. *Dowell D, Ragan KR, Jones CM, Baldwin GT, Chou R. CDC clinical practice guideline for prescribing opioids for pain – United States, 2022. MMWR Recomm Rep. 2022;71(3):1–95. https://doi.org/10.15585/mmwr.rr7103a1.
45. Shah A, Hayes CJ, Martin BC. Characteristics of initial prescription episodes and likelihood of long-term opioid use – United States, 2006–2015. MMWR Morb Mortal Wkly Rep. 2017;66(10):265–9. https://doi.org/10.15585/mmwr.mm6610a1.
46. Argoff CE, Alford DP, Fudin J, et al. Rational urine drug monitoring in patients receiving opioids for chronic pain: consensus recommendations. Pain Med. 2018;19(1):97–117. https://doi.org/10.1093/pm/pnx285.
47. Kirsh KL, Heit HA, Huskey A, Strickland J, City KE, Passik SD. Trends in drug use from urine drug testing of addiction treatment clients. J Opioid Manag. 2015;11(1). https://doi.org/10.5055/jom.2015.0253.
48. Mahajan G. Role of urine drug testing in the current opioid epidemic. Anesth Analg. 2017;125(6):2094–104. https://doi.org/10.1213/ANE.0000000000002565.
49. Kroenke K, Alford DP, Argoff C, et al. Challenges with implementing the Centers for Disease Control and Prevention opioid guideline: a consensus panel report. Pain Med. 2019;20(4):724–35. https://doi.org/10.1093/pm/pny307.
50. Veiga DR, Monteiro-Soares M, Mendonça L, Sampaio R, Castro-Lopes JM, Azevedo LF. Effectiveness of opioids for chronic noncancer pain: a two-year multicenter,

prospective cohort study with propensity score matching. J Pain. 2019;20(6):706–15. https://doi.org/10.1016/j.jpain.2018.12.007.

51. Shaw E, Braza DW, Cheng DS, et al. American Academy of Physical Medicine and Rehabilitation position statement on opioid prescribing. PM&R. 2018;10(6):681–3. https://doi.org/10.1016/j.pmrj.2018.05.004.

52. Fischer DJ, Villines D, Kim YO, Epstein JB, Wilkie DJ. Anxiety, depression, and pain: differences by primary cancer. Support Care Cancer. 2010;18(7):801–10. https://doi.org/10.1007/s00520-009-0712-5.

53. Chessa F, Moreno F. Ethical and legal considerations in end-of-life care. Prim Care. 2019;46(3):387–98. https://doi.org/10.1016/j.pop.2019.05.005.

54. Maher DP, Walia D, Heller NM. Suppression of human natural killer cells by different classes of opioids. Anesth Analg. 2019;128(5):1013–21. https://doi.org/10.1213/ANE.0000000000004058.

55. Herzig SJ, Calcaterra SL, Mosher HJ, et al. Safe opioid prescribing for acute noncancer pain in hospitalized adults: a systematic review of existing guidelines. J Hosp Med. 2018;13(4):256–62. https://doi.org/10.12788/jhm.2979.

56. Kwong TC, Magnani B, Moore C. Urine and oral fluid drug testing in support of pain management. Crit Rev Clin Lab Sci. 2017;54(6):433–45. https://doi.org/10.1080/10408363.2017.1385053.

57. Herring C, Muzyk AJ, Johnston C. Interferences with urine drug screens. J Pharm Pract. 2011;24(1):102–8. https://doi.org/10.1177/0897190010380463.

58. Savage SR, Joranson DE, Covington EC, Schnoll SH, Heit HA, Gilson AM. Definitions related to the medical use of opioids: evolution towards universal agreement. J Pain Symptom Manag. 2003;26(1):655–67. https://doi.org/10.1016/s0885-3924(03)00219-7.

59. Fleming MF, Balousek SL, Klessig CL, Mundt MP, Brown DD. Substance use disorders in a primary care sample receiving daily opioid therapy. J Pain. 2007;8(7):573–82. https://doi.org/10.1016/j.jpain.2007.02.432.

60. Webster LR. Risk factors for opioid-use disorder and overdose. Anesth Analg. 2017;125(5):1741–8. https://doi.org/10.1213/ANE.0000000000002496.

61. Ballantyne JC. Opioid analgesia: perspectives on right use and utility. Pain Physician. 2007;10(3):479–91.

62. Webster LR, Webster RM. Predicting aberrant behaviors in opioid-treated patients: preliminary validation of the Opioid Risk Tool. Pain Med. 2005;6(6):432–42. https://doi.org/10.1111/j.1526-4637.2005.00072.x.

63. Belgrade MJ, Schamber CD, Lindgren BR. The DIRE score: predicting outcomes of opioid prescribing for chronic pain. J Pain. 2006;7(9):671–81. https://doi.org/10.1016/j.jpain.2006.03.001.

64. Butler SF, Budman SH, Fernandez K, Jamison RN. Validation of a screener and opioid assessment measure for patients with chronic pain. Pain. 2004;112(1–2):65–75. https://doi.org/10.1016/j.pain.2004.07.026.

65. Butler SF, Budman SH, Fernandez KC, et al. Development and validation of the current opioid misuse measure. Pain. 2007;130(1–2):144–56. https://doi.org/10.1016/j.pain.2007.01.014.

66. Cheatle MD, Compton PA, Dhingra L, Wasser TE, O'Brien CP. Development of the revised opioid risk tool to predict opioid use disorder in patients with chronic nonmalignant pain. J Pain. 2019;20(7):842–51. https://doi.org/10.1016/j.jpain.2019.01.011.

67. *Bell J, Strang J. Medication treatment of opioid use disorder. Biol Psychiatry. 2020;87(1):82–8. https://doi.org/10.1016/j.biopsych.2019.06.020.

68. Krantz MJ, Lewkowiez L, Hays H, Woodroffe MA, Robertson AD, Mehler PS. Torsade de pointes associated with very-high-dose methadone. Ann Intern Med. 2002;137(6):501–4. https://doi.org/10.7326/0003-4819-137-6-200209170-00010.

69. Faggiano F, Vigna-Taglianti F, Versino E, Lemma P. Methadone maintenance at different dosages for opioid dependence. Cochrane Database Syst Rev. 2003;(3):CD002208. https://doi.org/10.1002/14651858.CD002208.

70. Chen KY, Chen L, Mao J. Buprenorphine-naloxone therapy in pain management. Anesthesiology. 2014;120(5):1262–74. https://doi.org/10.1097/ALN.0000000000000170.
71. Kuhlman JJ, Levine B, Johnson RE, Fudala PJ, Cone EJ. Relationship of plasma buprenorphine and norbuprenorphine to withdrawal symptoms during dose induction, maintenance and withdrawal from sublingual buprenorphine. Addiction. 1998;93(4):549–59. https://doi.org/10.1046/j.1360-0443.1998.93454910.x.
72. Tucker K, Thamizan AJR. Naltrexone in the treatment of heroin dependence: a literature review. Drug Alcohol Rev. 2000;19(1):73–82. https://doi.org/10.1080/09595230096174.

Educational Guidelines for Multidisciplinary Pain Medicine Fellowship: Cancer Pain, Procedural and Surgical Interventions for Chronic and Cancer Pain, Practice Management, Legal and Research Matters

Cancer Pain and Supportive Care: Assessment, Evaluation, and Treatment

7

Gina Votta-Velis, Bhuvaneswari Sandeep Ram,
Nancy Beckman, Monica Malec, Ariana Nelson,
Joshua Russell, Vasyl Hereha, Amy Siston,
Adaobi Tochukwu Ibe, Tian Yu, and Magdalena Anitescu

Abbreviations

CBT	Cognitive behavioral therapy
CIPN	Chemotherapy induced peripheral neuropathy
EMLA	Eutectic mixture of lidocaine and prilocaine
HFS	Hand foot syndrome
IrAE	Immunotherapy related adverse events
ORN	Osteoradionecrosis
PMPS	Post mastectomy pain syndrome

G. Votta-Velis
Department of Anesthesiology, University of Illinois at Chicago College of Medicine, Chicago, IL, USA

B. S. Ram (✉) · N. Beckman · M. Malec · V. Hereha · A. Siston · A. T. Ibe
University of Chicago, Chicago, IL, USA
e-mail: bsandeep@bsd.uchicago.edu; nbeckman1@uchicagomedicine.org; mmalec@bsd.uchicago.edu; cwy6966@bsd.uchicago.edu; asiston@bsd.uchicago.edu; tochukwu.ibe@uchicagomedicine.org

T. Yu
Department of Anesthesia & Critical Care, University of Chicago Medicine, Chicago, IL, USA
e-mail: tian.yu@uchicagomedicine.org

A. Nelson
Department of Anesthesiology, University of California, Irvine, CA, USA
e-mail: arianamn@hs.uci.edu

J. Russell
Kaiser Permanente, Renton, WA, USA

M. Anitescu
Department of Anesthesia & Critical Care, University of Chicago Medicine, Chicago, IL, USA
e-mail: manitescu@bsd.uchicago.edu

RIBP　　　Radiation induced brachial plexopathy
SBRT　　　Stereotactic body radiation therapy
SNM　　　Sacral neuromodulation

Introduction: Definition of Cancer Pain

Tochukwu Ibe and Bhuvaneswari Sandeep Ram

Cancer-related pain is a significant and pervasive issue affecting a large proportion of cancer patients. While current literature suggests that the prevalence and severity of cancer pain have declined over the years, approximately 44% of cancer patients still experience pain at some point during their disease trajectory, with higher rates in advanced stages [1]. Cancer pain can arise from the tumor itself, treatment-related interventions, or secondary conditions unrelated to the neoplasm. The complex and multifaceted nature of cancer pain makes it challenging to manage effectively, requiring a multidimensional approach that addresses both physical and psychosocial aspects.

Cancer pain is unique in that it may be related to the specific pathophysiology of the tumor, anatomical location of the tumor, or the treatment of the tumor. As a result, cancer pain is diverse and can be broadly classified into *nociceptive pain* (somatic or visceral), *neuropathic pain, or even mixed in nature*. Given this complexity, understanding the pathophysiology of cancer pain is critical, as it directly influences the expected outcome and intensity of pain and guides more targeted management and as a result can improve patient satisfaction and treatment adherence [2].

Beyond the physical dimensions, cancer pain has a profound impact on psychological well-being. Psychological factors such as depression, anxiety, and emotional distress are strongly associated with cancer pain during diagnosis, treatment, and survivorship [3]. Some survivors are able to overcome these psychological challenges, particularly with adequate pain management, while others continue to struggle with emotional adjustment during and after treatment. For this reason, the interplay between physical pain and psychological distress highlights the importance of integrating mental health support into the overall pain management strategy to help patients improve their quality of life [4].

The approach to cancer pain management continues to evolve as new therapies and insights into pain mechanisms emerge. Advancements in pharmacology, including the development of targeted therapies for neuropathic pain, and in interventional procedures, offer new avenues for relieving cancer-related pain while minimizing adverse effects. Despite these advancements, cancer pain management remains multifaceted and requires an individualized, multimodal approach incorporating pharmacological treatments, psychological support, and interventional therapies. A comprehensive understanding of the various dimensions of cancer pain is essential for improving patient outcomes, enhancing quality of life, and alleviating the suffering associated with this debilitating symptom.

Types of Cancer Pain

Ariana Nelson and Josh Russell

Cancer Related

Pain that is directly related to the neoplasm can be distinctly identified as somatic, visceral, and/or neuropathic, but the impact on the patient may be experienced in an array of dimensions. Cancer-related pain may be anatomically or physiologically mediated but also affects other dimensions [5]. The organic etiology of pain often occurs because the neoplasm has invaded or affected pain-sensitive tissues, but the process of experiencing cancer-pain often increases likelihood of depression or anxiety (the affective dimension) and interferes with mental processing (cognitive dimension). These factors result in changes to the patient's behavior and are all influenced by the sociocultural dimensions of the patient's experience, which has long been identified as a dimension neglected by clinicians [6].

Treatment Related

Cancer treatments cause pain symptoms and other adverse effects such as nausea, anorexia, hair loss, and fatigue. Treatments that most often result in these symptoms include radiotherapy, chemotherapy, hormonal therapy, and procedural interventions such as surgical excision of primary or metastatic cancerous lesions [7]. Addressing the side effects of treatment-related pain is paramount as the resultant reduction in quality of life for the patient can reduce patient adherence to these treatments, with potential impact on survival [8].

Independent of Cancer

Although pain is often the presenting symptom of cancer, in approximately 10% of patients, the pain is ultimately found to be unrelated to the disease process. After treatment of the incidentally discovered neoplasm, patients may continue to have the initial pain, which is most often caused by muscles and connective tissues [9]. Breakthrough pain that is not adequately controlled by the treatments that at baseline have controlled a patient's background pain can be more severe in those patients with other non-cancer related pains. This type of severe pain is more common in the cancer patient population with the following attributes: English speaking country of origin, presence of more than one pain generator, co-existing plexopathy, or co-existing spinal pain syndrome [10].

Chronic Pain After the Cure of the Disease

Immediately following treatment, most cancer survivors experience a degree of pain, but this is reduced over time. However, 5–10% of cancer survivors experience levels of pain that interfere with function in the long-term, a rate that is even higher in certain sub-populations [11]. In breast cancer survivors, the rate of chronic pain is 19–41% and 27% in colorectal cancer survivors [12].

In patients with non-terminal cancer or a prognosis longer than 6 months, the pain specialist should adhere to the principles of the World Health Organization's "analgesic ladder" and utilize non-opioid options and multimodal analgesia before initiating opioid therapy [13]. In patients with longer prognoses, it is important to regularly assess for signs of substance misuse or opioid use disorder and wean opioids if there is disease response or remission [14]. While opioids are the mainstay of therapy among analgesic options for patients with cancer-related pain, it is still worthwhile to consider the type of pain (i.e., neuropathic vs. visceral vs. somatic) and tailor the choice of agents accordingly. While opioids are most effective for somatic pain related to cancer, adjuvant medications (e.g., gabapentinoids) are indicated for neuropathic pain related to cancer or chemotherapy induced neuropathy and have a more desirable side effect profile [15, 16]. Visceral pain is also exceptionally difficult to control with opioids alone, while adjuvant medications (e.g. corticosteroids, antispasmodics) and procedural approaches, such as celiac plexus neurolysis, often provide superior palliation of symptoms while limiting adverse effects of high-dose opioids [17].

Evaluation of Patient with Cancer Pain

Functional Assessment

Bhuvaneswari Sandeep Ram

Assessment of functional status is an integral factor in oncological assessment. Functional impairment directly correlates with pain, complications with cancer treatments and survival.

It is imperative to delineate patients ADLs (bathing, self-transferring, eating, etc.) and instrumental ADLs (driving, buying groceries). Functional decline can occur with the disease process and treatment-related side effects. Functional resilience (ability to recover functional status back to baseline) has also been studied.

Functional assessment tools can be either self-reported (patient or caregiver) or healthcare provider-based objective assessment.

- Self-Reported Measurements include ADL (Katz index), IADL (Lawton scale), Barthel index (any version), and Patient-Reported Outcomes Measurement Information System (PROMIS)—global to name a few.
- Performance Measurements include Timed Up and Go test, Hand grip strength, Short Physical Performance Battery, Gait speed, gait assessment, Chair stand test, and 6-minute walk.

- Pain disability index is used as a tool to evaluate pain in patients with malignancy. FACT-G is a self-reported tool which is used to assess healthcare related QOL [18] and ECOG PS (Eastern Cooperative Oncology Group (ECOG) Performance Status (PS) scale) is used to assess functional status and ability to tolerate treatment.

Prehabilitation is initiation of functional improvement and targeted exercise therapy at the time of diagnosis, typically prior to surgery and is known to prevent the impact of treatment and improve functional recovery. Patients with breast, colorectal, and lung cancer showed shorter LOS and improved functional status after surgical treatment when they were assigned to Prehabilitation programs [19]. Prehabilitation can likely treat functional decline if it occurs.

Psychiatric Evaluation of Patients with Cancer Pain

Nancy Beckman and Amy Siston

Pain is a common side effect of cancer and its treatment and often most distressing to patients [20]. Multiple biological, psychological, and social variables contribute to the development and maintenance of cancer pain. Inadequate pain control leads to increased anxiety, depression, hopelessness, other affective distress, e.g., anger, frustration [3, 21, 22], and in some cases wish for death and suicide. For many patients, pain represents progression of disease [3, 23, 24] and causes fear of increased dependence or disability, or fear of a painful death [25]. Quality of social support may also impact pain, distress, and disability. To better understand psychological and social variables, initial evaluation should include assessment of (1) affective distress; (2) pain severity, coping, and functional impact; (3) behavioral observation; and (4) type of social support.

Affective Distress
Evaluation of affective distress can be obtained through clinical interview of symptoms or standardized assessment, such as with the Patient Health Questionnaire [26] which screens for symptoms of depression and includes a question about suicidal thoughts and the Generalized Anxiety Disorder scale [27] which screens for anxiety. Screening can help pain providers quickly identify patients at risk of having a comorbid psychiatric disorder or suicidal thoughts and appropriately manage and/or triage to a mental health specialist. It is important to identify and treat comorbid psychiatric disorders because they are associated with more pain and disability, poorer treatment response, greater complications, and lower quality of life [28, 29].

Pain
Evaluation of pain can be obtained by patient report and history during initial clinical and/or follow-up appointments. A brief screening instrument (e.g., Pain, Enjoyment, General Activity scale (PEG-3) [30], or the Distress Thermometer and Problem List (DT & PL) [31]) can facilitate discussion of the presence and impact of pain. Additional questions—i.e., "What does the patient think the pain signifies?" or "How much control does the patient think they have?"—may lead to greater

understanding of a patient's pain perception and adjustment [32]. Research suggests that patients who report benign causes to new or increased pain have reported less adjustment issues than patients who perceive their pain as an indicator of disease progression [3]. Patients who report that pain is unrelenting and overwhelming, who feel helpless in the face of it, and cannot stop thinking about it also tend to report higher pain and disability [22]. When assessing pain, it is helpful to set SMART specific, measurable, achievable realistic, and time-limited functional goals (e.g., walk for 15 minutes) to measure progress.

Behavioral Observation

The clinician should be sensitive to behaviors that signify non-disclosure of pain, non-adaptive coping, or underlying affective distress. Facial grimacing, guarding, rocking or fidgeting, moaning, and/or tearfulness may all be indictors of persistent pain and accompanied distress that is not being disclosed. Assessment, which may include identifying behaviors as typical of persistent pain, should be undertaken, discussed, and appropriately managed.

Social Support

Caregiver response may also influence a patient's perception and adjustment to pain. For example, caregivers may respond to a patient's pain by being dismissive, overwhelmed themselves, or overly solicitous, e.g., taking over patient roles, which in turn may inadvertently reinforce pain-related distress and disability [22]. On the other hand, caregiver support is vital in helping patients adapt to their illness. The clinician can best understand the role of family/caregiver support through clinical interview and when appropriate directly asking the family/caregiver to describe how they respond to the patient's pain. Caregivers should be included in pain education and psychosocial interventions to minimize caregiver strain and optimize the benefit of social support on the patient's pain management and functioning [33].

Effects of Cancer Treatments on Pain Progression

Monica Malec and Vasyl Herera

Chemotherapy-Associated Pain Syndromes

Chemotherapeutic agents may result in pain progression through administration-related complications or in relation to the cytotoxic side effects of the agents.

Chemotherapy Infusion-Related Pain (e.g., Extravasation)

Chemotherapy extravasation remains a concerning administration complication, which can result in burning pain, induration, erythema, and more grievously—necrosis of the subcutaneous tissues or even more superficial structures. Although most chemotherapeutic agents have the potential to cause some degree of detriment related to extravasation, agents can be further classified based on their vesicant potential—or the ability to cause severe tissue blistering and necrosis. Management includes immediate cessation of the infusion and may include attempts at aspirating the extravasated contents [34].

Cytotoxicity-Related Pain
(i) Chemotherapy-Induced Peripheral Neuropathy (CIPN)

Chemotherapy-induced peripheral neuropathy (CIPN) is a common cytotoxic complication of chemotherapy on the peripheral nervous system, which results in sensory-predominant deficits and pain, and may lead to chronic neuropathy. Certain chemotherapeutic agents—platinum agents, vinca alkaloids, and taxanes—are well-established in causing CIPN, although other agents have been implicated. CIPN typically develops within 2 months of initiating chemotherapy and develops in a dose-dependent fashion. If identified, it usually leads to treatment dose reduction or discontinuation. A comprehensive review by Staff et al. (2017) describes well-established causative agents, presentation, differential diagnosis, prevention, and treatment [35].

Use of duloxetine for CIPN (related to platinum and taxane chemotherapy) has been evidenced to improve function and pain-related quality-of-life scores in a randomized controlled Phase 3 clinical trial [36]. Other neuropathic-pain medications (e.g., gabapentin, tricyclics) are used off-label [35].

(ii) Hand-Foot Syndrome and Nail-Changes

Hand-foot syndrome (HFS), also known as palmoplantar erythrodysesthesia, can likewise present as neuropathic pain but is distinguishable from CIPN by dermatologic findings from direct capillary microtrauma of cancer treatments. Skin lesions usually manifest as painful and well-demarcated erythematous plaques. The most common causative chemotherapeutic agents include pegylated liposomal doxorubicin, capecitabine, and 5-fluorouracil, while a similar skin reaction has been noted with multikinase inhibitors [37]. Dose reduction and treatment interruption or discontinuation are the only reliable management options, with treatment discontinuation typically leading to lesion resolution and skin regeneration in 1–2 weeks. Supportive therapy such as cold compresses and wound care may be utilized for pain management [38].

Radiation Therapy-Radiation Therapy-Associated Pain Syndromes

Radiation therapy or radiotherapy (RT) is a mainstay of cancer treatment for the majority of cancer patients but may be associated with unintended radiation-induced DNA damage to non-cancerous tissue. This may occur via direct irradiation or the bystander effect—the concept that irradiated cells release radical oxygen species, which will alter the metabolic activities and cell signaling pathways of neighboring cells [39]. RT can lead to multiple pain syndromes depending on the adjacent healthy tissue that sustained DNA damage. The following narrative will touch upon some radiation-induced pain syndromes but is not exhaustive and does not include important entities like radiation-induced dermatitis, lymphedema, cystitis, and others. For further reading, please see a review on radiation therapy-associated toxicities by Wang et al. (2021) [40].

Chest Wall Pain and Fractures

Radiation-induced chest wall pain may be a late complication of stereotactic body radiotherapy (SBRT) for inoperable neoplastic lesions. Toxicity typically occurs at a median of 6–9 months after SBRT [41, 42] and may include pain and rib fractures with varying grades of severity [43]. The severity of chest wall toxicity has been linked with the irradiated volume to radiation dose relationship [41–43], which may be considered for treatment planning purposes. If pain develops, it may be focal or neuropathic in nature [41]. Moderate pain may be targeted with acetaminophen or anti-inflammatory medications, while severe pain may require opioid medications or nerve block interventions [44].

Pelvic Fractures

Use of external-beam RT may contribute to incidence of symptomatic insufficiency pelvic fractures in patients receiving RT for gynecologic malignancies, with a calculated incidence of 13% in one study [45]. This study also noted that most patients showed good symptomatic response to bedrest and analgesics.

Bone Pain Flares

RT is used for the treatment of painful bone metastases but may precipitate acute pain flares as treatment is initiated. These flares are likely due to local release of cytokines, rather than the direct effect of RT, and therefore, dexamethasone has been demonstrated as an appropriate prophylaxis for radiation-induced pain flares [46].

Osteoradionecrosis

Radiation can cause serious and painful damage to osseous tissue—described by several terms including radiation osteitis, radiation necrosis, and osteoradionecrosis (ORN). ORN is characterized by exposed irradiated bone, through fistulization with mucosa or skin. The wound remains non-healing for 3 or more months post-radiation, with symptoms of pain and drainage. The mandible is most commonly affected, with preceding trauma or dental procedures contributing to greater incidence [47]. Other risk factors include radiation doses of greater than 60 Gy and use of brachytherapy [47, 48].

Prevention of ORN is important given the identified risk factors. Historically, patients who required multiple dental extractions or surgically extensive extraction could be treated with hyperbaric oxygen before and after the procedure. Although a regimen of pentoxifylline with tocopherol has shown success for prevention and can be continued (+/− clodronate) as treatment if ORN develops. Use of antibiotics in ORN is appropriate with clinical signs of infection [49]. Most patients improve with conservative measures like chlorhexidine rinses, pain medications, and sequestrectomy—the surgical removal of loose bone fragments [49]. For severe or refractory cases, free tissue transfer can be considered, while rigid fixation may be an option for those unfit for reconstructive surgery [50].

Brachial Plexopathy

Radiation-induced neuropathies are less common complications of RT but should be noted given their late onset. Radiation-induced brachial plexopathy (RIBP) is a well-described delayed neuropathy, which may arise months to years after RT, with a mean incidence of 1.8–2.9% per year. RIBP is most commonly seen in patients who had received radiation for breast cancer but is also found in patients treated for head and neck cancer, lung cancer, and Hodkin's disease. It is important to consider cancer recurrence as the etiology of plexopathy, using modalities like magnetic resonance imaging (MRI) and positron emission tomography (PET). Patients usually develop paresthesia or dysesthesia, although neuropathic pain is possible and may be managed with non-opioid analgesics, benzodiazepines, and neuropathic agents like tricyclic antidepressants or anti-epileptics [51].

Chemotherapy or Radiation Therapy Associated Syndromes

Mucositis

Oral and gastrointestinal mucositis is a common and potentially devastating side effect occurring in patients receiving high-dose chemotherapy, radiation therapy, or both [52–54]. In broad terms, mucositis is characterized by inflammation, erythema, and ulceration of any mucous membrane. Therefore, radiation-induced esophagitis, enteritis, and proctitis are all manifestations of GI mucositis. Oral mucositis is a common complication of head and neck cancer treatment—termed as stomatitis [52]. The pathophysiology of mucositis is complex—nearly all cell types and the extracellular matrix are believed to be involved in mucosal barrier injury, and proinflammatory cytokines also play a major role in amplifying injury [53].

For patients receiving high-dose chemotherapy with hematopoietic stem cell transplantation, the incidence of mucositis is close to 100%, while it is around 80% for patients receiving radiotherapy for head and neck cancer [52]. The severity of mucosal injury can be classified on internationally recognized scales, with incidence and severity varying greatly based on treatment regimen and modality [53].

Elad et al. (2020) can be referenced for the latest consensus mucositis prevention and treatment guidelines. The panel recommended use of multi-agent combination oral care protocols with emphasis on basic oral care for prevention, rather than endorsing particular agents. Previous panel reviews favored use of transdermal fentanyl and doxepin mouthwashes in specific patient populations with mucositis, although this was downgraded to "no guidance possible" in the latest guideline [54].

Surgery-Cancer-Related Surgery-Associated Pain Syndromes

Post-mastectomy Pain

Breast cancer is the most commonly diagnosed cancer in women in the United States (excluding skin cancers), and advances in breast cancer treatment have led to improved trends in 5-year survival [55]. Post-mastectomy pain has therefore emerged as a clinically significant complication of breast cancer treatment, with an incidence between 20% and 50% in patients that have undergone the procedure [56, 57].

Post-mastectomy pain syndrome (PMPS) is defined as pain persisting beyond 3 months after the mastectomy procedure [58], although it may persist for years after treatment [59]. Classically, PMPS is considered to be a neuropathic pain syndrome with distribution of pain in the anterolateral thorax, the axilla, or the medial upper arm. Pain is characteristically burning, shooting, or pressure like, and paresthesias may also occur [58], although a broader definition may include pain with nociceptive characteristics. The syndrome is correlated with myriad other quality of life complications, such as reduced function, mood disorders, and problems with sleep and fatigue [56].

Prevention of acute and chronic post-mastectomy pain may benefit from use of perioperative regional anesthesia. Additionally, local anesthesia (intraoperative intravenous lidocaine and perioperative EMLA cream) has been demonstrated to reduce chronic post-mastectomy pain [60]. Treatment of PMPS should integrate physical therapy, given that multifactorial physical therapy (active exercises and stretching) has been demonstrated to improve range-of-motion and pain outcomes [61]. Self-management strategies like group-based education, relaxation training, and cognitive restructuring may also be helpful [56].

Pharmacotherapy for persistent pain should focus on targeting multiple post-mastectomy symptoms—like concurrent mood disorders or insomnia—with a foundation on neuropathic agents like gabapentinoids, SNRIs (e.g., duloxetine, venlafaxine), or tricyclic antidepressants. Acetaminophen or NSAIDs may be useful adjuncts, while long-term opioids are generally not recommended [56]. There is also evidence for use of injection therapy in reduction of chronic pain scores in post-mastectomy pain, such as single-injection thoracic paravertebral block and continuous paravertebral nerve block [62, 63].

Post-head and Neck Postoperative Pain

Acute and chronic postoperative orofacial or musculoskeletal pain may result from numerous surgical procedures for head and neck cancer—the scope of which is outside of this review. Maxillectomy has been associated with significant pain in up to 60% of recipients—especially those treated with prosthetic obturation [64]. Neck dissection surgery is associated with greater pain and function complications with resection of the spinal accessory nerve (CN XI) [65]. Opioid analgesics are a mainstay of treatment for nociceptive pain arising postoperatively. Although there is great variability, pain tends to be the most severe 1–2 months after surgery and gradually improves over time [66].

Post-thoracotomy Pain

Chronic post-thoracotomy pain may occur at an even greater incidence than chronic post-mastectomy pain, with an observed incidence of 30–50% [57]. Intercostal nerve injury may be the driving insult for post-thoracotomy pain due to rib retraction when entering the intercostal space or during chest closure [67, 68]. Thoracotomy surgery is associated with acute postoperative pain, while post-thoracotomy pain syndrome (PTPS) is defined as persistent pain greater than 2 months after the surgical procedure [69]. Novel pain may arise in individuals with adequate postoperative pain control and may persist for months to years [69, 70]. The mechanism of PTPS is likely a combination of neuropathic and myofascial pain [69]. Similarly to post-mastectomy pain, use of regional and local anesthesia may help to prevent severe acute and chronic post-thoracotomy pain, while a multidisciplinary and multimodal approach of pain management may be necessary for management [60, 69].

Immunotherapy

Bhuvaneswari Sandeep Ram

In cancer patients, the primary and the metastatic lesions cause immunosuppression to survive the immune system. One of the novel therapies against cancer, immune therapy is used to trigger the immune system against malignant cells. Immune system can be stimulated actively or passively.

Immunotherapy is known to regulate tumor microenvironment and reduce neoantigens, hence reduce recurrence [71]. Various forms of immunotherapy include immune check point inhibitors, adoptive cell therapy, monoclonal antibodies, immunomodulators, and treatment vaccines. Immunotherapy-related adverse events, known as IrAEs, can involve multiple systems. Pain related symptoms can be fatigue, arthralgias, myalgias, and neuropathy.

Most of these are temporary. Treatments include pausing or discontinuation of immunotherapy for a short term allowing cooling period, administering methyl-prednisolone and providing immunesuppression [72]. Pain management therapy includes anti-inflammatory medications, neuropathic agents, and infusion therapy.

Treatments for Cancer Pain

Non-interventional Therapies

Pharmacological Treatments
Tochukwu Ibe and Bhuvaneswari Sandeep Ram

Pharmacological therapies form the foundation of cancer pain management, particularly when the pain is moderate to severe or when interventional treatments are not suitable. The World Health Organization (WHO) developed a three-step "analgesic ladder," which remains a guiding principle for treating cancer-related pain. This approach involves using non-opioid analgesics, such as acetaminophen and NSAIDs, as the first line of treatment for mild cancer pain, while opioids serve as the mainstay therapy for moderate to severe pain or for mild pain that is persistent or unresponsive to non-opioid medications [73].

Acetaminophen can be used alone or in combination with an opioid. However, its use in oncology patients may be limited due to hepatotoxicity concerns, especially in those with liver disease. NSAIDs are another common choice, often prescribed alone, but their use requires careful consideration due to potential side effects like renal impairment, bleeding, and gastrointestinal upset. The development of selective COX-2 inhibitors, such as meloxicam and celecoxib (Celebrex), helps to minimize some of the gastrointestinal side effects, although these drugs still require careful monitoring during initiation.

For neuropathic cancer pain or pain that is resistant to opioids alone, adjuvant analgesics can provide additional relief when used either alone or in combination with opioids and non-opioid medications [24, 73]. These adjuvants include anticonvulsants, such as gabapentin and pregabalin, as well as antidepressants like duloxetine or amitriptyline, particularly in patients with concurrent depression or anxiety. While corticosteroids are sometimes used as adjuvants in the management of cancer pain, evidence supporting their long-term efficacy is weak, with pain relief—if any—typically being short-lived [74]. Nevertheless, corticosteroids may be considered in patients with poor overall clinical status where other options are limited.

Ultimately, pharmacological treatments should be tailored to the individual patient, taking into account the specific pain mechanisms and potential side effects.

Psychological Treatments for Cancer Pain
Nancy Beckman and Amy Siston

Psychological treatments help patients manage cancer pain and the distress that commonly accompanies it. Cognitive Behavioral Therapy (CBT) teaches patients about their condition and strategies to manage it such as reframing negative thoughts about the meaning of cancer and/or pain, problem-solving, goal-setting, and relaxation. A promising single, 2-hour class called Empowered Relief (ER), which teaches pain self-management skills, has shown comparable benefits to CBT [75]. In one study, patients who watched an ER video prior to breast cancer surgery stopped using opioids 5 days sooner than controls [76]. The use of relaxation with imagery as part of CBT or alone, as well as hypnosis, is associated with less pain and distress among cancer patients [77, 78]. Additionally, mindfulness-based therapies encourage purposeful, non-judgmental, present moment awareness and have shown to reduce stress, depression, fatigue, insomnia, pain perception, and disability [79]. Finally, Acceptance and Commitment Therapy (ACT) fosters values-consistent behavior with the use of acceptance and mindfulness skills [80]. There is support for the use of ACT for reducing distress and helping people live a meaningful life despite their cancer and pain [81].

Palliative Interventional Therapies

Tian Yu and Bhuvaneswari Sandeep Ram

Kyphoplasty/Radiofrequency Ablation for Vertebral Malignancies
Kyphoplasty and radiofrequency ablation are minimally invasive therapies aimed at stabilizing vertebral compression fractures caused by metastatic bone disease. Indications include painful vertebral fractures from cancers like breast, lung, or prostate cancer. Kyphoplasty restores vertebral height using bone cement, while radiofrequency ablation techniques can be utilized to destroy tumor cells and provide structural support [82]. Patient selection includes individuals with recent, symptomatic fractures that affect mobility. Side effects include rare complications like cement leakage or nerve damage. Contraindications involve spinal canal compromise, severe vertebral destruction, or uncorrected coagulopathy.

Radiation Therapy for Pain Palliation
Radiation therapy is often used for palliating bone pain due to metastatic cancer, particularly when tumors press on bones or nerves. Indications include patients with painful bone metastases, such as those found in the spine, pelvis, or ribs. Patient selection focuses on those who may not respond well to systemic treatments. Side effects include fatigue, skin irritation, and potential nerve damage. Contraindications involve poor performance status or nearby organs at risk from radiation exposure.

Intrathecal Pumps for Intractable Cancer Pain
Intrathecal pumps deliver pain medications directly into the cerebrospinal fluid, significantly reducing systemic opioid use [83]. Indications include intractable cancer pain in patients who fail systemic treatments due to excessive side effects. Patient selection involves those with longer life expectancy and severe pain from abdominal or pelvic malignancies. Side effects include infections, catheter dislodgement, and drug-related complications like respiratory depression. Contraindications include active infection, coagulopathy, or very limited life expectancy.

Spinal Cord Stimulation (SCS) for Refractory Cancer Pain
SCS modulates pain signals at the spinal level, using electrical impulses to interfere with the perception of pain. Indications include refractory neuropathic pain from cancer, particularly post-surgical pain or nerve compression [84]. Patient selection includes those with a longer prognosis and intact cognitive function to manage the device. Side effects include lead migration and infection. Contraindications are systemic infections, bleeding disorders, or poor cognitive function.

Sacral Neuromodulation for Pelvic Organ Dysfunction
Sacral neuromodulation (SNM) is used to treat pelvic organ dysfunctions such as bladder or bowel incontinence caused by cancer or its treatments. Indications include refractory organ dysfunction due to pelvic malignancies. Patient selection focuses on those with longer life expectancy and severe incontinence. Side effects

include pain, infection, and device malfunction. Contraindications include active infections or anatomical abnormalities that prevent device implantation.

Neurolytic Celiac Plexus Blocks for Visceral Malignancies
Neurolytic celiac plexus blocks involve chemical ablation of the celiac plexus with ethanol or phenol to disrupt pain transmission from abdominal organs. Indications are severe, unremitting visceral pain, particularly in pancreatic, gastric, or hepatic cancers [85]. Patient selection includes those with significant pain unresponsive to opioids. Side effects include transient hypotension, diarrhea, or inadvertent nerve damage. Contraindications include coagulopathies, local infections, or altered anatomy from prior surgeries.

Sympathetic Blocks for Pelvic Malignancies
Sympathetic nerve blocks such as superior hypogastric plexus and ganglion impart blocks are used to manage deep pelvic cancer pain [86, 87]. Indications include patients with refractory pain from pelvic malignancies such as prostate, bladder, or rectal cancers. Patient selection includes those who fail systemic treatments or cannot tolerate higher opioid doses. Side effects include transient hypotension, leg weakness, or bowel/bladder dysfunction. Contraindications include infection, coagulopathy, or distorted anatomy from previous surgery.

Peripheral Nerve Blocks and Stimulators
Peripheral nerve blocks can be effective for managing localized cancer pain, particularly in patients with somatic pain, such as those with extremity sarcomas or localized tumor invasion [88]. Indications include patients who experience somatic pain from cancer that cannot be adequately controlled with systemic medications. Peripheral nerve stimulators (PNS) can also be utilized in these cases, providing continuous low-voltage electrical stimulation to the nerve, modulating pain perception. PNS indications include patients with persistent neuropathic pain that is resistant to nerve blocks or systemic analgesics. The non-opioid nature of this approach can make it appealing for patients looking to minimize systemic medication use. Patient selection focuses on individuals with localized pain or neuropathic pain in the extremities. Side effects of nerve blocks include localized infection, hematoma, or nerve damage, while peripheral nerve stimulators carry risks like lead migration and infection. Contraindications include active infection at the site or coagulopathy that prevents safe application of nerve blocks or implantation of nerve stimulators.

Head and Neck Malignancies: Nerve Blocks
Nerve blocks like sphenopalatine ganglion blocks and cervical nerve blocks are used for patients with head and neck cancers experiencing severe cranial or facial pain. Indications include refractory pain caused by tumor invasion or compression of cranial nerves. Patient selection focuses on those with severe, localized pain. Side effects include temporary facial numbness or infection. Contraindications include local infections, coagulopathy, or distorted anatomy.

Trunk Pain from Malignancies: PECS and TAP Blocks

PECS and TAP blocks targeting localized cancer pain in the chest wall and abdomen, respectively, have been described in case reports. PECS blocks are particularly useful for patients with breast cancer [89], while TAP blocks can be effective for abdominal malignancies [90]. Indications include localized pain in the chest or abdomen unresponsive to systemic medications. Patient selection focuses on patients with localized pain from malignancies or post-surgical complications. Side effects are rare but may include infection or local anesthetic toxicity. Contraindications include active infection or distorted local anatomy from extensive tumor invasion.

Addressing Pain at End of Life and During Active Dying Process

Josh Russell and Ariana Nelson

For any patient with cancer-related pain, an early referral to a trained palliative care physician is beneficial. Importantly, in patients with newly diagnosed incurable cancers, early integration of palliative care into their treatment improved quality of life measures, decreased rates of depression, and even increased lifespan [91, 92]. Outside of medication management, palliative care physicians are trained to facilitate discussions to clarify goals of care, code status, and optimal timing for hospice enrollment. Improving comfort and functionality are the objectives of palliative plans of care. Therefore, referral to these specialists should be conducted early in the disease course, while the patient retains capacity to maximize comfort and preserve functional status.

Ethical Considerations

The management of a patient with cancer-related pain differs markedly from that of patients with chronic non-cancer pain, namely, because the expected trajectory is for increasing pain with disease progression. However, ethical considerations related to the patient and greater society must be considered when making treatment plans. While desires of the patient are paramount, preventing or alleviating suffering should be the principal goal of the clinician while counseling patient and family [93]. The benefit or burden of the treatment must also be considered with respect to patient's quality of life and costs of treatment that must be shouldered by patients or their estates. Similarly, family wishes and ability to care for the debilitated patient (fiscally and physically) must be assessed [94]. When treating patients with terminal cancer diagnoses, regimens including opioids are often unavoidable if palliation of pain is to be achieved. In such cases, liberal up titration of opioids to achieve symptom control is preferable, and clinicians and patients should expect the development of tolerance as well as dose-dependent side effects (e.g., constipation). However, use of intrathecal (IT) pump devices, commonly reserved for baclofen therapy in patients with chronic non-cancer pain due to spasticity, is a desirable option in patients with intractable cancer pain despite high doses of systemic opioids. Opioid-delivering IT pumps are especially beneficial in select patients with known terminal diagnosis but a prognosis of sufficient survival to maintain a functional status consistent with carrying out their activities of daily living independently, usually at least 3–6 months. IT delivery will reduce the side effect burden (namely, sedation and constipation) that patients would experience with high-dose systemic opioids and can deliver more consistent analgesia due to continuous nature of drug administration [95].

Admission to Hospice

Qualifying for hospice: Typically, patients must meet the criterion of an abbreviated prognosis of fewer than 6-month survival and express the desire to prioritize comfort over survival. Patients with cancer will experience undesirable pain symptoms and non-pain symptoms as they approach death. Hospice care has been shown in qualitative studies to reduce suffering in both pain and non-pain dimension of QOL [96].

There are four levels of hospice care (medicare.gov):

1. Routine home care: This is the most common level of care in hospice. At this level, patients are generally stable with adequate control of pain and other symptoms.
2. General inpatient care: Patients may be admitted for short-term management of poorly controlled pain of symptoms during an acute crisis. This is generally provided at either a hospital or a skilled nursing facility.
3. Continuous home care: As an alternative to admission for general inpatient care, patients may receive short-term continuous management of pain or other symptom crises at home.
4. Respite care: Temporary admission of the patient to a hospital, inpatient hospice facility, or a skilled nursing facility to provide the primary caregivers of the patient with a reprieve from their duties in caring for the patient. All other levels are predicated on patient needs and presentation, but this level of care is dependent on caregiver requirements.

Opioid management during hospice care: If a patient has established that their principal goal of care is comfort, it is appropriate, based on the principle of double effect, to rapidly escalate doses of opioids to achieve desired analgesia, accepting that there may be excessive sedation and/or respiratory depression. If the intent of increasing opioid dosing is to treat uncontrolled pain and not to accelerate death, the practice is ethically sound. Liability for consequences of opioid overdose in such patients is minimal, and this is standard practice for patients enrolled in hospice. Most patients prioritize comfort over longevity at the end of life, and the general opinion of patients with terminal diseases is to receive end-of-life care in their homes rather than at the hospital [97].

Hospital Death

It is challenging to qualitatively assess the experience of patients that unexpectedly deteriorate while in the inpatient setting. On occasion the patient may have capacity to decide to forgo care and pursue hospice, but often this decision will fall to the person designated as the patient's durable power of attorney [98]. If the patient has not made such designations and bereaved family members do not achieve a consensus on the desires of the patient to forgo treatment, it may be necessary to consult the ethics committee of the healthcare institution. Communication regarding the treatment, expected prognosis, and honest predictions of the patient's likely disease progression are paramount for both the patient and family if the patient has reported a desire for family to be involved in care [99]. Possessing dual insurance from Medicare and Medicaid is a risk factor for the undesirable outcome of hospital death versus death at home [100]. All patients should receive counseling regarding goals of care during hospice, but special attention is required in this at-risk group.

Death at Home Considerations

The ability of patients to elect to die at home has been available for all of modern healthcare history and is channeled by the comfort a patient will feel in familiar surroundings during the end-of-life processes that can cause clouded sensorium [101]. Funding for hospice care at home has been supported internationally by governments as most patients with subacute clinical deterioration wish to spend their final days in a familiar location [102]. Patients and families that elect to receive end-of-life care are more likely to die while at home rather than in the hospital compared to patients receiving usual care. Re-admission to the hospital while receiving hospice care at home does occur on occasion, but different study populations have shown different rates [97].

Summary

Ibe Tochukwu and Bhuvaneswari Sandeep Ram

Cancer-related pain is multifaceted and requires a comprehensive approach to management. Effective treatment involves not only addressing the physical dimensions of pain but also the emotional, cognitive, and sociocultural factors that influence the patient's experience. Pharmacological management remains a cornerstone of treatment, with non-opioid analgesics, opioids, and adjuvant therapies playing essential roles depending on the type and severity of the pain. Non-interventional therapies such as these can provide substantial relief, especially when applied in a multimodal fashion. In cases where pharmacological therapies are insufficient or side effects become intolerable, interventional therapies offer an additional avenue for relief. These interventional strategies are valuable for reducing opioid requirements, enhancing pain control, and improving the patient's quality of life. Given the multidimensional nature of cancer pain, psychological and social support must also be integrated into the treatment plan. Ultimately, the goal of cancer pain management is to alleviate suffering through individualized treatment plans that combine pharmacological, interventional, and psychosocial therapies. By addressing the full spectrum of pain—from its physical causes to its emotional impacts—clinicians can help patients achieve better functional outcomes and a higher quality of life during their cancer journey.

References

1. Snijders RAH, et al. Update on prevalence of pain in patients with cancer 2022: a systematic literature review and meta-analysis. Cancers (Basel). 2023;15(3):591.
2. Beck SL, et al. Core aspects of satisfaction with pain management: cancer patients' perspectives. J Pain Symptom Manag. 2010;39(1):100–15.
3. Syrjala KL, et al. Psychological and behavioral approaches to cancer pain management. J Clin Oncol. 2014;32(16):1703–11.
4. Yi JC, Syrjala KL. Anxiety and depression in cancer survivors. Med Clin North Am. 2017;101(6):1099–113.
5. McGuire DB. Occurrence of cancer pain. J Natl Cancer Inst Monogr. 2004;(32):51–6.
6. Ahles TA, Blanchard EB, Ruckdeschel JC. The multidimensional nature of cancer-related pain. Pain. 1983;17(3):277–88.
7. Ripamonti CI, et al. Pain related to cancer treatments and diagnostic procedures: a no man's land? Ann Oncol. 2014;25(6):1097–106.
8. Paice JA. Chronic treatment-related pain in cancer survivors. Pain. 2011;152(3 Suppl):S84–9.
9. Marcus NJ. Pain in cancer patients unrelated to the cancer or treatment. Cancer Investig. 2005;23(1):84–93.
10. Caraceni A, et al. Breakthrough pain characteristics and syndromes in patients with cancer pain. An international survey. Palliat Med. 2004;18(3):177–83.
11. Glare PA, et al. Pain in cancer survivors. J Clin Oncol. 2014;32(16):1739–47.
12. van den Beuken-van Everdingen M. Chronic pain in cancer survivors: a growing issue. J Pain Palliat Care Pharmacother. 2012;26(4):385–7.
13. Yang J, et al. The modified WHO analgesic ladder: is it appropriate for chronic non-cancer pain? J Pain Res. 2020;13:411–7.
14. Paice JA, et al. Management of chronic pain in survivors of adult cancers: American Society of Clinical Oncology clinical practice guideline. J Clin Oncol. 2016;34(27):3325–45.
15. Swarm RA, et al. Adult cancer pain, version 3.2019, NCCN clinical practice guidelines in oncology. J Natl Compr Cancer Netw. 2019;17(8):977–1007.
16. Fallon MT. Neuropathic pain in cancer. Br J Anaesth. 2013;111(1):105–11.
17. Lee DY, Lee JJ, Richeimer SH. Cancer pain syndromes. Cancer Treat Res. 2021;182:17–25.
18. Cella DF, et al. The Functional Assessment of Cancer Therapy scale: development and validation of the general measure. J Clin Oncol. 1993;11(3):570–9.
19. Piraux E, Caty G, Reychler G. Effects of preoperative combined aerobic and resistance exercise training in cancer patients undergoing tumour resection surgery: a systematic review of randomised trials. Surg Oncol. 2018;27(3):584–94.
20. van den Beuken-van Everdingen MH, et al. Update on prevalence of pain in patients with cancer: systematic review and meta-analysis. J Pain Symptom Manag. 2016;51(6):1070–1090.e9.
21. Mitchell AJ, et al. Prevalence of depression, anxiety, and adjustment disorder in oncological, haematological, and palliative-care settings: a meta-analysis of 94 interview-based studies. Lancet Oncol. 2011;12(2):160–74.

22. Porter LS, Keefe FJ. Psychosocial issues in cancer pain. Curr Pain Headache Rep. 2011;15(4):263–70.
23. Sun V, et al. Barriers to pain assessment and management in cancer survivorship. J Cancer Surviv. 2008;2(1):65–71.
24. Scarborough BM, Smith CB. Optimal pain management for patients with cancer in the modern era. CA Cancer J Clin. 2018;68(3):182–96.
25. Turk DC. Remember the distinction between malignant and benign pain? Well, forget it. Clin J Pain. 2002;18(2):75–6.
26. Kroenke K, Spitzer RL, Williams JB. The PHQ-9: validity of a brief depression severity measure. J Gen Intern Med. 2001;16(9):606–13.
27. Spitzer RL, et al. A brief measure for assessing generalized anxiety disorder: the GAD-7. Arch Intern Med. 2006;166(10):1092–7.
28. Maizels M, Smitherman TA, Penzien DB. A review of screening tools for psychiatric comorbidity in headache patients. Headache. 2006;46(Suppl 3):S98–109.
29. Wang HL, et al. Predictors of cancer-related pain improvement over time. Psychosom Med. 2012;74(6):642–7.
30. Krebs EE, et al. Development and initial validation of the PEG, a three-item scale assessing pain intensity and interference. J Gen Intern Med. 2009;24(6):733–8.
31. NCCN practice guidelines for the management of psychosocial distress. National Comprehensive Cancer Network. Oncology (Williston Park). 1999;13(5A):113–47.
32. Gatchel RJ, et al. The biopsychosocial approach to chronic pain: scientific advances and future directions. Psychol Bull. 2007;133(4):581–624.
33. Porter LS, et al. Caregiver-guided pain coping skills training for patients with advanced cancer: results from a randomized clinical trial. Palliat Med. 2021;35(5):952–61.
34. Kreidieh FY, Moukadem HA, El Saghir NS. Overview, prevention and management of chemotherapy extravasation. World J Clin Oncol. 2016;7(1):87–97.
35. El-Saghir N, et al. Dexrazoxane for anthracycline extravasation and GM-CSF for skin ulceration and wound healing. Lancet Oncol. 2004;5(5):320–1.
36. Smith EM, et al. Effect of duloxetine on pain, function, and quality of life among patients with chemotherapy-induced painful peripheral neuropathy: a randomized clinical trial. JAMA. 2013;309(13):1359–67.
37. Miller KK, Gorcey L, McLellan BN. Chemotherapy-induced hand-foot syndrome and nail changes: a review of clinical presentation, etiology, pathogenesis, and management. J Am Acad Dermatol. 2014;71(4):787–94.
38. Gressett SM, Stanford BL, Hardwicke F. Management of hand-foot syndrome induced by capecitabine. J Oncol Pharm Pract. 2006;12(3):131–41.
39. Hubenak JR, et al. Mechanisms of injury to normal tissue after radiotherapy: a review. Plast Reconstr Surg. 2014;133(1):49e–56e.
40. Wang K, Tepper JE. Radiation therapy-associated toxicity: etiology, management, and prevention. CA Cancer J Clin. 2021;71(5):437–54.
41. Stephans KL, et al. Prediction of chest wall toxicity from lung stereotactic body radiotherapy (SBRT). Int J Radiat Oncol Biol Phys. 2012;82(2):974–80.
42. Dunlap NE, et al. Chest wall volume receiving >30 Gy predicts risk of severe pain and/or rib fracture after lung stereotactic body radiotherapy. Int J Radiat Oncol Biol Phys. 2010;76(3):796–801.
43. Andolino DL, et al. Chest wall toxicity after stereotactic body radiotherapy for malignant lesions of the lung and liver. Int J Radiat Oncol Biol Phys. 2011;80(3):692–7.
44. Din SU, et al. Impact of fractionation and dose in a multivariate model for radiation-induced chest wall pain. Int J Radiat Oncol Biol Phys. 2015;93(2):418–24.
45. Ikushima H, et al. Pelvic bone complications following radiation therapy of gynecologic malignancies: clinical evaluation of radiation-induced pelvic insufficiency fractures. Gynecol Oncol. 2006;103(3):1100–4.

46. Chow E, et al. Dexamethasone in the prophylaxis of radiation-induced pain flare after palliative radiotherapy for bone metastases: a double-blind, randomised placebo-controlled, phase 3 trial. Lancet Oncol. 2015;16(15):1463–72.
47. Teng MS, Futran ND. Osteoradionecrosis of the mandible. Curr Opin Otolaryngol Head Neck Surg. 2005;13(4):217–21.
48. Schwartz HC, Kagan AR. Osteoradionecrosis of the mandible: scientific basis for clinical staging. Am J Clin Oncol. 2002;25(2):168–71.
49. Frankart AJ, et al. Osteoradionecrosis: exposing the evidence not the bone. Int J Radiat Oncol Biol Phys. 2021;109(5):1206–18.
50. Lyons A, Ghazali N. Osteoradionecrosis of the jaws: current understanding of its pathophysiology and treatment. Br J Oral Maxillofac Surg. 2008;46(8):653–60.
51. Delanian S, Lefaix JL, Pradat PF. Radiation-induced neuropathy in cancer survivors. Radiother Oncol. 2012;105(3):273–82.
52. Rubenstein EB, et al. Clinical practice guidelines for the prevention and treatment of cancer therapy-induced oral and gastrointestinal mucositis. Cancer. 2004;100(9 Suppl):2026–46.
53. Sonis ST, et al. Perspectives on cancer therapy-induced mucosal injury: pathogenesis, measurement, epidemiology, and consequences for patients. Cancer. 2004;100(9 Suppl):1995–2025.
54. Elad S, et al. MASCC/ISOO clinical practice guidelines for the management of mucositis secondary to cancer therapy. Cancer. 2020;126(19):4423–31.
55. DeSantis CE, et al. Breast cancer statistics, 2017, racial disparity in mortality by state. CA Cancer J Clin. 2017;67(6):439–48.
56. Tait RC, et al. Persistent post-mastectomy pain: risk factors and current approaches to treatment. J Pain. 2018;19(12):1367–83.
57. Kehlet H, Jensen TS, Woolf CJ. Persistent postsurgical pain: risk factors and prevention. Lancet. 2006;367(9522):1618–25.
58. Alves Nogueira Fabro E, et al. Post-mastectomy pain syndrome: incidence and risks. Breast. 2012;21(3):321–5.
59. Gartner R, et al. Prevalence of and factors associated with persistent pain following breast cancer surgery. JAMA. 2009;302(18):1985–92.
60. Humble SR, Dalton AJ, Li L. A systematic review of therapeutic interventions to reduce acute and chronic post-surgical pain after amputation, thoracotomy or mastectomy. Eur J Pain. 2015;19(4):451–65.
61. De Groef A, et al. Effectiveness of postoperative physical therapy for upper-limb impairments after breast cancer treatment: a systematic review. Arch Phys Med Rehabil. 2015;96(6):1140–53.
62. Karmakar MK, et al. Thoracic paravertebral block and its effects on chronic pain and health-related quality of life after modified radical mastectomy. Reg Anesth Pain Med. 2014;39(4):289–98.
63. Ilfeld BM, et al. Persistent postmastectomy pain and pain-related physical and emotional functioning with and without a continuous paravertebral nerve block: a prospective 1-year follow-up assessment of a randomized, triple-masked, placebo-controlled study. Ann Surg Oncol. 2015;22(6):2017–25.
64. Rogers SN, et al. Health-related quality of life after maxillectomy: a comparison between prosthetic obturation and free flap. J Oral Maxillofac Surg. 2003;61(2):174–81.
65. Terrell JE, et al. Pain, quality of life, and spinal accessory nerve status after neck dissection. Laryngoscope. 2000;110(4):620–6.
66. Epstein JB, et al. Oral complications of cancer and cancer therapy: from cancer treatment to survivorship. CA Cancer J Clin. 2012;62(6):400–22.
67. Rogers ML, et al. Preliminary findings in the neurophysiological assessment of intercostal nerve injury during thoracotomy. Eur J Cardiothorac Surg. 2002;21(2):298–301.
68. Cerfolio RJ, et al. Intracostal sutures decrease the pain of thoracotomy. Ann Thorac Surg. 2003;76(2):407–11; discussion 411–2.
69. Karmakar MK, Ho AM. Postthoracotomy pain syndrome. Thorac Surg Clin. 2004;14(3):345–52.

70. Gotoda Y, et al. The morbidity, time course and predictive factors for persistent post-thoracotomy pain. Eur J Pain. 2001;5(1):89–96.
71. Akkin S, Varan G, Bilensoy E. A review on cancer immunotherapy and applications of nanotechnology to chemoimmunotherapy of different cancers. Molecules. 2021;26(11):3382.
72. Okwundu N, et al. The dark side of immunotherapy. Ann Transl Med. 2021;9(12):1041.
73. World Health Organization. WHO guidelines for the pharmacological and radiotherapeutic management of cancer pain in adults and adolescents. Geneva: WHO; 2018.
74. Haywood A, et al. Corticosteroids for the management of cancer-related pain in adults. Cochrane Database Syst Rev. 2015;2015(4):CD010756.
75. Darnall BD, et al. Comparison of a single-session pain management skills intervention with a single-session health education intervention and 8 sessions of cognitive behavioral therapy in adults with chronic low back pain: a randomized clinical trial. JAMA Netw Open. 2021;4(8):e2113401.
76. Darnall BD, et al. "My surgical success": effect of a digital behavioral pain medicine intervention on time to opioid cessation after breast cancer surgery-a pilot randomized controlled clinical trial. Pain Med. 2019;20(11):2228–37.
77. Montgomery GH, Schnur JB, Kravits K. Hypnosis for cancer care: over 200 years young. CA Cancer J Clin. 2013;63(1):31–44.
78. Syrjala KL, Cummings C, Donaldson GW. Hypnosis or cognitive behavioral training for the reduction of pain and nausea during cancer treatment: a controlled clinical trial. Pain. 1992;48(2):137–46.
79. Carlson LE. Mindfulness-based interventions for coping with cancer. Ann N Y Acad Sci. 2016;1373(1):5–12.
80. Fashler SR, et al. The use of acceptance and commitment therapy in oncology settings: a narrative review. Psychol Rep. 2018;121(2):229–52.
81. Mathew A, et al. Acceptance and commitment therapy in adult cancer survivors: a systematic review and conceptual model. J Cancer Surviv. 2021;15(3):427–51.
82. Angileri SA, et al. Cooled radiofrequency ablation technology for painful bone tumors. Acta Biomed. 2020;91(10-S):e2020007.
83. Shah N, Di Napoli R, Padalia D. Implantable intrathecal drug delivery system. In: StatPearls. Treasure Island: StatPearls Publishing; 2024. Disclosure: Raffaela Di Napoli declares no relevant financial relationships with ineligible companies. Disclosure: Devang Padalia declares no relevant financial relationships with ineligible companies.
84. Crowther JE, et al. Spinal cord stimulation in the treatment of cancer pain: a retrospective review. Neuromodulation. 2022;25(5):693–9.
85. Ambai VT, et al. Celiac plexus neurolysis for abdominal cancers: going beyond pancreatic cancer pain. Pain Rep. 2021;6(1):e930.
86. Rocha A, et al. Effectiveness of superior hypogastric plexus neurolysis for pelvic cancer pain. Pain Physician. 2020;23(2):203–8.
87. Ferreira F, Pedro A. Ganglion impar neurolysis in the management of pelvic and perineal cancer-related pain. Case Rep Oncol. 2020;13(1):29–34.
88. Sudek EW, et al. Use of temporary percutaneous peripheral nerve stimulation in an oncologic population: a retrospective review. Neuromodulation. 2024;27(1):118–25.
89. Elshanbary AA, et al. Efficacy and safety of pectoral nerve block (Pecs) compared with control, paravertebral block, erector spinae plane block, and local anesthesia in patients undergoing breast cancer surgeries: a systematic review and meta-analysis. Clin J Pain. 2021;37(12):925–39.
90. Hung JC, et al. Neurolytic transversus abdominal plane block with alcohol for long-term malignancy related pain control. Pain Physician. 2014;17(6):E755–60.
91. Temel JS, et al. Early palliative care for patients with metastatic non-small-cell lung cancer. N Engl J Med. 2010;363(8):733–42.
92. Temel JS, et al. Effects of early integrated palliative care in patients with lung and GI cancer: a randomized clinical trial. J Clin Oncol. 2017;35(8):834–41.

93. Akdeniz M, Yardimci B, Kavukcu E. Ethical considerations at the end-of-life care. SAGE Open Med. 2021;9:20503121211000918.

94. Zimbelman J. Good life, good death, and the right to die: ethical considerations for decisions at the end of life. J Prof Nurs. 1994;10(1):22–37.

95. Ma K, et al. Intrathecal delivery of hydromorphone vs morphine for refractory cancer pain: a multicenter, randomized, single-blind, controlled noninferiority trial. Pain. 2020;161(11):2502–10.

96. Black B, et al. The relationships among pain, nonpain symptoms, and quality of life measures in older adults with cancer receiving hospice care. Pain Med. 2011;12(6):880–9.

97. Shepperd S, et al. Hospital at home: home-based end-of-life care. Cochrane Database Syst Rev. 2016;2(2):CD009231.

98. Faber-Langendoen K. A multi-institutional study of care given to patients dying in hospitals. Ethical and practice implications. Arch Intern Med. 1996;156(18):2130–6.

99. Haugen DF, et al. Good quality care for cancer patients dying in hospitals, but information needs unmet: bereaved relatives' survey within seven countries. Oncologist. 2021;26(7):e1273–84.

100. Herrel LA, et al. Intensity of end-of-life care for dual-eligible beneficiaries with cancer and the impact of delivery system affiliation. Cancer. 2021;127(24):4628–35.

101. Martinson IM, et al. Home care for children dying of cancer. Pediatrics. 1978;62(1):106–13.

102. Gomes B, Higginson IJ. Factors influencing death at home in terminally ill patients with cancer: systematic review. BMJ. 2006;332(7540):515–21.

Procedural Interventions in Pain Medicine

8

Christine Hunt, Paul Scholten, Dmitri Souza, Rene Przkora,
Jason S. Eldridge, Yashar Eshraghi, Sahil Gupta, Terry Hunt II ⓘ,
Eva Kubrova, and Susan M. Moeschler

Abbreviations

ACGME	Accreditation Council for Graduate Medical Education
ASIPP	American Society for Interventional Pain Procedures
ASRA Pain	American Society for Regional Anesthesiology and Pain Medicine
CBP	Chronic back pain
CDC	Centers for Disease Control and Prevention
CMS	Centers for Medicare and Medicaid Services
DDD	Degenerative disc disease
ESI	Epidural steroid injection
FDA	Food and Drug Administration
HA	Hyaluronic acid

C. Hunt (✉) · J. S. Eldridge · S. Gupta · E. Kubrova
Department of Pain Medicine, Mayo Clinic, Jacksonville, FL, USA
e-mail: Hunt.christine@mayo.edu; eldrige.jason@mayo.edu; gupta.sahil@mayo.edu;
kubrova.eva@mayo.edu

P. Scholten
Department of Physical Medicine and Rehabilitation, Mayo Clinic, Rochester, MN, USA
e-mail: scholten.paul@mayo.edu

D. Souza
Department of Anesthesiology, Western Reserve Hospital, Cuyahoga Falls, OH, USA

R. Przkora
Department of Anesthesiology, University of Florida College of Medicine, Gainesville, FL, USA

Y. Eshraghi
Department of Anesthesiology & Critical Care Medicine, Oschner Medical,
New Orleans, LA, USA

T. Hunt II · S. M. Moeschler
Department of Anesthesiology & Perioperative Medicine, Mayo Clinic, Rochester, MN, USA
e-mail: hunt.terry@mayo.edu; moeschler.susan@mayo.edu

© The Author(s), under exclusive license to Springer Nature Switzerland AG 2025
M. Anitescu (ed.), *Multidisciplinary Pain Medicine Fellowship*,
https://doi.org/10.1007/978-3-031-88357-6_8

IACS	Intra-articular corticosteroid
LAs	Local anesthetics
LBP	Low back pain
MBB	Medial branch blocks
MPC	Mesenchymal precursor cell
MPE	Methylprednisolone equivalents
MRI	Magnetic resonance imaging
NSAIDs	Nonsteroid anti-inflammatory drugs
OA	Osteoarthritis
PRP	Platelet rich plasma
RCT	Randomized controlled trial
RFA	Radiofrequency ablation
SC	Stem cells
SNRB	Selective nerve root block
TFESI	Transforaminal epidural steroid injection
US	United States

Introduction

Interventional pain management is a key pillar of comprehensive, multimodal pain care. A key aspect of high-quality fellowship training includes comprehensive exposure to common interventional pain procedures. This includes didactic-style lectures, observation, and significant hands-on experience to provide safe, effective high-quality care to patients. Although there can be some variability in terms of approach, there are comprehensive guidelines and standardized approaches for most common, foundational interventional procedures. The following section will discuss medications and products utilized for interventional pain procedures, approaches to spine procedures, musculoskeletal injections and nerve blocks, and lesioning procedures involving neurolytic agents and radiofrequency ablation. The goal of this section is to provide an overview of procedures taught in most fellowship programs and to orient trainees to the breadth of training that can be expected in most accredited training programs.

Corticosteroids and Local Anesthetics

Paul M. Scholten

Corticosteroids and local anesthetics (LAs) are commonly delivered to intra-articular, epidural, perineural, and peritendinous locations to manage and diagnose pain [1–6]. Understanding the pharmacologic properties and risks associated with these agents is important for optimizing outcomes.

Corticosteroids

Injected corticosteroids are structurally similar to cortisol and mimic its inhibitory effects on inflammatory cytokines and immune function [7]. Formulations having larger particle size and lower solubility (methylprednisolone, triamcinolone, beta-methasone acetate) are thought to have slower onset and longer duration of action compared to freely soluble agents (betamethasone sodium phosphate, dexametha-sone) with quicker onset and shorter duration of action. However, no studies directly comparing them have shown any significant clinical differences [8].

Given the immunosuppressives properties of corticosteroids, they are contraindi-cated when injection site infection or bacteremia is present. Additionally, they nega-tively impact fracture healing and should not be used intra-articularly when fracture is present. Systemic steroid effects including decreased bone mineral density and adrenal suppression occur with repeated chronic exposure [7]. Therefore, sites should not be injected more frequently than every 6 weeks or more than 3 times in a year [9].

Potential adverse events of steroid use include allergic reactions, infection, flush-ing, and increased blood glucose levels [7, 8]. Risks specific to the use of triamcino-lone include local tissue necrosis and tendon rupture and, therefore, its use is limited to intra-articular procedures [10, 11]. Furthermore, brain and spinal cord infarct following transforaminal epidural steroid injection (TFESI) have been reported [12–15], likely due to particulate steroid aggregation and embolization, although a recent report of infarction following the use of dexamethasone (non-particulate) [16] suggests that other mechanisms such as direct vascular injury or vasospasm may play a role. Although rare, the consequences of using particulate steroids for TFESI appear to be more often catastrophic than when using non-particulate agents, and given a lack of superiority over non-particulate steroids [17–19], their use should be avoided.

Local Anesthetics

Amide LAs such as short-acting lidocaine and long-acting bupivacaine and ropiva-caine are commonly administered to provide periprocedural cutaneous analgesia, short-term pain relief, and diagnostic information. Adverse events associated with the use of LAs include allergic reaction and toxicity.

The incidence of true allergy to amide LAs is low [20]; however, patients often mistake side effects of epinephrine containing LAs such as racing heart rate and palpitations as an allergic reaction. Careful history taking is essential to establishing the presence of a true allergy.

The risk of life-threatening systemic LA toxicity is dose-dependent and not expected with typical doses used in interventional pain procedures. However, even small amounts of LA injected intrathecally can lead to total spinal anesthesia and if delivered intraarterially can cause generalized seizures.

Bupivacaine- and epinephrine-containing LA formulations are chondrotoxic [20]. Ropivacaine offers a safer (albeit more expensive) long-acting LA alternative for intra-articular injections. While safe for intra-articular use, ropivacaine should not be used for epidural injections due to its vasoconstrictive properties and increased risk of CNS infarction [8, 21].

The properties of commonly used steroids and LAs for pain procedures described here provide a basic framework for selecting the most appropriate agent. Knowledge gained should help refine these decisions over time.

Blood-Based and Cell-Based Biological Therapies for Back Pain

Dmitri Souza

After decades of basic research, blood- and cell-based biological therapies, also commonly referred to as Regenerative Medicine, are entering the clinical realm and becoming one of the most innovative and extraordinary trends in pain medicine [22]. In the past, successful tissue restoration was believed to require the presence of polypotent cellular material [23]. In the last decade, however, the role of blood- and cell-based therapies was found to differ significantly from what was initially thought. Beyond the traditional stem cell role of producing replicated cells, researchers discovered the signaling functions of biological agents [24]. Blood- and cell-based biological therapies serve as a "toolbox" for tissue repair, delivering a customized library of signaling factors rather than simply a self-dividing entity leading to tissue restoration [25]. It is essential to mention that currently, there is no blood- or cell-based biological treatment that is FDA approved for the treatment of pain, including chronic back pain (CBP) [26, 27]. However, assessment of current clinical research suggests that approval of clinical applications is forthcoming [27, 28]. Herein, we will discuss blood- and cell-based biological therapies for CBP. Chronic back pain is a widespread problem [29, 30]. It is one of the most encountered chronic pain conditions in the USA and throughout the world [31–33]. It affects young and older adults, the elderly, and even children [34–37]. It is associated with persistent opioid use [38]. Chronic back pain is a common trigger for emergency department visits, hospitalizations, and surgery [39]. It is commonly associated with significant functional and psychological impairment and disability [29, 30, 36, 39, 40].

A recent systematic review and meta-analysis investigated regenerative properties of intradiscal injections of platelet-rich plasma (PRP), stem cells (SC), and other biologic agents [41]. The patient sample included subjects with discogenic low back pain (LBP) confirmed by provocation discography or clinical and imaging findings consistent with discogenic pain. The primary outcome was the proportion of patients with ≥50% pain relief after intradiscal biologic injection at 6 months.

Secondary outcomes included ≥2-point pain score reduction, patient satisfaction, functional improvement, decreased utilization of other health care including analgesics and surgery, and structural disc changes determined with MRI. The study examined biologic therapies including PRP, SC, microfragmented adipose tissue, autologous conditioned serum, and amniotic membrane-based injectates. Twelve studies met established inclusion criteria. The quality of evidence was very low. One randomized controlled trial (RCT) evaluating PRP was positive but had significant methodological flaws [41]. A single trial that evaluated mesenchymal stem cells was negative. In aggregate, 6-month success rates for PRP were 55% and for SC—53.5%. The worst-case analysis decreased SC success rate to 40.7%. More than 30% functional improvement was achieved in 74.3%, but the worst-case analysis decreased it to 44.1%. The authors of the systematic review concluded that some observational data support the use of intradiscal biologic agents to treat discogenic LBP. However, the quality was very low [41]. No studies included in this systematic review reported any serious complications.

Several important RCTs were published after this review [28, 42–45]. One high-quality multicenter RCT evaluated the safety and efficacy of a single intradiscal injection of adult allogeneic mesenchymal precursor cells (MPCs) combined with hyaluronic acid (HA) in a total of 100 subjects with LBP with moderate degenerative disc disease (DDD) for at least 6 months and failing 3 months of conventional conservative treatment [28]. The patients were randomized to receive six million MPCs with HA, 18 million MPCs with HA, HA vehicle control, or placebo (saline control) injections. There were significant differences between the MPCs groups and control. The MPC therapy was superior to controls in improvement of pain and function at various time points through 36 months. Both the injection and the treatment were well tolerated, and there were no clinical symptoms of immune reaction to allogeneic MPCs. One case of severe back pain was potentially related to the study agent, and one implantation site infection was probably related to the study intervention. The study demonstrated that intradiscal injection of MPCs "could be a safe, effective, durable, and minimally invasive therapy for subjects associated with moderate DDD [28]." Therefore, recent data suggest that intradiscal biologic agents may be effective treatments for discogenic LBP [46].

Several studies evaluated blood- and cell-based biological therapies on facetogenic CBP and radicular pain [43, 44, 47–49]. One RCT demonstrated the superiority of PRP over steroid injections for sacral LBP [50]. A case series and a case report showed the effectiveness of PRP for coccydynia [51, 52]. Several studies evaluated prolotherapy for CBP [53–56]. While the studies seem promising, the presented level of evidence was, overall, low. Studies focused on the safety of blood- and cell-based biological therapies support safety of this type of treatment [57]. Many suggest, and we agree, that research should focus on developing high-quality clinical evidence and evaluating safety and long-term outcomes [41, 58–61].

Spine Injections: Selective Nerve Root Block, Epidural Steroid Injection, and Transforaminal Epidural Steroid Injection

Jason S. Eldrige

When considering the neuraxial procedures of selective nerve root block (SNRB), epidural steroid injection (ESI), and transforaminal epidural steroid injection (TFESI) is it best to first clarify nomenclature. By definition, a SNRB generally involves targeting of an individual spinal nerve and utilizes a specific technique designed to provide useful diagnostic information (as opposed to a longer-lasting therapeutic effect). The goal is to precisely identify which spinal nerve is responsible for causing painful symptoms, typically in the context of understanding what sort of surgical intervention will be most helpful to the patient. As such, there needs to be careful consideration of precision and procedural specificity; the interventionalist must use a method to target an identified spinal nerve and ONLY that identified nerve. The first step is applying appropriate skill using guidance to deploy the needle safely to the nerve root of interest, including demonstration of anticipated medication spread with contrast along the nerve root up to the lateral foraminal opening without evidence of more medial epidural transgression which would allow medication exposure to additional adjacent anatomy. A further consideration is constraining injection volume to minimize spread to adjacent anatomy (often 0.5 cc or less) and utilizing medication types that are focal in their mechanism of action (potent local anesthetic, such as 2% lidocaine, instead of steroid which may have broad/systemic effect). Lastly, though the needle is typically more laterally located and less obliquely angulated than traditional TFESI technique (see below), it is important to follow the same safety protocols to avoid transgression of blood vessels which may perfuse the spinal cord. Failure to consider these factors will at a minimum decrease the specificity of the procedure, thereby reducing its clinical utility.

ESI and TFESI may be considered together, despite technical differences and unique safety considerations, since the goal of steroid-containing neuraxial procedure is primarily therapeutic instead of diagnostic. ESI generally refers to a midline or parasagittal needle placement between spinal laminae, whereas TFESI directs the needle to the lateral foraminal opening with a goal of targeting a specific spinal nerve or nerves with medication spread that travels medially through the foramen and into the epidural space. Given these technical considerations, ESI generally deposits medication in the dorsal epidural space and may facilitate "bilateral" epidural medication spread patterns. Distinctly, TFESI aims at more precise anatomic localization to facilitate medication spread into the ipsilateral and ventral epidural space, which includes the spinal nerve DRG and also often the area of physical contact from a disc or other impinging/sensitizing anatomy. The unique needle positioning of a TFESI requires unfaltering adherence to certain safeguards to ensure the most effective and safe outcomes. Particular attention is given to needle positioning in the dorsal aspect of the foramen primarily to avoid radicular medullary arteries which anastomose with segmental blood supply to the cord parenchyma via the anterior spinal artery. Mitigation of this concern is further assured by the location of the needle being lateral to the pedicular midpoint in AP fluoroscopic views (which also minimizes risk of inadvertent intrathecal spread) and use of a 2% lidocaine test dose and gross neurological testing prior to steroid administration. Consideration of using digital subtraction angiography prior to steroid administration is an additional safety factor worthy of consideration for TFESI.

In closing, let me pass along a few words of wisdom imparted to me during my own residency training from a prominent anesthesiologist and regional proceduralist. While performing a routine intercostal nerve block, Dr. DW advised to aspirate every 2 cc aliquot—her point was not about systemic toxicity, but rather about something much more philosophically expansive and clinically important. The rationale, and further discussion that ensued, highlighted the necessity for developing best practice habits which are adhered to with absolute consistency.The self-discipline, and intentionality, to demand exacting technique and be meticulously attentive to detail for all procedures performed (no matter how simple or routine an individual procedure may appear) ensures that the highest standard of care is always maintained, even when tired, post-call, or responding to a stressful/unexpected situation. Aspiring to Dr. DW's sage advice has served me well, and I hope "paying it forward" provides a modicum of benefit to other providers committed to offering their absolute best to patients every day.

Regenerative Treatment Options for Tendinopathy

Yashar Eshraghi

Tendinopathies are common conditions treated in chronic pain clinics in both athletic and elderly patient populations. The resulting pain and functional deterioration due to tendinopathy can have a significant negative impact on patients' ability to exercise and work. This condition is caused by repetitive microtrauma resulting in failure of tendon cells to regenerate normal tendon tissue. Histological findings showed necrotic tenocytes, collagen disarray, and neovascularization in injured tendons [62]. Common standard treatment includes the use of the PRICE principle: Protection, Rest, Ice/cold, Compression, and Elevation. Other traditional treatment options include rehabilitation programs, analgesics/nonsteroidal anti-inflammatory drugs (NSAIDs), corticosteroid injections, and surgical interventions [63]. Historical and recent evidence increasingly refute the commonly used treatments for tendinopathies [64]. The application of regenerative biological treatments for ailments of the musculoskeletal system emerged in the 1930s [65]. The purpose of regenerative medicine is to heal a pathologic process by augmenting the body's physiology by nature or by means of bioengineering. In contrast to conventional steroid injections, which are used to modulate pain, these emerging options are being explored to eliminate/minimize degenerative tissue changes and to encourage regeneration [66]. The current practice of regenerative medicine encompasses prolotherapy and biological agents [67]. The most common chemical procedure is called prolotherapy, where an irritant such as dextrose or other chemicals is used to initiate an inflammatory cascade, which is considered to enable a healing process [68]. Biological agents include autologous agents such as platelet-rich plasma (PRP), various types of cells (mainly stem cells from bone marrow and adipose), or tissue derived from placenta [69].

Platelet-rich plasma is obtained by centrifugation of autologous blood and collecting concentrated platelets in plasma. It is considered to apply regenerative effect by targeted delivery of growth factors and is a promising new treatment for refractory tendinopathy [65]. Currently, the best indication is chronically painful tendinopathy that has failed to improve despite proper conservative therapy [65]. Currently, the strongest evidence for the efficacy of PRP remains for common extensor tendinopathy and patellar tendinopathy [70]. However, the evidence for the benefit of PRP for Achilles, rotator cuff, gluteal, and proximal hamstring tendinopathies is limited and sometimes controversial [70]. Several factors need to be considered to optimize the outcome of PRP injection. Current research suggests that age, platelet counts with leukocytes, and pH of the injected product may play an important role in optimizing the results of PRP [67]. The use of stem cells in tendon injury treatment is relatively new and is inspired by in vitro research that mesenchymal stem cells may differentiate into tenocytes, but clinical studies are inconsistent [64]. Stem cells can be obtained from bone marrow, adipose tissue, or skin [69].

Research in this field has been progressing rapidly though there remains much controversy surrounding the efficacy of these therapies, as few large randomized controlled trials (RCTs) exist [64]. The emerging evidence for prolotherapy, PRP, cellular injections, and, more recently, exosomes have added novel options that appear to be safe and potentially effective, which patients can consider prior to contemplating an invasive surgical intervention [66]. Large variability in procedural protocol should be standardized. However, for such standardization, well-designed studies need to be continued to characterize targeted and individualized regenerative treatments for tendinopathies [63].

Sympathetic Blocks

Sahil Gupta

The sympathetic nervous system has been connected to multiple types of pain syndromes ranging from neuropathic pain to visceral pain to complex regional pain syndrome [71]. Blockade of the corresponding sympathetic ganglia has become a common mode of treatment for diagnosing and treating sympathetically mediated pain. If the patient experiences pain relief from an initial local anesthetic blockade, then neurolysis or neuromodulation can be performed to provide long-term pain relief [72].

Multiple sympathetic ganglia including the sphenopalatine, stellate, paravertebral (thoracic and lumbar), celiac plexus, superior hypogastric plexus, and ganglion impar are targeted by pain physicians for a variety of pain-related conditions [73]. These ganglions are targeted with the help of imaging techniques including ultrasonography and fluoroscopy [73]. The first step in management of sympathetically mediated pain is to have an accurate diagnosis for such conditions. This is the most challenging step at times because of the nebulous and varying presentation of such pain. Sympathetically mediated pain can present with allodynia, muscle atrophy and loss of function, abnormal circulation, and temperature and sweat pattern changes. Diagnosing such conditions can be difficult as these symptoms mimic various other disorders [74].

Sympathetically mediated pain can be helped in its initial stages with conservative measures including physical therapy, psychological therapy, and medications. If the above treatment measures are unsuccessful, then interventions like sympathetic blocks and neuromodulation are considered [75, 76]. Injection of local anesthetic for a sympathetic block was first described more than a century ago when a temporary sphenopalatine block was performed in 1908 for chronic headache syndrome by Sluder et al., and by 1912, reports of neurolysis with phenol for prolonged relief were published [77]. Since then, various sympathetic ganglion targets have been identified and successfully treated with the use of local anesthetics like lidocaine, bupivacaine, and ropivacaine, as well as corticosteroids at times for temporary blockade. Permanent neurolysis with the help of alcohol and phenol is also performed for a more long-term treatment if initial blockade is successful [78].

To perform temporary or permanent blockade of sympathetic ganglions, imaging techniques like fluoroscopy and ultrasonography is used. Safe execution of such injections can only be performed with the help of a detailed understanding of flouroantomy and sonoanatomy. Most of the sympathetic ganglions reside close to important anatomical structures like major blood vessels and, therefore, identification of such structures under ultrasound guidance or recognition of appropriate contrast patterns under fluoroscopy guidance is imperative for ensuring safe outcomes [71, 79]. After a sympathetic block, repeat physical examination is useful in confirmation of an appropriate block by recognizing signs and symptoms like Horner's syndrome in stellate ganglion block, or lower limb temperature changes after a successful lumbar sympathetic block [80].

In conclusion, a high degree of suspicion from a trained pain physician is necessary for early recognition and treatment of sympathetic-mediated pain. Once the decision is made to treat such conditions with sympathetic blocks, a sound anatomical foundation is needed to safely and accurately perform such injections to provide the highest standard of care.

Spinal Facet Procedures: Medial Branch Blocks and Radiofrequency Ablations

Rene Przkora

Rationale

The spinal facet joints can be a common source of spine-related pain. There are options in interventional pain medicine to test the diagnosis as well as to treat this condition. Most common diagnostic injections are medial branch blocks (MBBs) followed by non-surgical radiofrequency ablations (RFAs) of the medial branch nerves if the blocks provided temporary relief. As this approach is one of the most common pain interventions in academic and private practice, pain medicine fellows should be competent in this approach including the cervical, thoracic, and lumbar spine.

The didactic experience can be designed at the discretion of the ACGME-accredited fellowship program. The fellow must perform cervical, thoracic and lumbar facet joint MBBs and RFAs in a lead function in patients with diverse comorbidities under the supervision of a board-certified faculty member over the course of the fellowship year to establish a longitudinal experience. The fellow should receive regular feedback and guidance of her or his progress in compliance with Accreditation Council for Graduate Medical Education (ACGME) Guidelines.

The skill set required to obtain competency in medial branch blocks and radiofrequency ablations can be divided into sub-competencies, as suggested below in the following examples:

Competencies

1. *Clinical Condition and Indications*

This sub-competency entails identification of patients suffering from a possible painful facet joint condition including cervicogenic headaches and axial lumbar back pain. There should be knowledge of the non-interventional diagnostic tools and differentials as well as the underlying anatomy of the corresponding facet joint and the medial branch innervation as potential treatment targets.

Understand the patient's comorbidities and how they can influence the procedures or may reveal a contra-indication. Anticoagulation management (e.g., ASRA Pain Anticoagulation Guidelines) and cardiac or stimulator devices have to be considered and managed appropriately (e.g. Cardiac Defibrillator or Spinal Cord Stimulator Systems).

2. *Principles of Medial Branch Blocks and Radiofrequency Ablations*

Next to the anatomy, understand how to perform the medial branch blocks, for example needle size and the volume of the injectate including adjustments if given for a cervical versus lumbar medial branch block.

Fellows should possess knowledge of the principles of non-surgical ablative procedures including chemical, cryoneurolysis, pulsed, and thermal radiofrequency including cooled RF with focus on thermal neurolysis, as treatment approaches to spinal facet joint pain. Technical knowledge is mandatory about the MBBs and RFAs, and insurance requirements need to be discussed (e.g., one or two successful MBBs prior to RFA for authorization and insurance coverage). Radiofrequency probe size, target temperature, and duration of the lesioning do affect the outcome of RFAs (Table 8.1).

Table 8.1 Modified Table 11 from Guidelines for Clinical Practice—Lumbar MBB and RFA [4]

Factor	Clinical practice
Patient selection	
Failure of conservative treatment	Preferably 3 months, but may be less in certain circumstances (e.g., incapacitating pain with strong suspicion of facetogenic origin, competitive athlete, military deployment)
Injectate volume:	
Medial branch block	≤0.5 mL
Imaging:	
Medial branch block	Fluoroscopy
Contrast	With or without contrast
Sedation	Not routinely
Patient-reported outcomes	
Pain relief cut-off	≥50%, with lower cut-offs considered in certain circumstances (and/or other metrics of improvement achieved, consider insurance requirements of necessary improvements)
Multiple blocks	Not routinely (consider insurance requirements)
Repeat diagnostic MBB for repeat RFA	No
RFA technique	
Stimulation	Motor strongly recommended; sensory at discretion of the physician
Needle size	Large
Temperature	80–90 °C
Duration	At least 1.5 min
Multiple lesions and/or other techniques to increase lesion size	Depends on circumstances

The fellow has to show knowledge of the published guidelines from our pain societies, such as ASRA Pain Medicine and ASIPP.

3. *Equipment and Facilities*

Understanding of and familiarity with the necessary equipment are requisite, including imaging modalities, emergency equipment, and policies. The fellow should demonstrate knowledge of an effective procedure suite/operating room setup to perform MBBs and RFAs.

4. *Preparation and Performing the Intervention*

The fellow has to demonstrate knowledge of the patient, the procedure, and expectations and instructions including obtaining consent, which requires a detailed understanding of the potential complications, ranging from post-ablation neuritis to neurological injury. The fellow has to demonstrate effective communication with the staff involved and their roles, knowledge and practice of setting up a sterile surgical field, patient positioning and monitoring, knowledge of the RFA generator and grounding electrode placement, knowledge and application of fluoroscopic needle guidance and radiation safety principles, sterile working conditions, performance of the procedures, and postoperative monitoring and follow-up.

5. *Compliance and Billing*

The fellow has to understand the documentation and billing requirements for MBBs and RFAs including the number of MBBs necessary per insurance requirements and obtained temporary pain relief.

6. *Outcomes*

The fellow has to demonstrate knowledge of the outcomes of MBBs and RFAs including the capability to formulate these to healthcare professionals as well as laypersons.

Facet joint interventions are well established for spinal facet joint pain with a record of accomplishment of efficacy and safety. Based on the nature of the procedure and the widespread utilization in diverse pain medicine practices, the fellow has to perform these interventions in person under supervision over the fellowship year to gain longitudinal experience including assessment of outcomes and management.

Steroid Injection and Joint Ablation of Large Joints (Shoulder, Hip, Knee)

D. O. Christy Hunt

Chronic joint pain is a prevalent problem, with knee and hip pain among the most common areas of pain in the estimated nearly 245 million patients with chronic pain in the United States [32]. Similar to low back pain, chronic joint pain is associated with disability and mood symptoms [81–83]. Surgery does not always definitively relieve pain symptoms: nearly 40% of patients continue to experience postoperative pain after knee replacement surgery [84], with persistent opioid use following joint surgery of particular concern [85].

When conservative management is inadequate for managing chronic joint pain and surgery is not indicated, interventional pain management should be considered. Herein we will discuss the use of techniques including intra-articular corticosteroid (IACS) injections and radiofrequency ablation (RFA) of the large joints for management of chronic pain of the hip, shoulder, and knee.

Injection of IACS has long been available for the treatment of joint pain due to arthritis including osteoarthritis (OA) and rheumatoid arthritis [86]. Such injections are relatively low risk when appropriate dosage and interval of methylprednisolone equivalents (MPE) are considered, and the physician is adequately trained in the performance of IACS injections. Risks include bleeding, infection, and post- procedural pain [87]. Certain types of anesthetics can be damaging to cartilage, thus the use of the least chondrotoxic agent, ropivacaine, is used in the injectate in combination with steroid [20]. Typically higher particulate steroid is used as this is thought to have longer-lasting effect than non-particulate steroid and there is no clear safety advantage to the use of non-particulate steroid in appendicular joint injections. Steroid injection can be performed with or without image guidance, although the use of ultrasound or fluoroscopy has been associated with better accuracy [88] and less procedural pain [89]. Long- term outcomes in combination with recommended conservative strategies including physical therapy and medications are generally favorable, with guidelines emphasizing the importance of exercise, weight loss, and self-management strategies for long-term improvement. Injection of IACS is generally avoided in the perioperative period, as injection within 3 months prior to joint surgery has been associated with increased risk of postoperative infection [90].

Radiofrequency neurotomy or radiofrequency ablation (RFA) of the hip, shoulder, and knee is a newer technique for the treatment of pain of the native large joint or in patients with chronic postoperative joint pain [91, 92]. This involves the creation of a thermal lesion inducing destruction of key sensory nerves supplying the large joints using image guidance following a positive response to prognostic nerve blocks using local anesthetic [93]. Risks of large joint RFA are rare but include bleeding, infection, and post- procedural pain [94]. In addition, injury to the skin has been described following knee RFA, a greater risk particularly in patients with very thin body habitus where the location of the probe against the periosteal target is very superficial [95]. Research is ongoing to identify optimal candidates for the procedure of RFA in post-surgical patients [96]. Of particular ongoing interest and study is the optimal approach for genicular RFA, given newer anatomical studies suggesting wide variability of the location and distribution of genicular nerves [97].

The Role of Telemedicine as Part of Pain Medicine Care

Terry Hunt II

The Centers for Medicare and Medicaid Services (CMS) announced the expansion of coverage and payment options for telemedicine services in response to the COVID-19 pandemic on March 17, 2020 [98], which rapidly disseminated virtual health services [99]. Telemedicine can be defined as using technologies and telecommunication systems to administer healthcare to patients geographically separated from providers [100]. The implementation of telemedicine in pain medicine practices and its effect on improving the patient experience by addressing social determinants of health and reducing disparities [101] suggests that there should be a role for telemedicine in pain medicine beyond the COVID-19 era.

Despite the limitations of conducting a physical exam virtually, pain medicine healthcare professionals interview, observe, and counsel patients with chronic pain through audiovisual technologies. Telemedicine services include consultations and return visits with established patients (which may necessitate only a limited physical examination), diagnostic tests and imaging review, medication management, pre-procedural education, and e-consults with colleagues. Pain medicine practices have successfully incorporated these virtual offerings [102, 103].

Advantages of telemedicine services in the chronic pain population include increased opportunities to address psychosocial and motivational factors, improved convenience and access to care, and the ability to provide comprehensive evaluations remotely while bridging gaps in medical care [104].

Behavioral and psychosocial support can be effectively provided through virtual clinical interactions. For example, opioid safety education and evidence-based behavioral therapies for chronic pain can be delivered by psychologists and social workers [105] through telemedicine consistent with evidence-based Centers for Disease Control and Prevention (CDC) guidelines [106].

Comprehensive evaluations can be offered through virtual office visits. Multidisciplinary consensus physical examination algorithms exist for headaches and lumbar and cervical pain [107]. Additionally, telemedicine has been used for managing chronic pain by utilizing mobile applications and wearable devices to monitor patient symptoms, physical activity, and adherence to care plans. Telemedicine interventions are at least moderately beneficial concerning patient outcomes [108].

Physical therapy can be offered virtually as an essential component of a pain medicine treatment plan. It has been reported that physical therapy services delivered via telehealth for select patients produced similar outcomes to in-person care with lower direct and indirect costs [109].

Patient satisfaction with telemedicine may be higher than face-to-face encounters when considering transportation challenges, time restrictions, financial limitations, and concerns regarding the medical risk of leaving their homes [110].

Despite the purported benefits of telemedicine in pain medicine practices, there are challenges and barriers to navigate. Commonly reported barriers from the patient's perspective include the need for a fast and stable internet connection, digital literacy, and engagement. Clinician buy-in and acceptance of telemedicine are crucial and often barriers to successful implementation. Commonly cited concerns include difficulties forming a therapeutic bond with the patient and communication challenges resulting in misunderstandings and misinterpretations [108].

The future of the successful integration of telemedicine in pain medicine practices appears promising, assuming the resolution of related regulatory and legal issues. There is potential for telemedicine to enhance patient experience and improve patient outcomes while reducing costs for both the patient and healthcare system— consistent with our collective pursuit of the quadruple aim.

Conclusion

The preceding sections have outlined foundational knowledge for pain medicine fellows and provided a "roadmap" for trainees and programs to consider when acquiring knowledge over the course of a critical year that moves quickly. Facet procedures, epidural steroid injections, and joint procedures are among the most common procedures that are performed or considered by pain physicians, and knowledge of the different types of steroid and local anesthetics, the emerging role of regenerative medicine, and the importance of navigating a successful telemedicine visit in the post-COVID-19 era should all be considered fundamental in the armamentarium of the pain physician. We hope that the preceding section provides a helpful summary of key points for consideration during pain medicine fellowship.

References

1. Crawford R, et al. Diagnostic value of intra-articular anaesthetic in primary osteoarthritis of the hip. J Bone Joint Surg Br. 1998;80(2):279–81.
2. Ravaud P, et al. Effects of joint lavage and steroid injection in patients with osteoarthritis of the knee: results of a multicenter, randomized, controlled trial. Arthritis Rheum. 1999;42(3):475–82.
3. Robinson P, Keenan A-M, Conaghan PG. Clinical effectiveness and dose response of image-guided intra-articular corticosteroid injection for hip osteoarthritis. Rheumatology. 2006;46(2):285–91.
4. Cohen SP, et al. Consensus practice guidelines on interventions for lumbar facet joint pain from a multispecialty, international working group. Reg Anesth Pain Med. 2020;45(6):424–67.
5. Hurley RW, et al. Consensus practice guidelines on interventions for cervical spine (facet) joint pain from a multispecialty international working group. Pain Med. 2021;22(11):2443–524.
6. Khoury NJ, et al. Intraarticular foot and ankle injections to identify source of pain before arthrodesis. Am J Roentgenol. 1996;167(3):669–73.
7. Rhen T, Cidlowski JA. Antiinflammatory action of glucocorticoids—new mechanisms for old drugs. N Engl J Med. 2005;353(16):1711–23.
8. MacMahon PJ, Eustace SJ, Kavanagh EC. Injectable corticosteroid and local anesthetic preparations: a review for radiologists. Radiology. 2009;252(3):647–61.
9. Ostergaard M, Halberg P. Intra-articular corticosteroids in arthritic disease: a guide to treatment. BioDrugs. 1998;9(2):95–103.
10. Nanno M, et al. Flexor pollicis longus rupture in a trigger thumb after intrasheath triamcinolone injections: a case report with literature review. J Nippon Med Sch. 2014;81(4):269–75.
11. Zhang B, Hu ST, Zhang YZ. Spontaneous rupture of multiple extensor tendons following repeated steroid injections: a case report. Orthop Surg. 2012;4(2):118.
12. Houten JK, Errico TJ. Paraplegia after lumbosacral nerve root block: report of three cases. Spine J. 2002;2(1):70–5.
13. Ludwig MA, Burns SP. Spinal cord infarction following cervical transforaminal epidural injection: a case report. Spine. 2005;30(10):E266–8.
14. Muro K, O'shaughnessy B, Ganju A. Infarction of the cervical spinal cord following multilevel transforaminal epidural steroid injection: case report and review of the literature. J Spinal Cord Med. 2007;30(4):385–8.
15. Suresh S, Berman J, Connell DA. Cerebellar and brainstem infarction as a complication of CT-guided transforaminal cervical nerve root block. Skeletal Radiol. 2007;36:449–52.

16. Gharibo CG, et al. Conus medullaris infarction after a right L4 transforaminal epidural steroid injection using dexamethasone. Pain Physician. 2016;19(8):E1211.

17. Smith CC, et al. The effectiveness of lumbar transforaminal injection of steroid for the treatment of radicular pain: a comprehensive review of the published data. Pain Med. 2020;21(3):472–87.

18. El-Yahchouchi C, et al. The noninferiority of the nonparticulate steroid dexamethasone vs the particulate steroids betamethasone and triamcinolone in lumbar transforaminal epidural steroid injections. Pain Med. 2013;14(11):1650–7.

19. Dreyfuss P, Baker R, Bogduk N. Comparative effectiveness of cervical transforaminal injections with particulate and nonparticulate corticosteroid preparations for cervical radicular pain. Pain Med. 2006;7(3):237–42.

20. Jayaram P, et al. Chondrotoxic effects of local anesthetics on human knee articular cartilage: a systematic review. PM&R. 2019;11(4):379–400.

21. Dahl J, et al. The effect of 0.5% ropivacaine on epidural blood flow. Acta Anaesthesiol Scand. 1990;34(4):308–10.

22. Souzdalnitski D. Regenerative medicine: invigorating pain management practice. Tech Reg Anesth Pain Manag. 2015;1(19):1–2.

23. DiMarino AM, Caplan AI, Bonfield TL. Mesenchymal stem cells in tissue repair. Front Immunol. 2013;4:201.

24. Rodríguez-Fuentes DE, et al. Mesenchymal stem cells current clinical applications: a systematic review. Arch Med Res. 2021;52(1):93–101.

25. Caplan AI, Correa D. The MSC: an injury drugstore. Cell Stem Cell. 2011;9(1):11–5.

26. Demetriades AK, Orpen NM. Unproven regenerative medicine "therapies" in spine. Pain Pract. 2020;21(5):607.

27. Krut Z, et al. Stem cells and exosomes: new therapies for intervertebral disc degeneration. Cells. 2021;10(9):2241.

28. Amirdelfan K, et al. Allogeneic mesenchymal precursor cells treatment for chronic low back pain associated with degenerative disc disease: a prospective randomized, placebo-controlled 36-month study of safety and efficacy. Spine J. 2021;21(2):212–30.

29. Tamrakar M, et al. Completeness and quality of low back pain prevalence data in the global burden of disease study 2017. BMJ Glob Health. 2021;6(5):e005847.

30. Fatoye F, Gebrye T, Odeyemi I. Real-world incidence and prevalence of low back pain using routinely collected data. Rheumatol Int. 2019;39:619–26.

31. Cohen SP, Vase L, Hooten WM. Chronic pain: an update on burden, best practices, and new advances. Lancet. 2021;397(10289):2082–97.

32. Yong RJ, Mullins PM, Bhattacharyya N. Prevalence of chronic pain among adults in the United States. Pain. 2022;163(2):e328–32.

33. Fayaz A, et al. Prevalence of chronic pain in the UK: a systematic review and meta-analysis of population studies. BMJ Open. 2016;6(6):e010364.

34. Santos EDS, et al. Prevalence of low back pain and associated risks in school-age children. Pain Manag Nurs. 2021;22(4):459–64.

35. Hoy D, et al. The global burden of low back pain: estimates from the global burden of disease 2010 study. Ann Rheum Dis. 2014;73(6):968–74.

36. Meucci RD, Fassa AG, Faria NMX. Prevalence of chronic low back pain: systematic review. Rev Saude Publica. 2015;49:73.

37. Wong CK, et al. Prevalence, incidence, and factors associated with non-specific chronic low back pain in community-dwelling older adults aged 60 years and older: a systematic review and meta-analysis. J Pain. 2022;23(4):509–34.

38. Jantarada C, Silva C, Guimarães-Pereira L. Prevalence of problematic use of opioids in patients with chronic noncancer pain: a systematic review with meta-analysis. Pain Pract. 2021;21(6):715–29.

39. Edwards J, et al. Prevalence of low back pain in emergency settings: a systematic review and meta-analysis. BMC Musculoskelet Disord. 2017;18:1–12.

40. Fett D, Trompeter K, Platen P. Prevalence of back pain in a group of elite athletes exposed to repetitive overhead activity. PLoS One. 2019;14(1):e0210429.
41. Schneider BJ, et al. The effectiveness of intradiscal biologic treatments for discogenic low back pain: a systematic review. Spine J. 2022;22(2):226–37.
42. Zielinski MA, et al. Safety and efficacy of platelet rich plasma for treatment of lumbar discogenic pain: a prospective, multicenter, randomized, double-blind study. Pain Physician. 2022;25(1):29.
43. Ruiz-Lopez R, Tsai YC. A randomized double-blind controlled pilot study comparing leucocyte-rich platelet-rich plasma and corticosteroid in caudal epidural injection for complex chronic degenerative spinal pain. Pain Pract. 2020;20(6):639–46.
44. Xu Z, et al. Ultrasound-guided transforaminal injections of platelet-rich plasma compared with steroid in lumbar disc herniation: a prospective, randomized, controlled study. Neural Plast. 2021;2021(1):5558138.
45. Tuakli-Wosornu YA, et al. Lumbar intradiskal platelet-rich plasma (PRP) injections: a prospective, double-blind, randomized controlled study. PM&R. 2016;8(1):1–10.
46. Sakai D, Schol J, Watanabe M. Clinical development of regenerative medicine targeted for intervertebral disc disease. Medicina. 2022;58(2):267.
47. Won SJ, Kim D-Y, Kim JM. Effect of platelet-rich plasma injections for chronic nonspecific low back pain: a randomized controlled study. Medicine. 2022;101(8):e28935.
48. Bise S, et al. Comparison of interlaminar CT-guided epidural platelet-rich plasma versus steroid injection in patients with lumbar radicular pain. Eur Radiol. 2020;30:3152–60.
49. Wu J, et al. A prospective study comparing platelet-rich plasma and local anesthetic (LA)/corticosteroid in intra-articular injection for the treatment of lumbar facet joint syndrome. Pain Pract. 2017;17(7):914–24.
50. Singla V, et al. Steroid vs. platelet-rich plasma in ultrasound-guided sacroiliac joint injection for chronic low back pain. Pain Pract. 2017;17(6):782–91.
51. Hazazi A. Platelet-rich plasma for refractory coccydynia: a case report. J Spine Pract. 2021;1(1):44.
52. Montero-Cruz F, Aydin S. Platelet-rich plasma injection therapy for refractory Coccydynia: a case series. Interv Pain Manag Rep. 2018;2(5):183–8.
53. Hauser RA, et al. Lumbar instability as an etiology of low back pain and its treatment by prolotherapy: a review. J Back Musculoskelet Rehabil. 2022;35(4):701–12.
54. Kim WM, et al. A randomized controlled trial of intra-articular prolotherapy versus steroid injection for sacroiliac joint pain. J Altern Complement Med. 2010;16(12):1285–90.
55. Yelland MJ, et al. Prolotherapy injections, saline injections, and exercises for chronic low-back pain: a randomized trial. LWW; 2004.
56. Giordano L, Murrell WD, Maffulli N. Prolotherapy for chronic low back pain: a review of literature. Br Med Bull. 2021;138(1):96–111.
57. Centeno CJ, et al. A multi-center analysis of adverse events among two thousand, three hundred and seventy two adult patients undergoing adult autologous stem cell therapy for orthopaedic conditions. Int Orthop. 2016;40:1755–65.
58. Cheng J, et al. Treatment of symptomatic degenerative intervertebral discs with autologous platelet-rich plasma: follow-up at 5–9 years. Regen Med. 2019;14(9):831–40.
59. Levi D, et al. Intradiscal platelet-rich plasma injection for chronic discogenic low back pain: preliminary results from a prospective trial. Pain Med. 2016;17(6):1010–22.
60. McDonnell JM, et al. Regenerative medicine modalities for the treatment of degenerative disk disease. Clin Spine Surg. 2021;34(10):363–8.
61. Noriega DC, et al. Treatment of degenerative disc disease with allogeneic mesenchymal stem cells: long-term follow-up results. Transplantation. 2021;105(2):e25–7.
62. Neph A, Onishi K, Wang JH. Myths and facts of in-office regenerative procedures for tendinopathy. Am J Phys Med Rehabil. 2019;98(6):500–11.
63. Barnett J, et al. The effects of regenerative injection therapy compared to corticosteroids for the treatment of lateral epicondylitis: a systematic review and meta-analysis. Arch Physiother. 2019;9:12.

64. Pas H, et al. No evidence for the use of stem cell therapy for tendon disorders: a systematic review. Br J Sports Med. 2017;51(13):996–1002.
65. Filardo G, et al. Platelet-rich plasma in tendon-related disorders: results and indications. Knee Surg Sports Traumatol Arthrosc. 2018;26:1984–99.
66. Carayannopoulos A, et al. Prolotherapy versus corticosteroid injections for the treatment of lateral epicondylosis: a randomized controlled trial. PM&R. 2011;3(8):706–15.
67. Dhillon MS, et al. Orthobiologics and platelet rich plasma. Indian J Orthop. 2014;48(1):1–9.
68. Baraniak PR, McDevitt TC. Stem cell paracrine actions and tissue regeneration. Regen Med. 2010;5(1):121–43.
69. Lalu MM, et al. Safety of cell therapy with mesenchymal stromal cells (SafeCell): a systematic review and meta-analysis of clinical trials. PLoS One. 2012;7(10):e47559.
70. Centeno C, et al. Efficacy of autologous bone marrow concentrate for knee osteoarthritis with and without adipose graft. Biomed Res Int. 2014;2014:370621.
71. Baig S, Moon JY, Shankar H. Review of sympathetic blocks: anatomy, sonoanatomy, evidence, and techniques. Reg Anesth Pain Med. 2017;42(3):377–91.
72. Day M. Sympathetic blocks: the evidence. Pain Pract. 2008;8(2):98–109.
73. Chaturvedi A, Dash HH. Sympathetic blockade for the relief of chronic pain. J Indian Med Assoc. 2001;99(12):698–703.
74. Wasner G, et al. Complex regional pain syndrome–diagnostic, mechanisms, CNS involvement and therapy. Spinal Cord. 2003;41(2):61–75.
75. Charlton JE. Management of sympathetic pain. Br Med Bull. 1991;47(3):601–18.
76. Perez RS, et al. Treatment of reflex sympathetic dystrophy (CRPS type 1): a research synthesis of 21 randomized clinical trials. J Pain Symptom Manag. 2001;21(6):511–26.
77. Lyman HW, XV. Some sphenopalatine syndromes: a review of Sluder's observations on the sphenopalatine ganglion. Ann Otol Rhinol Laryngol. 1936;45(2):362–72.
78. Gungor S, Aiyer R, Baykoca B. Sympathetic blocks for the treatment of complex regional pain syndrome: a case series. Medicine (Baltimore). 2018;97(19):e0705.
79. Ryu JH, et al. Ultrasound-assisted versus fluoroscopic-guided lumbar sympathetic ganglion block: a prospective and randomized study. Anesth Analg. 2018;126(4):1362–8.
80. Cheng J, et al. Outcomes of sympathetic blocks in the management of complex regional pain syndrome: a retrospective cohort study. Anesthesiology. 2019;131(4):883–93.
81. Fujii T, et al. Disability due to knee pain and somatising tendency in Japanese adults. BMC Musculoskelet Disord. 2018;19(1):23.
82. Martinez-Calderon J, et al. The association between pain beliefs and pain intensity and/or disability in people with shoulder pain: a systematic review. Musculoskelet Sci Pract. 2018;37:29–57.
83. Hampton SN, et al. Pain catastrophizing, anxiety, and depression in hip pathology. Bone Joint J. 2019;101(7):800–7.
84. Drosos GI, et al. Persistent post-surgical pain and neuropathic pain after total knee replacement. World J Orthop. 2015;6(7):528–36.
85. Degen RM, et al. Persistent post-operative opioid use following hip arthroscopy is common and is associated with pre-operative opioid use and age. Knee Surg Sports Traumatol Arthrosc. 2021;29(8):2437–45.
86. Benedek TG. History of the development of corticosteroid therapy. Clin Exp Rheumatol. 2011;29(5 Suppl 68):5–12.
87. Ayub S, et al. Efficacy and safety of multiple intra-articular corticosteroid injections for osteoarthritis-a systematic review and meta-analysis of randomized controlled trials and observational studies. Rheumatology (Oxford). 2021;60(4):1629–39.
88. Hoeber S, et al. Ultrasound-guided hip joint injections are more accurate than landmark-guided injections: a systematic review and meta-analysis. Br J Sports Med. 2016;50(7):392–6.
89. Sibbitt WL Jr, et al. Does sonographic needle guidance affect the clinical outcome of intraarticular injections? J Rheumatol. 2009;36(9):1892–902.

90. Kolasinski SL, et al. 2019 American College of Rheumatology/Arthritis Foundation guideline for the management of osteoarthritis of the hand, hip, and knee. Arthritis Care Res (Hoboken). 2020;72(2):149–62.
91. Kallas ON, et al. Cooled radiofrequency ablation for chronic joint pain secondary to hip and shoulder osteoarthritis. Radiographics. 2022;42(2):594–608.
92. Davis T, et al. Prospective, multicenter, randomized, crossover clinical trial comparing the safety and effectiveness of cooled radiofrequency ablation with corticosteroid injection in the management of knee pain from osteoarthritis. Reg Anesth Pain Med. 2018;43(1):84–91.
93. Eckmann MS, et al. Peripheral joint radiofrequency ablation. Phys Med Rehabil Clin N Am. 2022;33(2):519–31.
94. Zhang H, et al. Efficacy and safety of radiofrequency ablation for treatment of knee osteoarthritis: a meta-analysis of randomized controlled trials. J Int Med Res. 2021;49(4): 3000605211006647.
95. McCormick ZL, et al. The safety of genicular nerve radiofrequency ablation. Pain Med. 2021;22(2):518–9.
96. Cheppalli N, et al. Safety and efficacy of genicular nerve radiofrequency ablation for management of painful total knee replacement: a systematic review. Cureus. 2021;13(11):e19489.
97. McCormick ZL, et al. Technical considerations for genicular nerve radiofrequency ablation: optimizing outcomes. Reg Anesth Pain Med. 2021;46(6):518–23.
98. Medicare CF, Services M. Medicare telemedicine health care provider fact sheet; 2020.
99. Hunt TL 2nd, Hooten WM. The effects of COVID-19 on telemedicine could outlive the virus. Mayo Clin Proc Innov Qual Outcomes. 2020;4(5):583–5.
100. Catalyst N. What is telehealth? NEJM Catal. 2018;4(1)
101. Simon DA, Shachar C. Telehealth to address health disparities: potential, pitfalls, and paths ahead. J Law Med Ethics. 2021;49(3):415–7.
102. Tauben DJ, et al. Optimizing telehealth pain care after COVID-19. Pain. 2020;161(11): 2437–45.
103. Alter BJ, et al. The use of telemedicine to support interventional pain care: case series and commentary. Pain Med. 2021;22(12):2802–5.
104. Emerick T, et al. Telemedicine for chronic pain in the COVID-19 era and beyond. Pain Med. 2020;21(9):1743–8.
105. Chen JA, et al. Telehealth and rural-urban differences in receipt of pain Care in the Veterans Health Administration. Pain Med. 2022;23(3):466–74.
106. Dowell D, Haegerich TM, Chou R. CDC guideline for prescribing opioids for chronic pain—United States, 2016. JAMA. 2016;315(15):1624–45.
107. Wahezi SE, et al. An algorithmic approach to the physical exam for the pain medicine practitioner: a review of the literature with multidisciplinary consensus. Pain Med. 2022;23(9):1489–529.
108. Fernandes LG, et al. At my own pace, space, and place: a systematic review of qualitative studies of enablers and barriers to telehealth interventions for people with chronic pain. Pain. 2022;163(2):e165–81.
109. Bailey V. Telehealth use yields successful post-op physical therapy results; 2021 [cited 2022 06/12]. Available from: https://www.techtarget.com/virtualhealthcare/news/366596705/Telehealth-Use-Yields-Successful-Post-Op-Physical-Therapy-Results.
110. Brown J, et al. In a pandemic that limits contact, can videoconferencing enable interdisciplinary persistent pain services and what are the patient's perspectives? Arch Phys Med Rehabil. 2022;103(3):418–23.

Surgical Interventions and Emerging Procedures in Pain Medicine

9

Rene Przkora, Joshua Pan, Sanjeev Kumar, Juan Mora, Ivan Samcam, Matthew Meroney, Tian Yu, Lee Tian, Joe Donnelly, and Magdalena Anitescu

Abbreviations

ACGME	Accreditation Council for Graduate Medical School
CGRP	Calcitonin gene-related peptide
CRPS	Complex Regional Pain syndrome
CSF	Cerebrospinal fluids
DRG	Dorsal root ganglion
EPG	External pulse generator
FBSS	Failed back surgery syndrome
GABA	Gamma-aminobutyric acid
IDDS	Intrathecal drug delivery system
IPG	Implantable pulse generator
LBP	Lumbar Back pain
LIS	Lumbar interspinous space

R. Przkora · S. Kumar · J. Mora · M. Meroney
Department of Anesthesiology, University of Florida College of Medicine, Gainesville, FL, USA
e-mail: rprzkora@anest.ufl.edu; skumar@anest.ufl.edu; jmora@anest.ufl.edu; mmeroney@anest.ufl.edu

J. Pan (✉)
University of Chicago, Department of Anesthesiology and Critical Care, Chicago, IL, USA

Department of Anesthesia and Critical Care, University of Chicago, Chicago, IL, USA
e-mail: jcpan@uchicagomedicine.org; jcpan@bsd.uchicago.edu

I. Samcam
Neuroscience and Spine associates P.L., Naples, FL, USA
e-mail: isamcam@apmss.net

T. Yu · L. Tian · J. Donnelly · M. Anitescu
Department of Anesthesia & Critical Care, University of Chicago Medicine, Chicago, IL, USA
e-mail: tian.yu@uchicagomedicine.org; lee.tian@uchicagomedicine.org; joseph.donnelly@uchicagomedicine.org; manitescu@bsd.uchicago.edu

© The Author(s), under exclusive license to Springer Nature Switzerland AG 2025
M. Anitescu (ed.), *Multidisciplinary Pain Medicine Fellowship*,
https://doi.org/10.1007/978-3-031-88357-6_9

201

LSS   Lumbar Spinal stenosis
MAC   Monitored anesthesia care
MILD   Minimally invasive Lumbar decompression
MRI   Magnetic resonance imaging
OVF   osteoporotic vertebral fracture
PMMA   polymethylmethacrylate
SCS   Spinal cord stimulation
SI   Sacroiliac
WDR   Wide dynamic Range

Introduction

Pain medicine unifies a broad spectrum of therapies to treat patients suffering from pain, ranging from integrative, medication, rehabilitative, and interventional approaches. One of our main advances is in the area of procedures and surgeries to treat pain. As we pain physicians have a very unique skill set and we provide longitudinal care for our patients, these advanced interventions are well embedded in our scope of practice. The fellow has to demonstrate proficiency in these procedures if there is an intent to practice them independently after graduation. The curriculum can be designed flexible to adjust to the circumstances of each individual fellowship. The curriculum should have didactic sessions and "hands-on" experiences. The "cross skill" set between most of the advanced interventions will aid tremendously in providing the necessary skill set. For example, many interventions require fluoroscopic guidance and/or tissue handling ranging from incision to dissection to hemostasis and layered wound closures.

This document contains suggestions of a curricula and educational experiences for the fellows to obtain the skill set to practice some or all of the advanced interventions independently at the end of their fellowship year.

We divided this chapter into a General Section and Specific Sections addressing certain interventions such as neuromodulation or intrathecal drug delivery.

Excursion: Definition Procedure versus Surgery:

One acceptable distinction is that "surgery" does require an incision, whereas a "procedure" does not. It is important to understand that an "incision" does not necessarily imply a riskier intervention or requiring a "higher" skill set.

General Section

Educational Approach to Advanced Procedures Surgeries and Competencies

Competency in the advanced pain interventions and surgeries such as lumbar decompressions (minimally invasive including endoscopically guided), implants, ablations, and fusions can be obtained employing a multilayered approach at the discretion of the ACGME-approved pain medicine fellowship program. Structured didactics including in-person or as independent study assignments as well as informal discussions are acceptable to gain subject knowledge.

Simulation can be used to supplement educational experience, for example, a simulation of a "patient consent" discussion or "emergency–code scenarios." Educational events provided by our pain societies such as ASRA Pain are acceptable in adding knowledge. Events sponsored by the industry or societies which are heavily depending on industry sponsoring should only be considered if the content has been reviewed by the ACGME-approved fellowship program faculty. It is recommended that the presenters of these events do not have any financial relationship to the sponsoring industry or device manufacturer (e.g., consultant or advisor to the device manufacturer). The application of the learned knowledge will happen in direct patient interactions; the longitudinal care provided to patients will assess the outcomes and will guide initiation of appropriate therapies pending patient's clinical coursse.

The manual skill set ("hands-on" experience) to perform advanced interventions safely and successfully can only be learned by direct patient care. Educational laboratories (cadaver and/or mannequin) can assist in this process, especially before the direct patient interaction to re-enforce the knowledge and gain familiarity with the necessary surgical tools or suturing techniques. However, these educational laboratories cannot replace the direct experience with patients.

Of note, especially the interactions with patients (clinic and procedure suite or operating room) should always happen under the supervision of a pain medicine board–certified faculty (e.g., American Board of Anesthesiology) as outlined in the ACGME guidelines about supervisory requirements. This supervision should be "direct" initially and can transition to "indirect" supervision per ACMG guidelines as the fellow demonstrates progress in his/her skill acquirement.

"Direct" supervision: The supervising physician is physically present with the fellow during the key portions of the patient interaction.

"Indirect" supervision: The supervising physician is not providing physical or concurrent visual or audio supervision but is immediately available to the fellow for guidance and is available to provide appropriate direct supervision. (ACGME).

Regular structured and informal feedback about the performance of the fellow and the progress is crucial to ensure a successful transition to independent practice by the end of the fellowship year.

Determinants of competency of each intervention are multitude of longitudinal experiences specific for a certain intervention as well as cross skills, which all should be considered when reviewing a fellow. The ultimate decision depends on the individual fellowship program as there are no specific guidelines (e.g., numbers) by the ACGME.

Indication of the Intervention

The fellow has to understand the clinical presentation of the patient in total as well as differentials. Appropriate diagnostic tools have to be employed including imaging. He/she has to formulate long-term expectations and options given the diverse portfolio of interventions we have in pain medicine. Additionally, Appropriate consultations and referrals should be ordered for surgical interventions in patients with acute neurological deficits. A multidisciplinary approach has to be integrated into the long-term care plan for our patients to maximize the outcomes of our interventions.

Patient Preparation for the Intervention

Knowledge of the entire medical history of the patient is vital. Discussion of the alternative therapy options, risks, benefits, and expectations including temporary or permanent postoperative restrictions is crucial in the indication, and finally, the consent process. The fellow has to demonstrate his/her competency under supervision until he/she can transition to be independent. Knowledge of the patient and the planned intervention will guide the fellow to make appropriate decisions regarding perioperative care, need for admission or anesthesiology services, and management of already implanted devices such as cardiac rhythm devices and stimulator systems. Postoperative management has to be discussed with the patient and his/her caregivers/family including postoperative pain control and monitoring for complications and contact management. Infection is one risk factor of our interventions and appropriate guidelines should be followed. A preoperative, intraoperative, and postoperative infection prophylaxis protocol should be implemented based on the guidelines of our pain societies such as ASRA Pain. Similar thoughts have to be given to the anticoagulation management of the patient based on his/her comorbidities, and guidelines should be followed, for example, from ASRA Pain or ASIPP.

Performing the Intervention

Appropriate supervision of the fellow as outlined in the ACGME guidelines (Pain Medicine) has to be provided by the training program. The responsible faculty has to have appropriate knowledge and experience in the intervention to be performed. The fellow has to demonstrate knowledge of the facility, and familiarity with resuscitation, emergency equipment, and policies is necessary prior to any intervention. The fellows have to demonstrate appropriate and effective communication with the team involved, for example, with the nursing staff and the surgical and fluoroscopy technicians and anesthesiology as deemed necessary to provide a safe and effective operating room environment. The fellow has to gain competency in setting up the procedure suite, for example, appropriate patient positioning and monitoring of the patient, setup and position of the required imaging equipment, and the sterile field. The fellow has to demonstrate competency in setting up a surgical sterile field and maintain a sterile surgical field throughout the procedure. It is important to recognize the indications of necessary surgical instruments and equipment including tools for incision, hemostasis, suturing materials, and wound closure options. The patient should be educated on appropriate adjustments to the intervention as necessary. For example, the expansion of an intervention or even the abandonment of the intervention pending the intra-operative course if this is in the best interest of the patient.

Cross Skill Set

Cross skills are skills that can be used during the different interventions. These cross skills are general concepts of patient preparation, positioning, operating room setup, staff communication, working in a sterile surgical environment, familiarity with the underlying anatomy, identification of pertinent anatomic points under imaging, setting up and using the endoscope and endoscopic instruments, tissue handling including dissection, hemostasis, "pocket creation," tissue closure, and many more concepts including infection prophylaxis, pain control, and postoperative wound assessment and complication management.

Follow-Up and Outcomes of the Intervention

The fellow has to demonstrate competency in the follow-up of the intervention, including determination of a successful outcome or identification and management of complications. The postoperative period also includes the implementation of eventual postoperative restrictions, even if temporarily.

Summary

Pain medicine and our ACGME-accredited fellowships have a record of accomplishment in procedures and surgeries to treat the most diverse pain conditions. Pain medicine is always on the forefront of developing, teaching, and implementing minimally invasive interventions combined with image-guidance to improve outcomes and safety by minimizing the tissue trauma. In addition, our longitudinal care approach makes pain medicine the most desired specialty to master the interventions and surgeries mentioned. Appropriate curricula for our fellowships and training of our fellows under board-certified pain physicians are therefore mandatory to maintain our excellent expertise.

Special Considerations

Intrathecal Drug Delivery Systems

Introduction

Intrathecal drug delivery systems (IDDS), or intrathecal pumps, are specialized devices designed for the management of chronic pain and severe spasticity by delivering medications directly into the cerebrospinal fluid (CSF) surrounding the spinal cord. This targeted delivery system allows for lower doses of medication, minimizes systemic side effects, and provides significant relief where other treatments have failed. This comprehensive summary explores the technology, mechanism, patient selection, medications, implantation techniques, complications, and MRI compatibility of intrathecal pumps.

Technology Involved

The core technology of intrathecal pumps involves a programmable pump and a catheter that delivers medication directly to the CSF. These pumps are typically implanted under the skin in the abdominal area and are connected by a catheter to the intrathecal space of the spine [1]. Modern pumps are battery-operated and programmable, allowing healthcare providers to adjust the medication dose as needed without further invasive procedures. Advances in pump technology have improved patient outcomes by increasing the precision of drug delivery and reducing the need for frequent surgical interventions [2].

Mechanism of Action

The efficacy of intrathecal pumps is primarily due to their ability to deliver medications directly into the CSF, bypassing the blood-brain barrier and reducing the required dose for pain relief or muscle spasm control. This direct delivery method impacts the pain-signaling pathways at the spinal level, which can lead to significant improvements in symptoms with reduced systemic side effects [2–5].

Patient Selection

Selecting appropriate candidates for intrathecal pump therapy is critical for its success. Ideal candidates are those with chronic pain or spasticity who have not responded to less invasive treatments. Conditions frequently treated with intrathecal pumps include severe chronic pain (non-cancer and cancer-related) and muscle spasticity due to neurological disorders such as multiple sclerosis or spinal cord injury. Prospective patients undergo a comprehensive evaluation including psychological assessment and a trial phase to gauge the potential effectiveness of the therapy before permanent pump implantation [1].

Common Medications Used

The types of medications delivered through an intrathecal pump can vary depending on the patient's condition and specific needs. There are three FDA-approved drugs for ITP: Morphine, Ziconotide, and baclofen. However, many other drugs are used on a regular basis. The most commonly used medications include:

1. Opioids: Morphine, hydromorphone, and fentanyl are the most frequently used opioids in intrathecal therapy. These drugs bind to mu-opioid receptors in the spinal cord, inhibiting the transmission of pain signals. Intrathecal opioids are particularly effective for managing severe cancer pain and chronic non-cancer pain that has not responded to oral or systemic opioids.
2. Local anesthetics: Bupivacaine and ropivacaine are local anesthetics used to block nerve conduction by inhibiting sodium channels. These medications are often used in combination with opioids to enhance pain relief and reduce opioid dosages, minimizing the risk of side effects.
3. Ziconotide: Ziconotide is a non-opioid analgesic derived from cone snail venom that blocks N-type calcium channels, reducing neurotransmitter release and pain transmission. It is used in patients who are intolerant to opioids or who require an alternative treatment for severe chronic pain.
4. Baclofen: Baclofen is a GABA-B receptor agonist used to treat severe spasticity by reducing the release of excitatory neurotransmitters in the spinal cord. Intrathecal baclofen is highly effective in patients with spasticity related to multiple sclerosis, cerebral palsy, or spinal cord injury, providing significant relief with lower doses compared to oral administration.
5. Clonidine: Clonidine is an alpha-2 adrenergic agonist that enhances the analgesic effects of opioids and local anesthetics by modulating pain pathways in the spinal cord. It is often used as an adjunct to other medications in patients with complex pain syndromes [5].

Trial and Implantation Techniques

The trial phase involves temporary intrathecal delivery of medication to confirm the effectiveness and appropriate dosing. Trials can either be done with a single injection of medication in the same fashion as a spinal anesthesia is administered, or a catheter can be placed intrathecally or epidurally with titration of the a medication infusion. If the trial is successful, indicating significant symptom relief with manageable side effects, the permanent pump is then implanted through a surgical procedure. This surgery typically requires general anesthesia and involves placing the pump in the abdomen and the catheter in the intrathecal space connected to the pump [2].

Complications

While intrathecal pumps are generally safe, they are not without risks. Complications can be categorized into surgical, device-related, and medication-related issues.

1. Surgical Complications: These include infection, bleeding, CSF leak, and catheter-related issues such as dislodgement or migration. Infections are a significant concern and can occur at the incision site, catheter entry point, or within

the intrathecal space. Most infections can be managed with antibiotics, but severe cases may require device explantation.
2. Device-Related Complications: These involve hardware issues such as pump malfunction, battery failure, or catheter kinking or breakage. Catheter-related complications can result in inadequate drug delivery, leading to loss of pain control or increased spasticity. Pump malfunctions, although rare, can occur and may require surgical intervention to replace or repair the device.
3. Medication-Related Complications: The use of intrathecal medications can lead to adverse effects, including respiratory depression, overdose, withdrawal symptoms, and neurotoxicity. Careful monitoring of drug dosage and patient response is essential to minimize these risks. Additionally, granuloma formation at the catheter tip can occur with long-term opioid use, potentially leading to catheter occlusion and loss of drug efficacy.
4. Granuloma Formation: Granulomas, which are inflammatory masses that can develop at the catheter tip, are a potential complication of long-term intrathecal opioid therapy. These masses can obstruct drug delivery and lead to loss of pain control. Regular imaging and monitoring are necessary to detect and manage granulomas early.
5. Overdose and Withdrawal: Because intrathecal pumps deliver medication continuously, there is a risk of overdose if the pump malfunctions or is programmed incorrectly. Conversely, abrupt discontinuation of intrathecal therapy can lead to withdrawal symptoms. Clinicians must carefully monitor and adjust drug delivery to avoid these complications [2].

MRI Compatibility

Given the prevalence of MRI in medical diagnostics, compatibility with MRI is essential. Most modern intrathecal pumps are designed to be MRI-conditional, meaning they can withstand certain MRI environments under specific conditions related to the magnetic field strength and type of MRI machine. Patients must consult healthcare providers to ensure MRI compatibility and proper settings of the pump before undergoing an MRI scan [6, 7].

Conclusion

Intrathecal pumps offer a significant improvement in quality of life for patients with severe chronic pain or spasticity, providing a targeted method of drug delivery that is both effective and efficient. Ongoing advancements in technology and a deeper understanding of the optimal application of these devices continue to enhance their efficacy and safety. However, careful patient selection, adherence to trial protocols, and management of potential complications are crucial for the success of intrathecal pump therapy. Healthcare providers must remain vigilant in monitoring these systems to maximize patient benefits and minimize risks.

Lumbar Interspinous Spacers

Introduction
Lumbar interspinous spacers (LIS) are minimally invasive devices used in the management of lumbar spinal stenosis (LSS), a degenerative condition where narrowing of the spinal canal leads to nerve compression, neurogenic claudication, and functional impairment. This condition commonly affects older adults and can significantly impact mobility and quality of life. Lumbar interspinous spacers provide an alternative to traditional decompressive surgeries, such as laminectomy, by offering a less invasive option that is particularly beneficial for patients with significant comorbidities who may not tolerate open surgery well. The primary goal of LIS is to maintain or increase the space between vertebrae, thereby alleviating pressure on spinal nerves and improving symptoms such as pain, numbness, and reduced walking tolerance.

Mechanism of Action
Interspinous spacers function by mechanically distracting the spinous processes of adjacent vertebrae, which increases the dimensions of the intervertebral foramen and the spinal canal. This distraction helps to decompress the neural elements without the need for extensive bone or soft tissue removal, as required in traditional decompressive surgeries. By limiting excessive lumbar extension—a movement that often exacerbates symptoms in patients with LSS—the spacers stabilize the affected spinal segment while preserving the overall biomechanics of the spine. This approach provides relief from neurogenic claudication and allows for improved mobility during activities like walking and standing, which are typically challenging for individuals with LSS [8].

Studies and meta-analyses have shown that interspinous spacers can reduce operation time and lower the likelihood of complications such as dural violations compared to more invasive decompressive surgeries [9]. The ability to perform these procedures under local anesthesia or with light sedation further enhances their appeal for patients with higher surgical risk profiles, making LIS a suitable choice for reducing perioperative risks in a broader range of patients.

Patient Selection
Selecting appropriate patients for interspinous spacer implantation is critical for achieving successful outcomes. Ideal candidates typically include those with mild to moderate lumbar spinal stenosis at one or two vertebral levels. These patients often present with neurogenic claudication that is relieved by forward flexion, such as sitting or leaning forward. Such symptoms are characteristic of lumbar spinal stenosis and are effectively managed by spacers. Patients who may benefit the most are often elderly and have comorbid conditions, such as cardiovascular disease, pulmonary conditions, or are on anticoagulant therapy, which elevate their risk for traditional open surgeries.

Contraindications for spacer use include significant spinal instability, high-grade spondylolisthesis (greater than grade I), multilevel stenosis beyond what can be managed with spacers, and severe osteoporosis, which could compromise the spine's structural integrity. Detailed preoperative imaging, such as MRI and CT scans, is essential to confirm the diagnosis and assess the suitability of the spacer based on the patient's specific anatomical characteristics. This thorough evaluation helps in tailoring the surgical approach to the patient's needs, optimizing the chances of a successful outcome [8].

Intraoperative Techniques
The insertion of lumbar interspinous spacers is typically performed under local anesthesia with sedation or general anesthesia, depending on the patient's health status and preferences. The procedure involves a small midline incision over the affected level of the spine, with minimal dissection required to expose the interspinous ligament. Specialized instruments are used to insert the spacer between the spinous processes, and intraoperative fluoroscopy is employed to confirm correct positioning. This minimally invasive approach is associated with shorter operative times and reduced risks of complications, such as dural tears or cerebrospinal fluid leaks, compared to traditional decompressive surgeries.

One of the key benefits of this procedure is the limited tissue disruption, which often results in quicker recovery times and lower overall morbidity. Patients undergoing spacer placement typically experience less postoperative pain, reduced need for opioid medications, and a faster return to normal activities compared to those undergoing more invasive spinal surgeries. The reduced impact on surrounding tissues also makes LIS an attractive option for patients who are looking for a less intensive intervention with a shorter recovery period [9].

Complications
While lumbar interspinous spacers are generally safe and effective, they are not without potential complications. Issues such as device migration, dislodgement, or fracture can occur, necessitating further intervention. Another consideration is adjacent segment disease, where increased stress on neighboring spinal levels may lead to new symptoms over time. However, these complications are relatively rare, and the overall safety profile of spacers remains favorable, particularly in populations at higher risk for traditional surgical approaches. Compared to open decompressive surgeries, spacers offer benefits such as reduced operation time, lower risk of dural violations, and decreased overall surgical morbidity [9].

Conclusion
Lumbar interspinous spacers offer a minimally invasive alternative for the treatment of lumbar spinal stenosis, especially in patients with significant comorbidities that preclude traditional open surgical options. By providing effective symptom relief with fewer intraoperative risks and a faster recovery, these spacers can greatly improve the quality of life for appropriately selected patients. As with any medical intervention, careful patient selection and thorough preoperative assessment are essential to optimize outcomes. Further research, particularly long-term

comparative studies, will help refine patient selection criteria and enhance the understanding of the spacers' efficacy in managing lumbar spinal stenosis.

Minimally Invasive Lumbar Decompression (MILD)

Introduction

Lumbar spinal stenosis (LSS) is a prevalent condition characterized by the narrowing of the spinal canal, leading to compression of neural and vascular elements in the lumbar spine. It often results in chronic pain, radiating leg pain, and neurogenic claudication, which significantly impair the quality of life. Traditional surgical treatments, such as laminectomy, can be invasive with considerable complications, making minimally invasive procedures an attractive alternative. Minimally invasive lumbar decompression (MILD) is a percutaneous procedure designed to relieve symptoms of LSS by removing portions of the hypertrophied ligamentum flavum, thus enlarging the spinal canal and reducing neural compression. MILD is particularly suitable for patients who are refractory to conservative treatments but are either unfit or unwilling to undergo more invasive surgeries.

Mechanism of Action

The primary goal of MILD is to reduce compression of neural elements by debulking the ligamentum flavum, a common contributor to LSS. The procedure involves the insertion of specialized instruments through a small incision under fluoroscopic guidance. An epidurogram is often used to identify the borders of the dural and epidural spaces, ensuring the safe removal of hypertrophic tissue. By targeting the thickened ligamentum flavum, MILD alleviates nerve compression without significant disruption to the surrounding structures, such as bone or muscles. This approach minimizes postoperative pain and preserves spinal stability, making it a viable option for patients with specific anatomical features of stenosis.

Long-Term Durability

Recent long-term studies have confirmed the durability of MILD over a 5-year follow-up period, demonstrating its efficacy in providing significant pain relief and reducing the need for further surgical interventions. A retrospective study at the Cleveland Clinic included 75 patients who underwent MILD for LSS with hypertrophic ligamentum flavum. The results showed that only 12% of these patients required subsequent open lumbar decompression surgery within 5 years, representing an annual incidence rate of 2.4% [10]. This finding underscores the long-term benefits of MILD, highlighting its ability to significantly reduce the need for more invasive surgeries while providing sustained symptomatic relief.

Additionally, the study reported statistically significant reductions in pain levels and opioid use at 3-, 6-, and 12-months post-procedure, further supporting the effectiveness of MILD in managing chronic pain associated with LSS [10]. The reduced reliance on opioids also suggests potential benefits in terms of quality of life and the broader implications of long-term opioid use in chronic pain management.

Patient Selection

Patient selection is crucial for the success of MILD. Ideal candidates are those with symptomatic LSS presenting with neurogenic claudication who have failed conservative treatments such as physical therapy, oral medications, or epidural steroid injections. Radiologic evidence of lumbar spinal stenosis, such as ligamentum flavum thickness greater than 2.5 mm, supports the use of MILD. Contraindications include prior surgery at the target level, lumbar spondylolisthesis greater than Grade 1, significant symptomatic disc protrusion, and inability to tolerate prone positioning during the procedure. Additionally, patients on anticoagulation therapy or those with bleeding disorders are generally excluded due to the increased risk of complications.

Intraoperative Considerations

The MILD procedure is typically performed under local anesthesia with sedation, which reduces the risks associated with general anesthesia, especially in elderly patients or those with multiple comorbidities. Intraoperatively, fluoroscopy is used to guide the insertion of specialized instruments, such as a bone rongeur and tissue sculptor, to remove hypertrophic ligamentum flavum through a small incision. The use of an epidurogram is recommended in many studies to ensure safe decompression by delineating the epidural space and monitoring the flow of contrast medium. The goal is to achieve sufficient decompression without compromising the integrity of the inner layer of the ligamentum flavum, which helps maintain the structural stability of the spine.

Complications

MILD is associated with a low complication rate, especially compared to more invasive spinal surgeries. Reported complications are typically minor and include localized soreness at the incision site and transient postoperative bleeding. Serious complications such as dural tears, significant hemorrhage, or nerve root injury are rare. The minimally invasive nature of the procedure reduces the risk of postoperative epidural fibrosis and adhesion, which are common issues in more extensive decompressive surgeries. Long-term complications are not well documented due to the relatively recent adoption of MILD, but current evidence suggests that it is a safe and effective option for properly selected patients.

Conclusion

Minimally Invasive Lumbar Decompression represents a valuable addition to the spectrum of treatments available for lumbar spinal stenosis. It offers significant pain relief and functional improvement with minimal risk and invasiveness, making it particularly suitable for patients who are not candidates for open surgery. While the procedure is not without its limitations, including a variable response rate and specific anatomical indications, the benefits of reduced recovery time, lower complication rates, and preservation of spinal stability make MILD a compelling option for many patients with LSS. Ongoing research is needed to further refine patient selection criteria and to compare MILD directly with other minimally invasive spinal interventions.

Neuromodulation: Spinal Cord Stimulation

Introduction
Spinal cord stimulation (SCS) is an established neuromodulation therapy used to manage chronic pain that has been refractory to conventional medical treatments. Since its introduction in the 1960s, SCS has evolved significantly with advancements in technology, patient selection criteria, and implantation techniques. The goal of SCS is to reduce pain, improve the quality of life, and decrease reliance on pain medications.

Technology Involved
The technology behind spinal cord stimulation involves a system that consists of three main components: an implanted pulse generator (IPG), electrodes (leads), and an external controller. The IPG, typically implanted in the gluteal region, generates electrical pulses that are transmitted to the spinal cord via the leads placed in the epidural space. These pulses modulate nerve activity to reduce the perception of pain [11].

Modern SCS devices have evolved to include rechargeable IPGs, feedback loops, multiple stimulation programs, and advanced waveform capabilities such as burst and high-frequency stimulation. Burst stimulation delivers electrical impulses in closely spaced groups followed by pauses, mimicking natural nerve firing patterns, which some studies suggest may be more effective in certain patients. High-frequency stimulation (10 kHz) pioneered pain relief without the paresthesia (tingling sensation) associated with traditional SCS [12]. There are many other waveforms that are paresthesia free.

Mechanism of Action
The exact mechanism by which SCS alleviates pain is not fully understood, but several theories have been proposed. The most widely accepted theory is the Gate Control Theory of Pain, introduced by Melzack and Wall in 1965. According to this theory, SCS works by activating the dorsal columns of the spinal cord, which in turn inhibits the transmission of pain signals through the spinothalamic tract. This process effectively "closes the gate" to pain signals before they reach the brain.

Additionally, SCS may induce the release of inhibitory neurotransmitters like gamma-aminobutyric acid (GABA) and serotonin, contributing to its analgesic effects. Recent research also suggests that SCS may modulate central sensitization and alter pain processing at the cortical level [13].

Patient Selection
Patient selection is crucial for the success of SCS therapy. Ideal candidates are those with chronic, intractable pain that has not responded to conservative treatments,

including physical therapy, medications, and less invasive interventions like nerve blocks. The most common indications for SCS include failed back surgery syndrome (FBSS), complex regional pain syndrome (CRPS), and peripheral neuropathy [11].

A multidisciplinary approach involving pain specialists, neurosurgeons, and psychologists is often employed to assess the suitability of patients for SCS. Psychological evaluation is particularly important, as conditions like depression, anxiety, or unrealistic expectations can negatively impact outcomes. Trial stimulation is a key component of the selection process, where temporary leads are placed to test the efficacy of the stimulation before committing to permanent implantation [14].

Trial and Implantation Technique

The trial phase involves the percutaneous placement of temporary leads in the epidural space under fluoroscopic guidance. The patient typically undergoes a one- to two-week trial period during which pain relief, functional improvement, and any side effects are closely monitored. Success in the trial phase, usually defined as at least a 50% reduction in pain and/or 50% increased functionality, is a prerequisite for permanent implantation [15, 16].

Permanent implantation involves a similar technique, with the placement of leads either percutaneously or through a laminotomy, depending on the specific case and physician preference. The leads are then connected to the IPG, which is implanted subcutaneously, usually in the lower abdomen or buttock. The entire procedure is typically done under local anesthesia with sedation or general anesthesia [17].

Postoperative programming of the IPG is critical, as the device needs to be tailored to the patient's specific pain patterns. Patients can adjust the stimulation settings using an external controller, allowing for individualized pain management.

Complications

While SCS is generally considered safe, it is not without risks. Complications can be categorized into surgical, device-related, and biological.

1. Surgical complications include infection, bleeding, CSF leak, and lead migration. Lead migration, in particular, can lead to loss of efficacy, requiring revision surgery.
2. Device-related complications involve hardware failure, such as battery depletion, lead fractures, or IPG malfunction. Advances in SCS technology, such as improved lead design and longer-lasting batteries, have reduced the incidence of these complications.
3. Biological complications encompass issues like painful stimulation, development of granulomas, or exacerbation of pain. Neuropathic pain at the IPG site, although rare, can also occur.

Infections remain a significant concern, with an incidence rate ranging from 3% to 10%. Most infections are managed with antibiotics, but in severe cases, device explantation may be necessary [18, 19].

MRI Compatibility

Traditionally, one of the major limitations of SCS has been the incompatibility of the implanted devices with magnetic resonance imaging (MRI), a diagnostic tool crucial for patients with chronic pain conditions. The presence of metallic components in the SCS system can lead to significant safety hazards during MRI, including heating of the device, movement of the leads, or image distortion.

However, recent advancements in SCS technology have led to the development of MRI-conditional devices. These devices are designed to be safe under specific MRI conditions, such as limiting the MRI scanner's power and ensuring the device is programmed to MRI-safe settings during the scan. Current MRI-compatible SCS systems allow for full-body scans, which is a significant advancement over earlier systems that restricted scanning to specific areas.

Clinical guidelines now recommend MRI-conditional SCS systems for patients who are likely to require MRI imaging in the future. These systems have undergone rigorous testing to ensure patient safety during MRI procedures, though certain precautions, such as constant monitoring during the scan, are still recommended [20–23].

Conclusion

Spinal cord stimulation has become an invaluable tool in the management of chronic pain, offering a viable option for patients who have exhausted other treatment modalities. The evolution of SCS technology, combined with a thorough understanding of patient selection, trial, and implantation techniques, has significantly improved patient outcomes. However, the potential for complications and the need for MRI compatibility must be carefully considered in the decision-making process. Ongoing research and technological advancements continue to refine the application of SCS, making it an ever more precise and effective therapy for chronic pain management.

Neuromodulation: Dorsal Root Ganglion Stimulation

Introduction

Dorsal root ganglion (DRG) stimulation is a relatively recent advancement in the field of neuromodulation, specifically designed to treat chronic, intractable pain that is often unresponsive to traditional therapies. Introduced in the early 2010s, DRG stimulation has garnered attention for its targeted approach and efficacy in treating conditions such as complex regional pain syndrome (CRPS) and chronic postoperative pain. Unlike spinal cord stimulation (SCS), which modulates pain by targeting the spinal cord, DRG stimulation specifically targets the dorsal root ganglion—a cluster of nerve cell bodies located at the junction of the spinal nerve and spinal cord. This focused approach allows for more precise pain relief, especially in areas that are traditionally difficult to treat.

Technology Involved

The technology behind DRG stimulation is similar in many ways to that of SCS but with some key differences. The DRG stimulation system comprises three main components: a pulse generator (IPG), leads with electrodes, and an external programmer.

1. Implanted Pulse Generator (IPG): The IPG is a battery-powered device that generates electrical pulses. These pulses are delivered to the dorsal root ganglion via the leads and electrodes. Modern IPGs are typically rechargeable and can be programmed to deliver a range of stimulation waveforms, including tonic, burst, and high-frequency stimulation, depending on the patient's needs.
2. Leads and Electrodes: The leads are thin, flexible wires with electrodes at their tips, which are placed near the dorsal root ganglia. Unlike traditional SCS, where the leads are placed in the epidural space, DRG leads are positioned closer to the spinal nerves, allowing for more precise targeting of specific pain areas. DRG leads are much thinner than traditional SCS leads.
3. External Programmer: This device allows the patient and clinician to adjust the stimulation parameters post-implantation. The ability to fine-tune the stimulation is crucial for achieving optimal pain relief while minimizing side effects.

DRG stimulation systems have evolved to include enhanced programming features and more sophisticated leads that minimize migration—a common issue in earlier neuromodulation devices. The ability to precisely target the DRG enables the system to address pain in specific body regions, such as the groin, knee, and foot, which are challenging to manage with SCS. This form of focused energy delivery reduces battery consumption up to 92.5% less than SCS and drastically extending pulse generator lifespan [24].

Mechanism of Action

The dorsal root ganglion plays a critical role in the transmission of sensory signals, including pain, from the peripheral nerves to the central nervous system. By targeting the DRG, this stimulation method can modulate the transmission of pain signals at a very focal level.

The exact mechanism by which DRG stimulation alleviates pain is not fully understood, but several hypotheses have been proposed:

1. Inhibition of Pathological Nerve Activity: Chronic pain is often associated with abnormal, spontaneous nerve activity. DRG stimulation may inhibit this pathological activity by stabilizing the electrical environment around the neurons in the DRG, thereby reducing pain.
2. Neuroplastic Changes: Similar to other forms of neuromodulation, DRG stimulation may induce neuroplastic changes in the nervous system, which can lead to

long-term alterations in pain perception. This effect may be due to the repetitive activation of certain neural pathways, which could reinforce non-painful sensations over time.

3. Modulation of Sensory Transmission: The DRG serves as a gateway for sensory information traveling from the peripheral nerves to the central nervous system. By applying electrical stimulation directly to the DRG, it is believed that the excitability of the neurons within the DRG is altered, which in turn reduces the transmission of pain signals [24, 25].

How It Differs from Spinal Cord Stimulation

While both DRG stimulation and spinal cord stimulation are forms of neuromodulation designed to treat chronic pain, there are key differences between the two modalities:

1. Target Area: The primary difference lies in the target of the stimulation. SCS targets the dorsal columns of the spinal cord, which modulates pain signals in a broad, often diffuse manner. In contrast, DRG stimulation specifically targets the dorsal root ganglia, allowing for more precise, localized pain control.
2. Paresthesia: SCS often produces a tingling sensation known as paresthesia, which overlaps with the painful area. Some patients find this sensation uncomfortable or unpleasant. DRG stimulation, on the other hand, can provide pain relief without paresthesia, which is a significant advantage for many patients.
3. Efficacy in Certain Pain Conditions: DRG stimulation has shown superior efficacy in treating certain types of pain that are difficult to manage with SCS, such as CRPS and pain in areas like the lower limbs and groin. This is likely due to the ability of DRG stimulation to target specific nerve roots that correspond to these pain regions [26].
4. Lead Placement: In SCS, leads are typically placed in the epidural space, while in DRG stimulation, the leads are positioned near the DRG, which is located at the intervertebral foramen. This difference in lead placement contributes to the more targeted nature of DRG stimulation.

Patient Selection

As with any neuromodulation therapy, patient selection is critical to the success of DRG stimulation. Ideal candidates for DRG stimulation are those with chronic, intractable pain that has not responded to conservative treatments such as medications, physical therapy, or less invasive procedures like nerve blocks.

1. Indications: DRG stimulation is particularly effective for treating CRPS, chronic post-surgical pain (such as groin or knee pain following surgery), peripheral causalgia, and neuropathic pain in the lower limbs. It is also considered for patients who have failed SCS therapy or those who require more targeted pain relief than SCS can provide.
2. Psychological Assessment: As with SCS, psychological evaluation is an important part of the patient selection process. Conditions such as depression, anxiety,

or catastrophizing behavior can negatively impact the outcomes of neuromodulation therapies, including DRG stimulation.

3. Trial Stimulation: A successful trial of DRG stimulation is a prerequisite for permanent implantation. During the trial, temporary leads are placed, and the patient is monitored for pain relief, functional improvement, and side effects. Typically, a successful trial is defined as a 50% or greater reduction in pain.

Additionally, patients should have realistic expectations about the therapy and be willing to participate in the trial phase, which is crucial for determining the likelihood of long-term success with DRG stimulation [27].

Trial and Implantation Technique
As with other neuromodulation therapies, DRG stimulation involves a trial phase to assess the effectiveness of the therapy before permanent implantation. The trial and implantation process involves several key steps:

- Trial Phase: During the trial, temporary leads are inserted into the epidural space and positioned near the dorsal root ganglia associated with the patient's pain. This procedure is typically performed under local anesthesia with fluoroscopic guidance to ensure precise placement of the leads. The leads are then connected to an external stimulator, and the patient is sent home to evaluate the level of pain relief over several days to a week. A successful trial is typically defined as at least a 50% reduction in pain and improvement in function.
- Permanent Implantation: If the trial phase is successful, the patient may proceed to permanent implantation. The permanent leads are positioned in the same location as the trial leads, and the IPG is implanted under the skin, usually in the lower back or abdomen. The procedure is typically performed under general or local anesthesia, depending on the patient's condition and the complexity of the surgery. The leads are tunneled subcutaneously to the IPG, and the system is programmed to deliver the desired level of stimulation.

The implantation procedure requires careful planning and precision, particularly in the placement of the leads, as the effectiveness of DRG stimulation is highly dependent on accurate targeting of the dorsal root ganglia. Post-operative care includes wound management, pain control, and the initiation of DRG stimulation programming. Patients may require several follow-up visits to optimize the device settings and achieve the best possible pain relief [27].

Complications
While DRG stimulation is generally safe, it is not without risks. Complications can be categorized into surgical, device-related, and patient-related.

1. Surgical Complications: These include infection, bleeding, and lead migration. The proximity of the leads to the spinal nerves and DRG can increase the risk of nerve irritation or injury. Lead migration is a particular concern with DRG

stimulation, as even slight shifts in lead position can significantly impact the efficacy of the therapy. Infection is a significant concern with any implanted device. The incidence of infection in DRG stimulation is similar to that in SCS, ranging from 3% to 10%. Most infections can be managed with antibiotics, but in severe cases, device explantation may be necessary. Given the close proximity of the leads to the spinal nerves and DRG, there is a risk of nerve injury during the implantation procedure. This can result in transient or permanent neurological deficits, depending on the severity of the injury.

2. Device-Related Complications: Common device-related issues include lead migration, lead fracture, and hardware malfunction. Lead migration, where the electrodes move from their intended position, can reduce the effectiveness of the stimulation and may require revision surgery. Advances in lead design and IPG technology have reduced the incidence of these complications, but they remain a potential concern.

3. Patient-Related Complications: Patients may experience discomfort at the IPG site, paresthesia, or pain due to improper lead placement. In rare cases, DRG stimulation may exacerbate pain, a phenomenon known as "stimulation-induced pain." Additionally, some patients may develop psychological dependence on the device, fearing the return of pain if the device is turned off. Long-term complications, while rare, can include fibrosis around the leads or IPG, which can impair device function and require revision surgery. Moreover, patients must be monitored for the potential development of tolerance to DRG stimulation, where the effectiveness of the stimulation diminishes over time [28–31].

MRI Compatibility

MRI compatibility is an important consideration for patients with implanted DRG stimulation systems, as many will require imaging for diagnostic purposes during their lifetime. The presence of implanted leads and the IPG can pose challenges for MRI, including the risk of lead heating, device malfunction, and patient injury. However, advancements in technology have led to the development of MRI-conditional DRG stimulation systems:

- MRI-Conditional Systems: These systems are designed to be safe for MRI under specific conditions, such as limiting the magnetic field strength (usually up to 1.5 Tesla) and following manufacturer-specific guidelines for patient positioning and scan duration. It is essential that the radiology team is aware of the presence of the DRG stimulation system and follows the recommended safety protocols to avoid complications.
- Precautions: Before an MRI scan, the DRG stimulation system should be set to a mode that minimizes risks, such as "MRI mode," or the device should be turned off entirely. After the scan, the DRG stimulation system should be thoroughly checked to ensure it is functioning correctly, and the settings should be restored to the patient's preferred parameters.
- Despite these advancements, not all patients with DRG stimulation implants can safely undergo MRI, particularly those with older or non-MRI-compatible

systems. Alternative imaging modalities, such as CT or ultrasound, may be necessary for these patients [22].

Conclusion

Dorsal root ganglion stimulation represents a significant advancement in the treatment of chronic pain, offering a more targeted approach than traditional spinal cord stimulation. The ability to selectively target specific areas of pain makes DRG stimulation particularly effective for conditions such as complex regional pain syndrome and chronic postoperative pain. While the technology and techniques involved in DRG stimulation are similar to those used in SCS, the key differences in target areas, efficacy, and potential complications highlight the unique advantages of DRG stimulation. Ongoing research and technological advancements continue to refine the application of DRG stimulation, making it an increasingly valuable option for patients suffering from chronic, intractable pain.

Neuromodulation: Peripheral Nerve Stimulation

Introduction

Peripheral nerve stimulation (PNS) is the application of electrical current to nerves for medical use. This concept was originated during the first century AD by Scribonius Largus with the Roman Empire, after incidentally finding that the electrical discharges of the torpedo fish were capable to provide analgesia for gout and headaches [32–34].

The first reported application of direct electrical stimulation of peripheral nerves was in 1859 by Althaus, used to relief postsurgical pain of the extremity [35]. A century later in 1960s, Wall and Sweet reported the use of percutaneous peripheral nerve stimulation; the initial techniques involved surgical dissection of the nerve, followed by a placement of bipolar leads on a "cuff-like" fashion around the nerve connected to an internal pulse generator (IPG) [34]. Due to reports of nerve damage due to scarring and compression, this method was later replaced in the 1970s by the positioning of paddle leads over a transposed fascial graft located right next to the nerve; however, this method fell out of favor as well due to the risks involved [34, 36, 37]. It was not until 1999 when Weiner and Reed used a percutaneous cylindrical lead in close proximity of the nerve, bypassing the need for extensive surgical dissection for its placement [36, 38–40].

The neuromodulation field has been exponentially growing for the past decades, proving to be extremely beneficial for the management of pain. Application of neuromodulatory current to the spinal cord has attracted most of the attention as the dorsal column has a high density of afferent fibers making it an appealing target for multiple painful neuropathic conditions. However, the development of smaller, more flexible, and better systems, combined with the improvement of ultrasound imaging, has allowed other anatomical structures to be used, allowing technologies like dorsal root ganglion (DRG) and PNS to be attractive alternatives for intractable pain.

PNS has received marked attention lately, because patients have a preference for less invasive procedures, requiring less incisions and smaller devices implanted. The technology has markedly advanced miniaturizing the equipment, improving the MRI compatibility, combating the risk of lead migration, and allowing the use of an external battery, able to power and wirelessly communicate to the implanted electrode (avoiding the implantation of a bulky IPG) [34, 38, 41]. Also, as mentioned above, these devices are able to be placed under sterile conditions with mostly ultrasound guidance, avoiding the need for extensive surgical dissection or solely relying on X-ray radiation and general anesthesia for lead positioning. As the depth of anesthesia does not need to be too deep, patient can provide feedback on nerve stimulation during the procedure, adding a safety feature and allowing verbal feedback that the lead is being placed at the correct location [34, 36].

Currently, there is no longer need to use the standard SCS systems to stimulate a peripheral nerve. In the market we can find different FDA-approved devices dedicated to PNS, some of them able to perform SCS+PNS: Freedom/StimQ (Stimwave Technologies) and Nalu (Nalu Medical Inc), while others are exclusively dedicated to peripheral nerve stimulation: StimRouter (Bioness), SPRINT (SPR therapeutics), and Reactiv8 (Mainstay Medical). Most of them consist of fully implantable leads, excluding SPRINT that offers a temporary 60 days, externalized leads placement. Most of these systems are MRI compatible with the exception of SPRINT, which is not MRI compatible.

StimRouter was one of the PNS systems obtaining earlier FDA clearance (2015) and comprises of a short fully implantable electrode connected to an external pulse generator (EPG) worn on the skin on an adhesive patch that should be replaced every 48–72 h. The cylindrical tined lead has 3 electrodes, measures 15 cm in length, and does come with a silicone anchor to reduce migration [34, 42].

The StimQ system gained FDA approval in 2016. The provider may choose between the 4 and 8 electrode Freedom PNS™ leads, which have a receiver and stimulator embedded. The energy is provided by a wearable external antenna/battery pad "Wearable Antenna Assembly" (WAA) worn on top of a layer of clothing [34, 43, 44].

In 2018, the SPRINT system gained FDA clearance as a temporary implant, indicated for 60 days of continuous use. This intervention has demonstrated in studies, sustained relief for 14 months (and potentially longer). Its electrode lead is stainless steel with a coiled design that enhance fibrotic ingrowth, reducing the risk of both migration and infection. This lead is externalized and directly connected to an EPG worn on the skin until the time of removal. Unfortunately, this device is not MRI compatible; however, due to its temporary design, it can be easily removed without a surgical intervention [34, 45–48].

Reactiv8 is a system that was approved by the FDA in 2020. This peripheral nerve stimulation system targets the multifidus muscles and, rehabilitates them to treat secondary low back pain. This treats more mechanical etiology of chronic low back pain. It uses two leads targeting the L2 medial branch nerves at the L3 transverse process, which are then connected to an IPG able to deliver two 30-min sessions of stimulation daily [34, 49].

Nalu is one of the recent systems on the market, obtaining FDA approval in 2020. The fully implantable electrode leads have a microstimulator (IPG) that is 27 times smaller than other standard IPGs used for SCS. This is powered by an external upgradeable therapy disc that requires to be worn with a single-use adhesive clip to the skin, or a belt [34].

A summary of PNS targets is given in Table 9.1.

Mechanism of Action

Peripheral nerve stimulation modulates peripheral factors and also affects the central nervous system.

Its main mechanism is based on the gate control theory which was first proposed by Melzack and Wall in 1965 [50]. The theory states that within the dorsal horn there exists a "gate" which allows the progression or inhibition of afferent impulses. The control of this gate can be modified by large diameter A-β fibers (carry afferent signals such as touch and pressure) as well as the small C -fibers (pain). For example, rubbing your knee after falling excites inhibitory neurons in the dorsal horn, thus impeding the progression of pain from the small fibers. A cat model has also shown that stimulating the A-β fibers of the pudendal nerve led to an increased activity of inhibitory input on bladder-related inter-neurons at the V1, v2 Rexed laminae in the S2 spinal region [51].

Endogenous neurotransmitters in the spinal cord are also modulated during PNS. For instance, sciatic nerve stimulation upregulates the "Arc" protein in a bone

Table 9.1 Summary of Common Peripheral Nerve Targets

Location	Nerves	Indication
Head and neck	Occipital nerve	Occipital neuralgia
	Cervical medial branch nerve	Cervical facet arthropathy
Upper extremity/ shoulder	Brachial plexus	CRPS
	Suprascapular nerve	Phantom limb/residual limb pain
	Axillary nerve	
	Median/ulnar/musculocutaneous/radial nerve	Shoulder pain
Truncal	Ilioinguinal/iliohypogastric/genitofemoral nerve	Post-inguinal herniorrhaphy neuralgia
	Intercostal	Intercostal neuralgia
Lumbar/thoracic spine	Thoracic/lumbar medial branch nerve	Lumbar/thoracic facet arthropathy
	Cluneal nerve	Cluneal neuralgia
		Multifidus atrophy
Lower extremity	Lateral femoral cutaneous	Meralgia paresthetica
	Femoral nerve and branches (saphenous nerve)	CRPS
		Phantom limb/residual limb
	Sciatic nerve and branches (tibial and peroneal nerve)	Knee/ankle pain
	Genicular nerves	

Less common targets include facial stimulation (V1,V2,V3), sphenopalatine, vagal nerve. Leads for these targets are more likely to be placed by a functional neurosurgeon cancer rat model. This Arc protein downregulates GluA1 transcription leading to decreases in allodynia and hyperalgesia [52].

Further modulation of receptor activity has been shown in humans with median nerve peripheral stimulation. These patients showed increased NMDA plasticity after stimulation [53]. NMDA activity is correlated with wind up activity [54]. In fact, it has been shown that there may be a reduction in the activation of WDR (wide dynamic range) neurons [55].The WDR neurons show increased excitability and response to peripheral stimuli after a nerve injury or tissue inflammation. Repeated noxious input of the same stimulus leads to a summative response of the WDR neurons, also known as "wind up." Studies have shown that this pathway leads to hyperalgesia. A study done by Yan, Fei et al. revealed the reduction of hypersensitivity and activation of the WDR neurons in the dorsal horn, after stimulating the dorsal root in L5 nerve root ligated mice [56].

PET scans taken during PNS stimulation has shown the supraspinal effects of PNS. Accessory nerve PNS has demonstrated increased activity of the dorsolateral pre-frontal cortex and sensorimotor cortex. These areas are associated with sensorimotor-discriminative and affective-motivational senses [57]. In addition, stimulation of the brachial plexus resulted in modulation of the primary sensory and motor regions of the cortex, S1 and M1 [58].

A human study evaluated the response of A and C fibers to repeated electrical stimulation. In the study, intradermal microelectrodes were inserted into nerves such as the saphenous nerve. Repeated stimulation of these nerves showed an increase in latency of the A and C fibers. This eventually stabilized, however, after a certain number of impulses. The same study also showed decreased conduction velocity and decrease excitability of C fibers at low frequencies such as 0.5/s [59]. Not only are A and C fibers modulated but various studies have also shown that peripheral nerve stimulation may accelerate axon regeneration in nerve injury [60, 61].

Furthermore, the local tissue environment during PNS is also modulated. In fact, a study showed increased macrophage activity and CGRP expression in Taxol-treated rats after sciatic nerve injury. The same study also demonstrated increased axon numbers after stimulation, thus displaying the effects PNS can have on the local inflammatory environment on nerve regeneration [62].

Location of Peripheral Nerve Stimulation

There is a vast array of peripheral nerve targets for PNS. Common targets include (Table 9.1):

Implantation of Peripheral Nerve Stimulators

Implantation of PNS depends on the device utilized. As described earlier, some devices are only temporary devices and others are permanent devices with an implantable IPG. Most permanent devices will trial a temporary device in a similar fashion to a SCS.

There are two imaging techniques routinely utilized for placement: Ultrasound and Fluoroscopy. Generally if the nerve can be clearly imaged on ultrasound, it is the preferred technique for implantation such as brachial plexus and it's respective individual nerves, and femoral and sciatic nerves and there respective branches and suprascapular nerve. Figures 9.1 and 9.2 demonstrate a femoral nerve target and lateral femoral cutaneous nerve target for a peripheral nerve stimulation, respectively. These are placed in a similar fashion to a peripheral nerve catheter placed by an anesthesiologist for perioperative pain control.

Some nerves are not clearly visualized on ultrasound and/or have very reliable fluoroscopic targets including medial branch nerves, genicular nerves, and cluneal nerves. Figures 9.3 and 9.4 demonstrate targets for genicular nerves. Some targets such as the intercostal may benefit from utilizing ultrasound in conjunction with fluoroscopy.

In lightly sedated or wake patients, stimulation can be confirmed with patient input to confirm appropriate coverage of stimulation.

Vertebral Augmentation

Introduction

Osteoporotic vertebral compression fractures (OVFs) are common among the elderly population, often resulting from reduced bone mineral density. These fractures can lead to significant pain, reduced mobility, and decreased quality of life. Most commonly, kyphoplasty and vertebroplasty are minimally invasive surgical interventions developed to treat OVFs by stabilizing the fracture, reducing pain, and in the case of kyphoplasty, attempting to restore vertebral height. Both procedures involve the percutaneous injection of bone cement into the vertebral body, though they differ in their approach and mechanism. This chapter will explore the mechanisms of action, patient selection criteria, intraoperative considerations, potential complications, and outcomes associated with kyphoplasty and vertebroplasty.

Fig. 9.1 Ultrasoudn image of Femoral nerve and artery, with sartorius muscle lateral to the femoral nerve

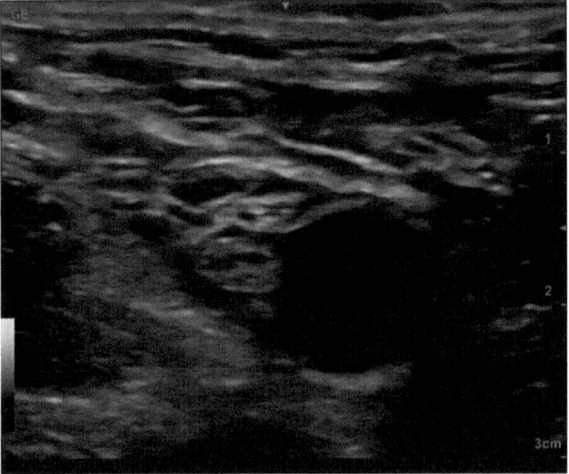

Fig. 9.2 Ultrasound Image of the Lateral Femoral Cutaneous Nerve

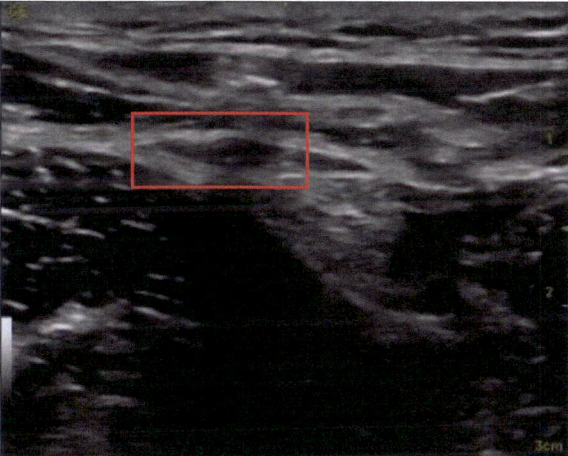

Fig. 9.3 AP fluoroscopic view of final PNS lead location at the inferior medial genicular nerve site

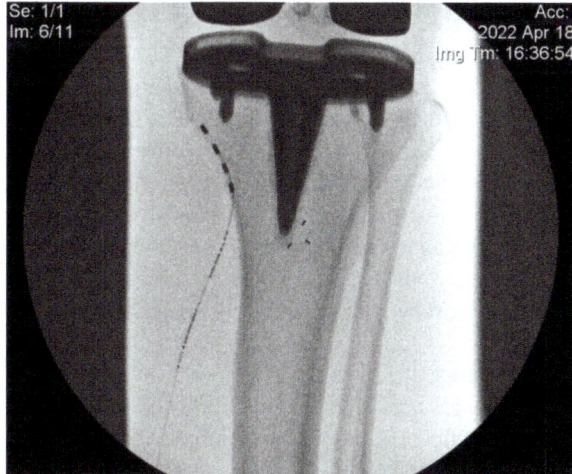

Mechanism of Action

Vertebroplasty involves the direct injection of polymethylmethacrylate (PMMA) cement into the fractured vertebra to stabilize the bone structure. This procedure aims to provide immediate pain relief by stabilizing the micro-movements of the fractured bone. Kyphoplasty, on the other hand, includes an additional step where a balloon is inflated within the vertebral body to create a cavity before cement injection, which may help restore some vertebral height and correct kyphotic deformity. The choice between these techniques often depends on the desired mechanical stabilization and the degree of vertebral height restoration needed.

Fig. 9.4 Lateral fluoroscopic view of final PNS lead location at the Inferior medial genicular nerve site; lead contacts are shown within the red rectangle

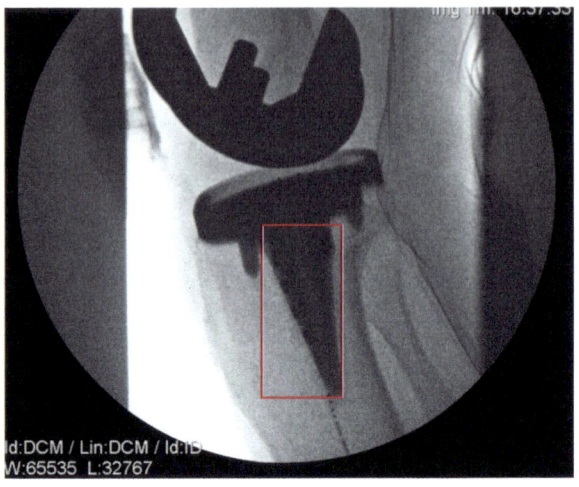

Patient Selection

Patient selection for kyphoplasty and vertebroplasty is critical to optimizing outcomes. Ideal candidates are those with painful OVFs that are refractory to conservative management, including analgesics, bracing, and physical therapy. Imaging studies, such as MRI, are used to confirm the presence of bone edema and to correlate the fracture with the patient's symptoms. Contraindications include fractures that are not associated with pain, extensive vertebral destruction, spinal instability, or an infection at the site of the procedure. Both techniques are generally reserved for patients who have experienced significant pain for several weeks to months and who exhibit functional impairment despite conservative treatment [63].

Techniques

The patient is positioned supine, followed by standard preparation and draping. AP and lateral fluoroscopic views are obtained to guide the procedure. After local anesthesia is administered to the skin superior and lateral to the target pedicle, a cannula is introduced. Under serial AP and lateral fluoroscopic guidance, the working cannula is advanced through the pedicle, aiming to access the vertebral body without breaching the medial border of the pedicle. In a bipedicular approach, both cannulas are positioned near the midline within the anterior third of the vertebral body. Alternatively, a curved system can be used for a unipedicular approach, advancing along a curved trajectory toward the medial border of the contralateral pedicle on the AP view. For kyphoplasty, a radiopaque balloon is inserted and inflated to create a void for cement placement—a step not included in vertebroplasty. Cement is then injected, with careful monitoring to prevent intravascular leakage and to avoid extravasation outside the vertebral body, especially retrograde flow toward the spinal canal. The equipment is subsequently removed, ensuring there is no cement leakage through the access pathway. Third-generation systems, such as the Spine Jack, involve additional implants and steps not covered in this review.

Intraoperative Considerations

Both procedures are typically performed under local anesthesia with sedation or general anesthesia, depending on the patient's condition and preferences. Fluoroscopic guidance is crucial for the accurate placement of the needles and cement injection to avoid complications such as cement leakage. In kyphoplasty, balloon inflation must be carefully monitored to avoid overexpansion, which can lead to fractures in adjacent vertebrae or cement extrusion. The viscosity and volume of the cement are also critical factors; cement should be injected slowly and under low pressure to reduce the risk of leakage. The procedures can be completed within an hour and generally allow patients to return home the same day, highlighting the minimally invasive nature of these treatments [63].

Outcomes

Both vertebroplasty and kyphoplasty have a significant improvement in pain relative to conservative management. Certain studies have shown that kyphoplasty outperforms vertebroplasty in measured disability, quality of life improvement, cement extravasation rate, and kyphosis correction [64–66], though the data varies on the significance of this improvement. Notably, mortality rate decreases s/p vertebral augmentation compared to medical management [67].

Complications

Complications of kyphoplasty include bleeding, infection, cement leakage, pulmonary embolism, adjacent fractures, and, rarely, death [68]. Bleeding can occur due to vascular injury during the procedure, while infections, though uncommon, can be severe, such as spondylitis requiring surgical intervention. Cement leakage is the most frequent complication, seen in about 8.1% of cases, and can lead to spinal cord compression or pulmonary embolism if the cement migrates into critical areas. Pulmonary embolism, though rare (0.17%), can be life-threatening [69].

Adjacent vertebral fractures are reported in 11.1% of cases, often due to altered spinal biomechanics or cement leakage into disc spaces. While the overall mortality rate is low, kyphoplasty still carries risks, including severe complications that require immediate intervention. Therefore, the procedure should be performed by skilled spine surgeons to minimize these risks and manage complications effectively [69].

Conclusion

Kyphoplasty and vertebroplasty offer effective pain relief and functional improvement for patients with OVFs that do not respond to conservative treatment. While both procedures share common benefits, kyphoplasty may provide the added advantage of vertebral height restoration and kyphotic angle correction. Careful patient selection and adherence to technical considerations during the procedure are essential to minimize complications. Ongoing research and advancements in technique may continue to refine these procedures, enhancing their safety and efficacy for patients with OVFs.

Basivertebral Nerve Ablation

Introduction

Basivertebral nerve (BVN) ablation is a minimally invasive procedure approved by the FDA in 2016 that targets the basivertebral nerve within the vertebral body to treat chronic axial low back pain (LBP) [70, 71]. LBP remains a leading cause of disability worldwide, with a substantial burden on healthcare systems due to its chronic nature and the frequent lack of effective long-term treatments. Identifying specific pain generators in the spine has historically been challenging, as the etiology of LBP is often multifactorial and non-specific. However, recent advances have highlighted the role of vertebral endplate damage and the associated basivertebral nerve as significant contributors to chronic vertebral pain, a distinct subset of LBP.

BVN ablation addresses this pain by interrupting nociceptive signals from the vertebral endplates, which are highly innervated and prone to inflammatory changes, fissuring, intraosseous edema, and degeneration [72]. This chapter explores the mechanism of action, patient selection criteria, intraoperative considerations, potential complications, and the overall clinical significance of BVN ablation in managing chronic axial LBP.

Mechanism of Action

BVN ablation aims to alleviate pain by creating a thermal lesion at the BVN terminus, effectively severing the nerve's capacity to transmit nociceptive information from damaged vertebral endplates. The basivertebral nerve arises from the sinuvertebral nerve and enters the vertebral body via the basivertebral foramen, where it branches to innervate the superior and inferior endplates of the vertebrae. These endplates are susceptible to Modic changes, which are pathological alterations visible on MRI that correlate with vertebral pain.

There are three types of Modic changes: type 1, characterized by inflammatory changes and fissuring within the endplates; type 2, marked by fatty degeneration of the bone marrow; and type 3, associated with subchondral bone sclerosis. Type 1 changes, in particular, have a strong association with severe, prolonged LBP and are considered the primary targets for BVN ablation. By ablating the nerve at its terminus, BVN ablation interrupts the flow of inflammatory mediators and pain signals, such as substance P and calcitonin gene-related peptide (CGRP), which are involved in chronic pain pathways [73, 74].

Patient Selection

Appropriate patient selection is paramount to the success of BVN ablation. The ideal candidates are those with chronic axial LBP persisting for more than 6 months, which has been refractory to conservative treatments, including physical therapy, oral analgesics, and non-steroidal anti-inflammatory drugs. Patients with vertebral endplate pain often experience significant functional impairment and severe pain that worsens when sitting, standing, or bending forward (spinal flexion), unlike during extension [75, 76]. The pain is typically described as a burning, deep, and achy sensation localized in the midline of the lumbar spine, without associated radicular symptoms, motor weakness, numbness, or tingling. These patients must also exhibit specific imaging findings, namely Modic type 1 or 2 changes on MRI at one or more vertebral levels from L3 to S1.

Patients with a history of spinal surgery, significant spinal stenosis, radicular symptoms, or other predominant sources of pain, such as sacroiliac joint dysfunction, are generally excluded. Additionally, contraindications include systemic infections, incomplete skeletal maturity, and proximity of the ablation zone to sensitive structures like the spinal canal or nerve roots. Safety concerns also preclude patients with implantable pulse generators, severe cardiopulmonary compromise, or conditions that increase the risk of intraoperative complications, such as morbid obesity or bleeding disorders.

Intraoperative Considerations

BVN ablation is performed using advanced image-guided technology to ensure precise targeting of the basivertebral nerve within the vertebral body. The procedure typically employs fluoroscopy or CT guidance to navigate instruments through a transpedicular approach. Key instruments include an introducer trocar with a diamond or bevel tip, a curved cannula assembly, and a bipolar radiofrequency ablation probe.

The procedure begins with the patient in a prone position under general anesthesia or monitored anesthesia care (MAC). The surgical site is prepared using a sterile technique, and imaging guidance is used to identify the target vertebral level. The surgeon first establishes an ideal anterior-posterior view of the pedicles at the level of interest, marking the skin entry point and confirming the correct trajectory for the transpedicular approach.

Local anesthesia is administered along the planned needle path, and a small incision is made to accommodate the introducer trocar. The trocar is advanced through the pedicle under continuous imaging, creating a pathway for the curved cannula. The cannula assembly, equipped with a straight stylet, allows for the creation of a channel within the vertebral body toward the BVN terminus. Accurate placement is verified with both anterior-posterior and lateral fluoroscopic views to avoid breaching the spinal canal or contacting nearby neural structures. The BVN is positioned 30% anteriorly into the vertebral body at 50% caudal from the superior endplate for lumbar levels, and 50% anterior into the vertebral body and 40% caudal from the superior endplate for the sacral levels [70, 71, 77].

Once the target site is confirmed, the stylet is removed, and the radiofrequency ablation probe is introduced. The probe is connected to a radiofrequency generator, which delivers controlled energy—typically at 85 degrees Celsius for 7 or 15 min—to create a spherical lesion at the nerve terminus. This ablation disrupts the nerve's ability to transmit pain signals from the vertebral endplates.

Upon completion of the ablation, the instruments are carefully withdrawn, and the incision is closed with minimal suturing or adhesive strips. Post-procedure, patients are monitored in a recovery area, where vital signs and neurological function are reassessed before discharge. Patients receive instructions on activity restrictions, incision care, and signs of potential complications, such as infection and neurological changes or deficits, to watch for after the procedure.

Complications

BVN ablation is generally considered safe, with a low incidence of serious complications. Most adverse events reported are mild and self-limiting, such as transient exacerbation of LBP or minor radiculitis that resolves with conservative treatment. Rare but notable complications include vertebral compression fractures, particularly in patients with underlying risk factors like osteoporosis or ongoing hormonal therapy. Other serious complications, such as retroperitoneal hemorrhage, have been documented but remain exceedingly rare.

The procedure's safety profile is bolstered by meticulous intraoperative technique and careful patient selection to minimize risks. Proper imaging guidance is essential to avoid unintended damage to nearby structures, and adherence to sterile protocols helps prevent infections. Overall, the low complication rate and favorable safety profile make BVN ablation a viable option for patients meeting the selection criteria.

Conclusion

Basivertebral nerve ablation offers a targeted, minimally invasive treatment option for patients with chronic axial low back pain attributed to vertebral endplate damage. By directly addressing the nociceptive pathways from these damaged endplates, BVN ablation provides significant pain relief and functional improvement in a subset of patients who have exhausted conservative therapies. The procedure's efficacy, combined with its safety profile and relatively straightforward technique, underscores its value in the comprehensive management of vertebral pain.

As our understanding of vertebral endplate pathology continues to evolve, BVN ablation may gain an increasingly prominent role in the interventional landscape for LBP. Future research and long-term outcome data will further refine patient selection criteria and procedural protocols, optimizing the therapeutic impact of this innovative approach to pain management.

Sacroiliac Joint Fusion

Introduction

It is estimated that 15–30% of low back pain can be attributed to sacroiliac (SI) joint pathology [78, 79] and that it may be the culprit in up to 40% of residual low back pain following lumbar fusion [80]. Minimally invasive SI joint fusion procedures to treat SI joint pain were first adopted by spine surgeons in the early 2000s and involved the placement of screws from lateral to medial, through the ilium, and across the SI joint [81]. The sacroiliac joint, located between the sacrum and ilium of the pelvis, plays a crucial role in transferring the weight from the upper body to the lower extremities and stabilizing pelvic movement. Dysfunction of this joint, often due to degenerative changes, trauma, or post-partum conditions, can lead to significant and persistent pain. Conservative treatments, including physical therapy, medications, and corticosteroid injections, are typically the first line of therapy. However, in patients with refractory symptoms, SIJ fusion can offer relief by stabilizing the joint and reducing pain.

Mechanism of Action

SIJ fusion aims to stabilize the sacroiliac joint by promoting bony fusion between the sacrum and ilium. This procedure is typically performed minimally invasively with implants or screws to immobilize the joint. By eliminating micro-motions within the joint, SIJ fusion reduces mechanical stress and irritation of the surrounding structures, alleviating the pain generator. Over time, the goal is for the bone to grow around the implanted hardware, leading to a permanent fusion. There are various surgical techniques, including percutaneous and open approaches, but the primary goal remains the same: joint stabilization. Different techniques are shown in Fig. 9.5.

Patient Selection

Treatment of SI joint pain is very similar to that of other osseous sources of low back pain—starting with conservative management via physical therapy and NSAIDs, escalating to steroid injections of the joint (Fig. 9.5), and then further to RFA of the lateral branch nerves innervating the SI joint. RFA does have the drawback of only being able to target the posterior nerves of the joint, and not the anterior [82]. Anterior innervation of the sacroiliac joint is from the ventral rami of the L5 to S2 nerve roots. The lateral branches of the dorsal rami of the S1 to S4 nerve roots innervate the posterior portion [83]. If none of these methods prove sufficient in achieving satisfactory pain control, then SI joint fusion may be considered.

Fig. 9.5 SI joint, as seen during fluoroscopy-guided contrast injection

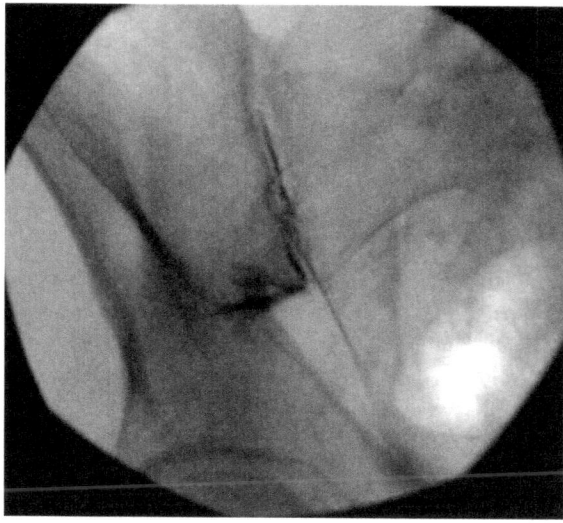

Intraoperative Considerations

There are several SI joint fusion devices currently on the market each with small differences in their surgical technique. However, the major steps of the procedures are fairly similar and will be described here.

Preparation

Patient is placed supine on the OR table, prepped and draped in standard sterile fashion. C-arm should be placed in a position where direct AP, lateral, and oblique images of the joint can be obtained.

Locating the Joint

The joint on the target side should first be identified on direct AP imaging. A guide-wire placed on the skin can be used to help mark the location of the PSIS and PIIS. A localizing device will then be placed into the joint under fluoroscopic guidance; this can be either guidewire(s) or a larger, handled device, depending on the specific product being used. Depth of advancement into the joint space should be checked on lateral and oblique imaging.

Bone Preparation

Once access to the SI joint has been established, the bony surfaces of the sacrum and ilium will need to be prepared to accept the implanted device. Some older devices relied on this step being done freehand using a bone curette, which required direct visualization of the joint, and even microscope utilization. Some newer devices (such as the Vyrsa Nevro1 and PainTEQ LinQ) achieve joint space preparation and decortication through proprietary percutaneous systems. Figure 9.6 demonstrates the introducer device placed in the lateral position. This generally involves placing a dilator over top of the original joint locating device, followed by a guide for either a drill, chisel, or rasp-like device that will clear soft tissue and a superficial layer of bone from the joint space.

Device Implantation

Many products will require the placement of trial, sizing devices into the joint prior to definitive fixation. Once a device size that fits snugly into the joint is found, the final implant can be placed using an administrator included in the device kit. These implants generally consist of either titanium or allogenic bone graft.

Efficacy

To date, outcome data for SI joint fusion through the posterior interpositional approach remains sparse and study quality is lacking. However, the limited studies available indicate a significant reduction in numerical pain scores following the procedure and possibly delay/avoidance of future procedures on the joint [84, 85].

A cadaveric study has also indicated that interpositional devices are able to achieve a comparable level of fixation to that of traditional lateral screw fixation [86], which have a longer track record of pain improvement [87].

Fig. 9.6 Implantation of the Vyrsa Nevro1 fusion device

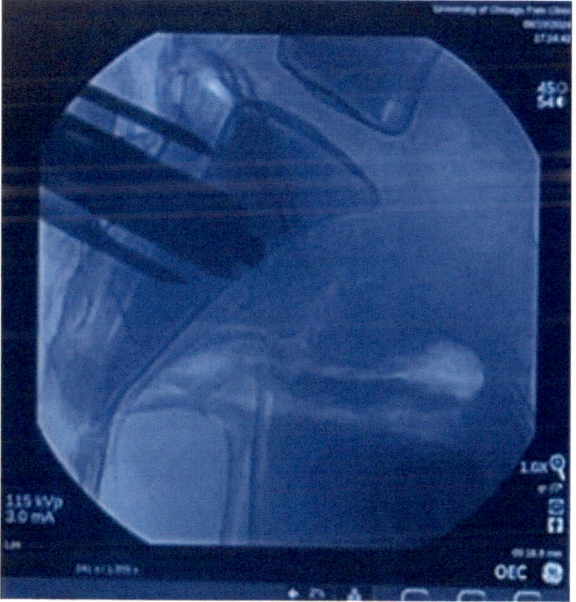

Complications

As with any surgical procedure, SIJ fusion carries a risk of complications, though it is generally considered safe when performed by experienced surgeons. Some potential complications include:

- Hardware-related issues: Implant migration or loosening can occur, especially if there is insufficient bone for proper fixation or if the procedure does not achieve adequate immobilization of the joint.
- Infection: As with any surgery, there is a risk of postoperative infection, which can range from superficial wound infections to deep infections that may necessitate hardware removal.
- Nerve injury: Though uncommon, there is a potential risk of injury to the nearby nerves, which could result in numbness, tingling, or motor weakness in the affected limb.
- Nonunion: Failure of the joint to fuse, also known as nonunion, may result in continued pain and potentially require revision surgery.
- Adjacent segment disease: Immobilizing the sacroiliac joint could potentially lead to increased stress on adjacent joints, such as the lumbar spine or hip, which may result in new pain or degeneration in these regions.

Conclusion

SIJ fusion can provide significant relief for patients with chronic sacroiliac joint dysfunction who have not responded to conservative treatment options. By promoting fusion of the sacrum and ilium, the procedure aims to stabilize the joint and reduce pain caused by micro-motions and mechanical stress. Careful patient selection is essential for successful outcomes, and while complications can occur, they are relatively rare when performed by experienced surgeons. As research continues to evolve and newer minimally invasive techniques are developed, SIJ fusion remains a promising solution for managing chronic sacroiliac joint pain.

Emerging Procedures/Surgical Interventions Including Endoscopic Interventions

Background

The specialty of pain medicine is seeing expansion in scope and upscaling of skill sets since the past few years. More and more advanced procedures are now being performed by well-trained pain medicine physicians, and the lines are getting blurred between spine surgery and the procedures or surgeries being performed by pain medicine physicians. The term "Pain Surgeon" has been getting traction due to the advancement in complexities of the procedures and surgeries being performed these days. Most of the advanced interventions like interspinous spacers (Vertiflex), MILD, and basivertebral nerve ablation (Intracept) utilize fluoroscopic guidance and the actual spinal canal is not directly visualized. Endoscopic spine decompression is done under direct endoscopic visualization, whereby a high-definition magnified image of the anatomical structures inside the spinal canal (ligamentum flavum, dura, nerve roots, posterior longitudinal ligament, intervertebral disc, etc.) can be viewed once the working channel and the endoscope with continuous irrigation is safely placed inside the spinal canal via the interlaminar window or via the neuroforamen.

Standardizing the Training

Endoscopic spine surgery is the least invasive form of spine surgery, has a minimal footprint, and has several advantages over traditional open and microscopic approaches to spine. It does have a steep learning curve even for trained spine surgeons and needs a master trainer initially [1]. Proper interpretation of MRI & CT images is essential to get a 3D perspective for pain medicine fellows before attempting to learn endoscopic spine techniques. The training for pain medicine fellows and practicing physicians should encompass cadaver sessions at the outset to get familiarity with holding the endoscope and wielding various surgical instruments as well as drills/burrs through the endoscope. The cadaver sessions should also focus on recognizing complications like a Dural tear at an early stage and, depending on the type of tear, taking a call on either leaving it alone or patching it with fibrin/surgicel or suturing it with 5–0 Prolene. The skill set of the pain medicine physician should be honed under direct supervision of a master trainer. A progressive increase in complexity of cases starting from transforaminal approach to foraminal disc herniations then progressing to paracentral and central herniations should give the trainee a good idea of the transforaminal technique of spine endoscopy. The trainee should simultaneously be coached about the interlaminar endoscopic approach starting out with L5-S1 disc herniations (largest interlaminar window) and then slowly advancing to disc herniations at higher levels in the lumbar spine, where bone work would be needed and getting experience in using drill/burr becomes necessary. Once the trainee feels comfortable in performing disc herniation surgeries under minimal supervision, he/she should then be exposed to foraminal stenosis and lateral recess decompression cases, where understanding spinal architecture and stabilizing forces becomes crucial in preserving integrity and stability of spine during decompression. Neuromonitoring with EMG for lumbar spine provides an added layer of safety for stenosis and more difficult cases in lumbar spine, and the trainee should have at least a basic understanding of interpretation of EMG waveforms and awareness to the audio feedback of the variations in continuous EMG recordings. Once adequate experience is gained with the above stenosis decompression techniques, subsequent exposure with central canal stenosis decompression starting on one side then going 'over the top' for bilateral central canal as well as lateral recess decompression. This should make the trainee gain expertise to handle any lumbar spine decompression cases utilizing the 'full endoscopic' technique. After enough experience with lumbar spine is gained and the trainee is confident about handling any complex cases or complications arising out of endoscopic decompression in the lumbar spine, an exposure to posterior cervical decompression as well as thoracic decompression would be the next logical step to expand on the skill sets of the trainee. Since every trainee is different with baseline skill sets, some can get well trained relatively quicker than others and the assessment by the master trainer should guide the progression of the complexities of the cases for the trainee. A completion certificate can be granted to the trainee upon satisfactory demonstration of diagnostic skills, image interpretation, and surgical skills.

References

1. Deer TR, et al. The polyanalgesic consensus conference (PACC): recommendations on intrathecal drug infusion systems best practices and guidelines. Neuromodulation. 2017;20(2):96–132.
2. Delhaas EM, Huygen F. Complications associated with intrathecal drug delivery systems. BJA Educ. 2020;20(2):51–7.
3. De Andres J, et al. Intrathecal drug delivery: advances and applications in the management of chronic pain patient. Front Pain Res (Lausanne). 2022;3:900566.
4. Bottros MM, Christo PJ. Current perspectives on intrathecal drug delivery. J Pain Res. 2014;7:615–26.
5. Deer TR, et al. The polyanalgesic consensus conference (PACC): recommendations for trialing of intrathecal drug delivery infusion therapy. Neuromodulation. 2017;20(2):133–54.
6. De Andres J, et al. The safety of magnetic resonance imaging in patients with programmable implanted intrathecal drug delivery systems: a 3-year prospective study. Anesth Analg. 2011;112(5):1124–9.
7. MedWatch Safety Alert. Implantable infusion pumps in the magnetic resonance (MR) environment: FDA safety communication—important safety precautions. Silver Spring: US Food and Drug Administration; 2017.
8. Hartman J, Granville M, Jacobson RE. The use of Vertiflex(R) Interspinous spacer device in patients with lumbar spinal stenosis and concurrent medical comorbidities. Cureus. 2019;11(8):e5374.

9. Xin JH, et al. Effectiveness and safety of interspinous spacer versus decompressive surgery for lumbar spinal stenosis: a meta-analysis of randomized controlled trials. Medicine (Baltimore). 2023;102(46):e36048.

10. Mekhail N, et al. The durability of minimally invasive lumbar decompression procedure in patients with symptomatic lumbar spinal stenosis: long-term follow-up. Pain Pract. 2021;21(8):826–35.

11. Garcia K, Wray JK, Kumar S. Spinal cord stimulation. In: StatPearls; 2024. Treasure Island ineligible companies. Disclosure: Joseph Wray declares no relevant financial relationships with ineligible companies Disclosure: Sanjeev Kumar declares no relevant financial relationships with ineligible companies.

12. Mekhail N, et al. Spinal cord stimulation 50 years later: clinical outcomes of spinal cord stimulation based on randomized clinical trials-a systematic review. Reg Anesth Pain Med. 2018;43(4):391–406.

13. Caylor J, et al. Spinal cord stimulation in chronic pain: evidence and theory for mechanisms of action. Bioelectron Med. 2019;5:1–41.

14. Malige A, Sokunbi G. Spinal cord stimulators: a comparison of the trial period versus permanent outcomes. Spine (Phila Pa 1976). 2019;44(11):E687–92.

15. Hagedorn JM, et al. The team approach to spinal cord and dorsal root ganglion stimulation: a guide for the advanced practice provider. Mayo Clin Proc Innov Qual Outcomes. 2021;5(3):663–9.

16. Burchiel KJ, et al. Prognostic factors of spinal cord stimulation for chronic back and leg pain. Neurosurgery. 1995;36(6):1101–10. discussion 1110–1

17. Deer TR, et al. The Neurostimulation Appropriateness Consensus Committee (NACC): recommendations for surgical technique for spinal cord stimulation. Neuromodulation. 2022;25(1):1–34.

18. North RB, et al. Spinal cord stimulation for chronic, intractable pain: experience over two decades. Neurosurgery. 1993;32(3):384–94. discussion 394–5

19. Rosenow JM, et al. Failure modes of spinal cord stimulation hardware. J Neurosurg Spine. 2006;5(3):183–90.

20. Nevro. 1.5 Tesla and 3 Tesla Magnetic Resonance Imaging (MRI) guidelines for the SENZA® neuromodulation systems. February 2024; Available from: https://www.nevro.com/English/us/providers/product-manuals/default.aspx.

21. Medtronic. Medtronic: instructions for use and product manuals for healthcare professionals. 2024-04-25; Available from: https://manuals.medtronic.com/manuals/.

22. Abbot. Abbot: MRI support for healthcare professionals. Available from: https://www.neuromodulation.abbott/us/en/healthcare-professionals/mri-support.html.

23. Scientific B. Boston Scientific: MRI technical guide.

24. Abd-Elsayed A, et al. Mechanisms of action of dorsal root ganglion stimulation. Int J Mol Sci. 2024;25(7):3591.

25. Graham RD, Sankarasubramanian V, Lempka SF. Dorsal root ganglion stimulation for chronic pain: hypothesized mechanisms of action. J Pain. 2022;23(2):196–211.

26. Deer TR, et al. Dorsal root ganglion stimulation yielded higher treatment success rate for complex regional pain syndrome and causalgia at 3 and 12 months: a randomized comparative trial. Pain. 2017;158(4):669–81.

27. Deer TR, et al. The neuromodulation appropriateness consensus committee on best practices for dorsal root ganglion stimulation. Neuromodulation. 2019;22(1):1–35.

28. Sivanesan E, Bicket MC, Cohen SP. Retrospective analysis of complications associated with dorsal root ganglion stimulation for pain relief in the FDA MAUDE database. Reg Anesth Pain Med. 2019;44(1):100–6.

29. Horan M, et al. Complications and effects of dorsal root ganglion stimulation in the treatment of chronic neuropathic pain: a nationwide cohort study in Denmark. Neuromodulation. 2021;24(4):729–37.

30. Hines K, et al. Single-center retrospective analysis of device-related complications related to dorsal root ganglion stimulation for pain relief in 31 patients. Neuromodulation. 2022;25(7):1040–4.
31. Kretzschmar M, Reining M, Schwarz MA. Three-year outcomes after dorsal root ganglion stimulation in the treatment of neuropathic pain after peripheral nerve injury of upper and lower extremities. Neuromodulation. 2021;24(4):700–7.
32. Kaye AD, et al. Peripheral nerve stimulation: a review of techniques and clinical efficacy. Pain Ther. 2021;10(2):961–72.
33. Nahm FS. From the torpedo fish to the spinal cord stimulator. Korean J Pain. 2020;33(2):97–8.
34. Strand NH, et al. Mechanism of action of peripheral nerve stimulation. Curr Pain Headache Rep. 2021;25(7):47.
35. Althaus J. A treatise on medical electricity, theoretical and practical: and its uses in the treatment of paralysis, neuralgia, and other diseases. London: Longmans, Green and Co; 1873.
36. Deer TR, et al. A review of the bioelectronic implications of stimulation of the peripheral nervous system for chronic pain conditions. Bioelectron Med. 2020;6:9.
37. Abd-Elsayed A, D'Souza RS. Peripheral nerve stimulation: the evolution in pain medicine. Biomedicines. 2021;10(1):18.
38. Goroszeniuk T, Pang D. Peripheral neuromodulation: a review. Curr Pain Headache Rep. 2014;18(5):412.
39. Chakravarthy K, et al. Review of recent advances in Peripheral Nerve Stimulation (PNS). Curr Pain Headache Rep. 2016;20(11):60.
40. Weiner RL, Reed KL. Peripheral neurostimulation for control of intractable occipital neuralgia. Neuromodulation. 1999;2(3):217–21.
41. Deer TR, et al. A systematic literature review of peripheral nerve stimulation therapies for the treatment of pain. Pain Med. 2020;21(8):1590–603.
42. Deer T, et al. Prospective, multicenter, randomized, double-blinded, partial crossover study to assess the safety and efficacy of the novel neuromodulation system in the treatment of patients with chronic pain of peripheral nerve origin. Neuromodulation. 2016;19(1):91–100.
43. Bolash R, et al. Multi-waveform spinal cord stimulation with high frequency electromagnetic coupled (HF-EMC) powered implanted electrode array and receiver for the treatment of chronic back and leg pain (SURF study). Pain Physician. 2022;25(1):67–76.
44. Hoang Roberts L, et al. Initial experience using a novel nerve stimulator for the management of pudendal neuralgia. Neurourol Urodyn. 2021;40(6):1670–7.
45. Gilmore CA, et al. Treatment of chronic axial back pain with 60-day percutaneous medial branch PNS: primary end point results from a prospective, multicenter study. Pain Pract. 2021;21(8):877–89.
46. Rauck RL, et al. Treatment of post-amputation pain with peripheral nerve stimulation. Neuromodulation. 2014;17(2):188–97.
47. Ilfeld BM, et al. Neurostimulation for postsurgical analgesia: a novel system enabling ultrasound-guided percutaneous peripheral nerve stimulation. Pain Pract. 2017;17(7):892–901.
48. Gilmore CA, et al. Percutaneous 60-day peripheral nerve stimulation implant provides sustained relief of chronic pain following amputation: 12-month follow-up of a randomized, double-blind, placebo-controlled trial. Reg Anesth Pain Med. 2019;44:637.
49. Gilligan C, et al. Long-term outcomes of restorative neurostimulation in patients with refractory chronic low back pain secondary to multifidus dysfunction: two-year results of the ReActiv8-B pivotal trial. Neuromodulation. 2023;26(1):87–97.
50. Melzack R, Wall PD. Pain mechanism: a new theory. Science. 1965;150(3699):971–9.
51. Yecies T, Li S, Zhang Y, Cai H, Shen B, Wang J, et al. Spinal interneuronal mechanisms underlying pudendal and tibial neuromodulation of bladder function in cats. Exp Neurol. 2018;308:100–10.
52. Sun KF, Feng WW, Liu YP, Dong YB, Gao L, Yang HL. Electrical peripheral nerve stimulation relieves bine caner pain by inducing arc protein expression in the spinal cord dorsal horn. J Pain Res. 2018;11:599–609.

53. Ceccanti M, Onesti E, Rubino A, Cambieri C, Tartaglia G, Miscioscia A, et al. Modulation of human corticospinal excitability by paired associative stimulation in patients with amyotrophic lateral sclerosis and effcts of riluzole. Brain Stimul. 2018;11(4):775–81.
54. Aguiar P, Sousa M, Lima D. NMDA channels together with L-type calcium currents and calcium actviated nonspecific cationic currents are sufficient to generate windup in WDR neurons. J Neurophysiol. 2010;104:1155.
55. Meyer-Friebem CH, Wiegand T, Eitner L, et al. Effects of spinal cord and peripheral nerve stimulation reflected in sensory profiles and endogenous pain modulatiom. Clin J Pain. 2019;35(2):111–20.
56. Yang F, Zhang T, Tiwari V, Shu B, Zhang C, Wang Y, Vera-Portocarrero LP, Raja SN, Guan Y. Effects of combined electrical stimulation of the dorsal column and dorsal roots on wide-dynamic-range neuronal activtity in nerve-injured rats. Neuromodulation. 2015;18(7):593–8.
57. Bandeira JS, Antunes LC, Soldatelli MD, Sato JR, Fregni F, Caumo W. Functional spectroscopy mapping of pain processing cortical areas during non-painful peripheral electrical stimulation of teh accessory spinal nerve. Front Hum Neurosci. 2019;13:200.
58. Schabrun SM, Ridding MC, Galea MP, Hodges PW, Chipchase LS. Primary sensory and motor cortex excitability are co-modulated in response to peripheral electrical nerve stimulation. PLOS One. 2012;7:e51298.
59. Torebjörk HE, Hallin RG. Responses in human A and C fibres to repeated electrical intradermal stimulation. J Neurol Neurosurg Psychiatry. 1974;37(6):653–64.
60. Gordon T, Udina E, Verge VM, de Chaves EI. Brief electrical stimulation accelerates axon regeneration in the peripheral nervous system and promotes sensory axon regeneration in the central nervous system. Mot Control. 2009;13(4):412–41.
61. Asensio-Pinilla E, Udina E, Jaramillo J, Navarro X. Electrical stimulation combined with exercise increase axonal regeneration after peripheral nerve injury. Exp Neuol. 2009;219(1):258–65.
62. Liao CF, Hsu ST, Chen CC, Yao CH, Lin JH, Chen YH, Chen YS. Effects of electrical stimulation on peripheral nerve regeneration in a silicone rubber conduit in taxol-treated rats. Materials (Basel). 2020;13(5):1063.
63. Halvachizadeh S, et al. Systematic review and meta-analysis of 3 treatment arms for vertebral compression fractures: a comparison of improvement in pain, adjacent-level fractures, and quality of life between vertebroplasty, kyphoplasty, and nonoperative management. JBJS Rev. 2021;9(10):e21.
64. Papanastassiou ID, et al. Comparing effects of kyphoplasty, vertebroplasty, and non-surgical management in a systematic review of randomized and non-randomized controlled studies. Eur Spine J. 2012;21(9):1826–43.
65. Wang B, et al. Balloon kyphoplasty versus percutaneous vertebroplasty for osteoporotic vertebral compression fracture: a meta-analysis and systematic review. J Orthop Surg Res. 2018;13(1):264.
66. Van Meirhaeghe J, et al. A randomized trial of balloon kyphoplasty and nonsurgical management for treating acute vertebral compression fractures: vertebral body kyphosis correction and surgical parameters. Spine (Phila Pa 1976). 2013;38(12):971–83.
67. Chandra RV, et al. Vertebroplasty and kyphoplasty for osteoporotic vertebral fractures: what are the latest data? AJNR Am J Neuroradiol. 2018;39(5):798–806.
68. Baerlocher MO, et al. Quality improvement guidelines for percutaneous vertebroplasty. J Vasc Interv Radiol. 2014;25(2):165–70.
69. Robinson Y, et al. Complications and safety aspects of kyphoplasty for osteoporotic vertebral fractures: a prospective follow-up study in 102 consecutive patients. Patient Saf Surg. 2008;2:2.
70. Kim HS, Wu PH, Jang IT. Lumbar degenerative disease part 1: anatomy and pathophysiology of intervertebral discogenic pain and radiofrequency ablation of basivertebral and sinuvertebral nerve treatment for chronic discogenic back pain: a prospective case series and review of literature. Int J Mol Sci. 2020;21(4):1483.
71. Tzika M, et al. Basivertebral foramina of true vertebrae: morphometry, topography and clinical considerations. Surg Radiol Anat. 2021;43(6):889–907.

72. Lotz JC, Fields AJ, Liebenberg EC. The role of the vertebral end plate in low back pain. Global Spine J. 2013;3(3):153–64.
73. Fras C, et al. Substance P-containing nerves within the human vertebral body: an immunohistochemical study of the basivertebral nerve. Spine J. 2003;3(1):63–7.
74. Bailey JF, et al. Innervation patterns of PGP 9.5-positive nerve fibers within the human lumbar vertebra. J Anat. 2011;218(3):263–70.
75. Kjaer P, et al. Modic changes and their associations with clinical findings. Eur Spine J. 2006;15(9):1312–9.
76. Kuisma M, et al. Modic changes in endplates of lumbar vertebral bodies: prevalence and association with low back and sciatic pain among middle-aged male workers. Spine (Phila Pa 1976). 2007;32(10):1116–22.
77. Shayota B, et al. A comprehensive review of the sinuvertebral nerve with clinical applications. Anat Cell Biol. 2019;52(2):128–33.
78. Sembrano JN, Polly DWJ. How often is low back pain not coming from the back? Spine. 2009;34(1):E27–32.
79. Schwarzer AC, Aprill CN, Bogduk N. The sacroiliac joint in chronic low back pain. Spine (Phila Pa 1976). 1995;20(1):31–7.
80. Liliang PC, et al. Sacroiliac joint pain after lumbar and lumbosacral fusion: findings using dual sacroiliac joint blocks. Pain Med. 2011;12(4):565–70.
81. Chip Routt ML, et al. Percutaneous iliosacral screws with the patient supine technique. Oper Tech Orthop. 1993;3(1):35–45.
82. Le Huec JC, et al. The sacro-iliac joint: a potentially painful enigma. Update on the diagnosis and treatment of pain from micro-trauma. Orthop Traumatol Surg Res. 2019;105(1s):S31–42.
83. Poilliot AJ, et al. A systematic review of the normal sacroiliac joint anatomy and adjacent tissues for pain physicians. Pain Physician. 2019;22(4):E247–74.
84. Sayed D, et al. A multicenter retrospective analysis of the long-term efficacy and safety of a novel posterior sacroiliac fusion device. J Pain Res. 2021;14:3251–8.
85. Calodney AK, et al. Six month interim outcomes from SECURE: a single arm, multicenter, prospective, clinical study on a novel minimally invasive posterior sacroiliac fusion device. Expert Rev Med Devices. 2022;19(5):451–61.
86. Cheng B. Preclinical characterizations of the camber SI and Siconus fixation systems. Vyrsa Tech; 2022.
87. Whang PG, et al. Minimally invasive SI joint fusion procedures for chronic SI joint pain: systematic review and meta-analysis of safety and efficacy. Int J Spine Surg. 2023;17(6):794–808.

Setting Up Fellows for Success

10

Rene Przkora, Ariana Nelson, Matthew Meroney, Nicholas Russo, and Magdalena Anitescu

Abbreviations

CPT®	Current Procedural Terminology
E/M	Evaluation and management
CMS	Centers for Medicare and Medicaid services
LCD	Local coverage determinants
ICD	International classification of disease
RVU	Relative value unit
SOS	Service sites
HMO	Health maintenance organization
FTE	Full time equivalent
OR	Operating room
APS	Acute pain service
ACGME	American college of graduate medical education
IT	Informational technology

R. Przkora (✉) · M. Meroney
Department of Anesthesiology, University of Florida College of Medicine, Gainesville, FL, USA
e-mail: rprzkora@anest.ufl.edu; mmeroney@anest.ufl.edu

A. Nelson
Department of Anesthesiology, University of California, Irvine, CA, USA
e-mail: arianamn@hs.uci.edu

N. Russo · M. Anitescu
Department of Anesthesia & Critical Care, University of Chicago Medicine, Chicago, IL, USA
e-mail: nicholas.russo@uchicagomedicine.org; manitescu@bsd.uchicago.edu

© The Author(s), under exclusive license to Springer Nature Switzerland AG 2025
M. Anitescu (ed.), *Multidisciplinary Pain Medicine Fellowship*,
https://doi.org/10.1007/978-3-031-88357-6_10

Introduction

While fellowship programs thoroughly educate trainees in the clinical aspects of medicine, practicing pain interventionalists require much more. Physicians must also be experienced in operating clinics, obtaining reimbursement from insurance, and obtaining employment. In the following guideline, we address topics for programs to integrate into their curricula, such as job search, contract negotiations, practice management, inpatient and outpatient pain services, and personal and professional wellness.

Basic Practice Management Principles

In addition to the clinical aspects of medicine, fellows will learn the following terminology related to basic practice management.

Current Procedural Terminology (CPT®) Codes Current Procedural Terminology (CPT®) codes are defined as a uniform language for coding medical services and procedures. CPT® codes are numeric or alphanumeric five-digit sequences [1]. For example, the code for percutaneous implantation of a peripheral nerve stimulator is 64,555 [2]. Universally, a procedure's medical necessity must be established before performing the procedure. Private insurance often requires that a procedure is explicitly authorized in writing before it is performed, whereas for most procedures, Medicare only requires proof of medical necessity if the clinic practice is audited. For most procedures, Medicare will state that there is "no auth required," but the proceduralist should carefully document medical necessity in the case of a future audit. The typical audit period is 6 years, and in the event of an improper payment, Centers for Medicare and Medicaid Services (CMS) will require that this be repaid within 60 days of identification [3]. Historically, no authorization was required for any procedure if the patient was insured by Medicare, but now certain procedures require authorization prior to completion. Notable exceptions to this are chemical denervation procedures such as the administration of botulinum toxin for migraine headaches and the implantation of spinal cord stimulator devices. Medicare billing and documentation requirements are established by local coverage determinants (LCDs) [4]. The ICD-11 diagnosis code associated with the procedure code must be an approved diagnosis code for a CPT to be covered by a given insurer. For example, insurers will only authorize medial branch blocks if the associated diagnosis is "lumbar spondylosis."

Global Period Most insurers will enforce a 10-day global period after neuromodulation procedures such as botulinum toxin injection or spinal cord stimulation. The physician providing the service will be restricted from charging a fee for the 10 days subsequent to that procedure, although the patient may be billed for healthcare services from other specialties [5].

Relative Value Units (RVUs) Instruction on RVUs will delineate the differences between work, practice expense, and malpractice RVUs and relate these RVU types to CPT codes. Work RVUs (wRVUs) account for the amount of time, skill, training, and intensity required of a given service. Practice expense RVUs capture the cost of maintaining a practice, including rent, equipment, and non-physician staff. Malpractice RVUs represent the payment for professional liability expenses [6]. For example, a spinal cord stimulation trial with epidural is associated with 66.47 non-facility RVUs and 12.15 facility RVUs, for a total of 78.62 RVUs on average [7].

Evaluation and Management (E/M) Visits Evaluation and Management (E/M) visits are cognitive services in which a physician diagnoses and treats illness or injury [8]. In these visits, typically, a patient is evaluated with a history and physical exam, and orders for diagnostic procedures are placed. Therapeutic methods such as medications, physical or behavioral therapies, or procedural treatments are also ordered. E/M visits for pain patients evaluated in a pain specialist office are typically billed at a "level 3" or a "level 4" wRVU level although in very complex cases a "level 5" billing may be appropriate. Higher levels of billing are associated with higher reimbursements from payers (i.e., insurance companies).

Time-Based Visits Time-based visits are defined by the portion of a medical visit allocated to counseling or coordination of care. If more than 50% of an encounter is dedicated to counseling and care coordination, an E/M visit may be listed under a time-based visit code [8]. These time units are very specific and are reimbursed at a variable rate for level 3, 4, and 5 visits, with higher time requirements for new patients than for follow-up patients.

Professional and Facility Fees Fellows should also be apprised of how facility and non-facility RVUs impact reimbursement [9]. Professional fees are paid directly to the health care provider. Facility fees are those that cover overhead costs, such as rent, electronic medical record systems, billing, and administrative expenses [10]. Although the pain physician is the entity contracted with each insurer, they may work at several clinical sites, and a payer may not cover services provided at certain service sites. If a pain physician works with an existing practice, that infrastructure will already be in place during the onboarding process to ensure that the physician is credentialed and contracted with the insurers. However, if the intention is to start a de novo new practice, it may be necessary to hire an administrator to assist in the burdensome legal task of obtaining contracts with target payers in the surrounding community while ensuring coverage of all service sites staffed by the physician.

Service Sites (10, 11, 19, and 22) Service sites are defined as the locations where services are provided. The codes associated with these sites specify the entity where services are rendered to individual payers for reimbursement policies. Several service sites relevant to pain management fellows include telehealth (SOS 10) provided in the patient's home, an office, and an off-campus-outpatient hospital, and on campus-outpatient hospital. Telehealth provided in a patient's home is defined as services given to a patient located in their home (a location other than a hospital or facility where the patient receives care in a private residence) through telecommunication technology. An office is a location other than a hospital, military treatment facility, nursing facility, public health clinic, or intermediate care facility where the health professional provides examinations, diagnosis, and treatment on an ambulatory basis. An off-campus-outpatient hospital provides diagnostic, therapeutic, and rehabilitation services to patients who do not require hospitalization. An on-campus-outpatient hospital (SOS 22) provides similar services but is part of a hospital's main campus [11]. A facility fee is paid for the on/off-campus-outpatient hospital places of service but is only exacted when the facility is a SOS 19 or 22 [4].

Job Search and Contract Negotiations A significant component of entering the workforce is understanding the various practice options available for pain management physicians. While fellows may have a clear picture of academic medicine, other forms of practice include private, part-time, locum tenens, group practice, and large health maintenance organizations (HMOs). Points to cover when initiating the job search include day-to-day responsibilities, salary compensation, working hours, and physician autonomy [12]. Fellows will also want to understand what their appointment percentage will entail. A full-time equivalent (FTE) may have variable hour requirements for clinical work at different institutions. In many academic practices, fellows will have the opportunity for day-to-day clinical variability and may divide time among multiple settings: operating room (OR), regional anesthesia, acute pain service (APS), or chronic pain outpatient clinic. However, in most private settings, the attending pain physician will work principally in the outpatient pain clinic, although there is the possibility of locum work with primary specialty-based practices to maintain skills.

Administrative Aspects of Pain Services

Private Practice or Academic Practice As pain fellowship is a single-year program, interventional pain fellows typically begin their employment search 6 months into their training. Community-based practices offer a career path that is conspicuously different from academic practices affiliated with university hospitals. Generally, there is greater opportunity for economic growth and freedom of fiscal diversification in community practices, but in an academic practice, the clinician will have the opportunity to continue to engage in educational exploits or research investigations. In the time frame immediately following graduation from fellowship, the number of clinical hours spent directly providing patient care is higher for private practice settings. However, this balance may shift if the provider in community practice adopts more administrative roles in their clinical practices as they gain experience. Although initially acute pain services (APS) were offered only in academic settings, the field is now expanding into private practice settings, where it is often integrated with regional pain services [13].

Chronic Pain Clinics Chronic pain clinics rely heavily upon a referral base to support a patient census that ensures a full or nearly full clinical template. This requires the chronic pain physician to market their skills, availability, and location to nearby referring clinics. The most common referral centers will be primary care clinics, either internal medicine or family practice, or surgical practices, especially orthopedic or spine surgery clinics. In rare circumstances, the interventionalist may wish to promote their services at emergency care or urgent care facilities, as often patients present with unexplained pain, but after concerning etiologies are ruled out, the patient still requires long-term or at least subacute management of their pain.

Inpatient Services for Acute on Chronic, Chronic, and Cancer Pain The field of acute pain medicine (APM) is growing in the United States and is becoming more standardized after the American College of Graduate Medical Education (ACGME) accreditation in 2017. However, at an institutional level, this specialty is staffed in a variable way. In some practices, APS is a standalone service, which is staffed by practitioners who do not have concomitant responsibilities in providing regional pain services or operating room services. However, in many smaller hospitals, these responsibilities will be combined, and a single faculty member will be responsible for two to three of these patient care assignments [14]. Of note, when acute pain management services are rendered outside of the OR, CMS will not permit the anesthesiologist providing these services to also bill for OR anesthetic supervision [3]. A hospital system may also have a palliative care inpatient consult team, which may have some overlap in duties with APS but generally treats patients with chronic cancer-related pain. Acute pain services for cancer patients would then be more specific to patients with acute pain post-operatively (e.g., after resection of a neoplasm) rather than pain from cancer itself.

Pain Surgical Services Integration Enhanced recovery after surgery protocols were originally developed to standardize the care of patients undergoing certain surgical procedures. Often, the goals include shorter hospitalization duration or decreased opioid requirements at the time of discharge. Many of these protocols are integrated into APS services, and entire societies now exist to develop these perioperative care guidelines. Some clinical trials have resoundingly supported their efficacy, but incomplete adherence to protocols can often mar the real-world efficiency of the practice [15–17]. Recognized barriers to compliance with protocols include individual surgeon preference, general resistance to change, and increased burden of interface with the electronic health record. Strong multi-disciplinary communication is the best method to reduce the impact of these barriers, although that requires significant buy-in from anesthesiologists, nurses, and surgeons, in addition to support from informational technology (IT) administrators.

Wellness and Burnout for Pain Physicians

Burnout is common among physicians across the nation. One study found that chronic pain anesthesiologists had significantly greater burnout than physicians from other anesthesiology subspecialties [18]. To prevent fellow and physician burnout and promote resilience, programs will inform trainees of wellness practices. Wellness and burnout prevention can manifest in either personal or professional manners. Curricula for personal wellness will include discussions on work-life balance, setting boundaries, nutrition, fitness, emotional health, financial literacy, and behavior adaptability [19]. Discourse on professional wellness will include methods to reduce physician workload, regular provider meetings focused on work-life issues, flexible or part-time work schedules, and solutions for covering unexpected leave [20].

References

1. Billing for Telehealth Encounters: An Introductory Guide on Fee-For-Service. 2021. Cchpca. org. Accessed 20 July 2022.
2. Slavitt AM, Burwell SM. Medicare program: payment policies under the physician fee schedule; Medicare advantage pricing data release; Medicare advantage and Part D Medical low ratio data release; etc. 2016. Regulation.gov. https://www.regulations.gov/document/CMS-2016-0116-0006
3. May KA, Craven JM, Wright C, Tran B. Regional anesthesia and the acute pain service: compliance and controversies. Curr Opin Anaesthesiol. 2022;35(2):224–9.
4. CMS Manual System. 2017. CMS.gov. Accessed 23 July 2022.
5. Global Surgery Booklet. 2018. https://www.cms.gov/outreach-and-education/medicare-learning-network-mln/mlnproducts/downloads/globalsurgery-icn907166.pdf
6. Introduction to Relative Value Units and How Medicare Reimbursement in Calculated. 2009. labor.alaska.gov. Accessed 23 July 2022.
7. Spinal Cord Stimulation (SCS). 2021 Physician Reimbursement and Coding Reference Guide. 2021.
8. Evaluation and Management Services Guide. 2022. CMS.gov. Accessed 23 July 2022.
9. AAPC. What are Relative Value Units (RVUs)? 2022. https://www.aapc.com/practice-management/rvus.aspx
10. Facility Fee Reporting. (n.d.). Washington State Department of Health. Accessed 23 July 2022.
11. Place of Service Code Set. 2021. CMS.gov. Accessed 23 July 2022.
12. MicroMD Hit Research Team. The 5 types of medical practices. blogMD. 2018. https://www.micromd.com/blogmd/5-types-medical-practices/
13. Webb CAJ, Kim TE. Establishing an acute pain service in private practice and updates on regional anesthesia billing. Anesthesiol Clin. 2018;36(3):333–44.
14. Missair A, Visan A, Ivie R, Gebhard RE, Rivoli S, Woodworth G. Daring discourse: should acute pain medicine be a stand-alone service? Reg Anesth Pain Med. 2021;46(6):529–31.

15. Lamm R, Woodward S, Creisher BA, et al. Toward zero prescribed opioids for outpatient general surgery procedures: a prospective cohort trial. J Surg Res. 2022;278:293–302.
16. Tong Y, Fernandez L, Bendo JA, Spivak JM. Enhanced recovery after surgery trends in adult spine surgery: a systematic review. Int J Spine Surg. 2020;14(4):623–40.
17. Birchall CL, Maines JL, Kunselman AR, Stetter CM, Pauli JM. Enhanced recovery for caesarean delivery leads to no difference in length of stay, decreased opioid use and lower infection rates [published online ahead of print, 2022 Sept 30]. J Matern Fetal Neonatal Med. 2022:1–9.
18. Hyman SA, Card EB, De Leon-Casasola O, Shotwell MS, Shi Y, Weinger MB. Prevalence of burnout and its relationship to health status and social support in more than 1000 subspeciality anesthesiologists. Reg Anesth Pain Med. 2021;46(5):381–7.
19. AMA. Preventing Burnout in medical residents and fellows: 6 keys for wellness. 2016. https://www.ama-assn.org/medical-residents/medical-resident-wellness/preventing-burnout-medical-residents-and-fellows-6-keys
20. AHRQ. Physician Burnout. 2017. https://www.ahrq.gov/prevention/clinician/ahrq-works/burnout/index.html

Enhancing Practice Value

11

Sayed Wahezi, Joshua Pan, Thelma Wright, Ryan Ference,
Daniel Pak, Aaron Calodney, Vivek Nagar, Timothy Deer,
Chong Kim, Tian Yu, Lee Tian, Fadi Farah,
and Susan M. Moeschler

S. Wahezi
Department of Physical Medicine & Rehabilitation, Montefiore Medical Center,
Bronx, NY, USA
e-mail: swahezi@montefiore.org

J. Pan (✉) · R. Ference · T. Yu · L. Tian
Department of Anesthesia & Critical Care, University of Chicago Medicine, Chicago, IL, USA
e-mail: jcpan@bsd.uchicago.edu

T. Wright
University of Maryland School of Medicine, Baltimore, MD, USA
e-mail: twright@som.umaryland.edu; tian.yu@uchicagomedicine.org;
lee.tian@uchicagomedicine.org

D. Pak
Department of Anesthesia, New York Presbyterian/Weill Cornell Medicine,
New York, NY, USA

A. Calodney
Precision Spine Care, Tyler, TX, USA

V. Nagar
Advent Health Medical Group, Spine Health, Altamonte Springs, FL, USA

T. Deer
The Spine and Nerve Center of the Virginias, Charleston, WV, USA

C. Kim
Metro Health/Case Western Reserve University, Cleveland, OH, USA
e-mail: ckim3@metrohealth.org

F. Farah
Beth Israel Deaconess Plymouth, Plymouth, MA, USA

S. M. Moeschler
Mayo Clinic, Rochester, MN, USA
e-mail: moeschler.susan@mayo.edu

Abbreviations

FDA   Food and Drug Administration
IME   Independent medical examination
IND   Investigational New Drug (application)
IRB   Institutional review board
PMA   Premarket approval
RCT   Randomized control trial

Introduction

The clinical practice of pain medicine is often the focal point of one's career with additional opportunities including research, consulting and teaching which can further enrich and inform a career in medicine. Pain medicine is one of the most dynamic fields of medicine secondary to active research and innovation. Pain physicians are uniquely positioned to make a significant contribution to healthcare and society given their background medical training in combination with the understanding of the impact of pain and therapies on patients. This chapter highlights these opportunities for outreach and career building beyond clinical practice.

Legal Consulting

Physicians, as members of society and as professionals, have a duty to testify in court as expert witnesses [1]. The American College of Physicians strongly encourages this participation by physicians in the administration of justice and as a component of their professional activities [1]. A physician should agree to participate as an expert only in cases they feel have strong merit, whether in support of the plaintiff or defendant [1].

Recommended qualifications for a physician expert witness include a valid and unrestricted license to practice in the state they practice, be certified by an appropriate American Board, have evidence of continuing medical education, and actively involved in the clinical practice of the specialty or the subject matter of the case for three of the five preceding years [1].

General guidelines recommend that the physician testify honestly, fully, and impartially to their qualifications and the medical information involved in the case. In addition, the physician should review standards of practice prevailing at the time of the alleged occurrence. Compensation of the physician expert witness should be reasonable and commensurate with the time and effort used for case preparation such as depositions and court appearances [1]. The acceptance of fees that are disproportionate to those customary for such professional endeavors is improper and may be construed as attempting to influence testimony given by a witness [2]. A physician should not accept compensation that is contingent upon the outcome of the litigation [2].

The physician expert witness must ensure that their testimony does not narrowly reflect their views about applicable standards to the exclusion of other acceptable and more realistic choices. The physician should make a clear distinction between medical malpractice and medical maloccurrence [2].

There are occasions when clinicians are summoned to court to testify. The physician may be served with a subpoena. The legal system is adversarial, and most clinicians do have feelings of dread, anxiety, and panic when they receive a subpoena [3]. Understanding the legal arena, court proceedings, and how to properly prepare can assist the clinician to stay calm under pressure if subpoenaed to testify. If unsure about the purpose of the subpoena, clinicians should ask for help from the legal counsel at the place of employment. In addition, the clinician should call the requesting attorney to find out exactly what is required and the likelihood that the clinician would indeed testify [3].

In preparation, the physician should furnish the attorney with a curriculum vitae. They should review questions that may be asked during direct examination in advance. The physician should also consider visiting the courthouse to familiarize themselves with the surroundings [3]. Speaking to other colleagues who have been through the process may help reduce the anxiety associated with testifying in a courtroom. A physician's appearance and dress are important as they will convey an impression with the desired one being one of professionalism and credibility [3]. Jurors ultimately rely on proxies such as appearance and demeanor to determine an expert's credibility [4]. A highly qualified expert with impressive professional credentials can buttress the jury's belief in the physician's opinion and even eliminate juror speculation regarding the appropriate standard of care [4]. On the other hand, evidence of a witness's past misconduct is admissible in narrow contexts. However, prior malpractice evidence is inadmissible in the courts [4].

Narratives and Case Review

Before entering an agreement to be an expert on a case, the physician witness must ensure that there is no conflict of interest between themselves and the case at hand [5]. The actual request, specified questions asked and expected to be fully answered, and reasons given for the answers should be clearly enunciated in writing [5]. The claimant must be made aware that the expert physician is acting as an evaluator not a treating physician [5]. The expert, during their case review, should not venture into areas that are not solicited. In the expert witness' report, they must be clear and concise in their report and if possible, give all the appropriate reasons for their medical diagnosis [5]. The physician must clearly state and distinguish what is said by the claimant, consultant, therapist, and by the nurse and under what circumstances. The narrative must be kept in order and the train of events recorded in a consecutive manner. No person's opinion should be infused in the discussion of facts—there should be a factual, objective, and non-judgmental expose of the case [5].

Depositions, Subpoenas, Trials

Experts may be subject to disciplinary sanctions from professional organizations and state medical boards due to the increased legal scrutiny being applied to expert witness testimony in medical malpractice litigation [6]. Under appropriate circumstances, state professional boards can revoke the medical license of a physician who is found to have delivered false testimony in a medical malpractice lawsuit [6]. It may be prudent for the expert to carry liability coverage that will support a legal defense in the event that expert witness work triggers a lawsuit against the testifying expert [6].

Independent Medical Examinations (IMEs)

IMEs have protected the rights of workers in the United States. IMEs represent a valuable mechanism for determining alleged impairment and/or disability [7]. Medical professionals must adhere to the same principles of impartial and ethical conduct that they uphold in general patient care when dealing with IMEs. A limited doctor-patient relationship may be forged during an IME [7].

Consulting for Industry

The relationship of clinicians partnering with industry is a collaboration that dates back to Earl Bakken and Wilson Greatbatch using engineering to partner with physicians to develop the pacemaker world of innovation [8]. This was followed in the arena of medical devices in the spine by leaders such as Dr. Richard Penn, a pioneer of baclofen pumps [9]. Similarly, cardiac pacemakers and other devices and medications were delivered to the clinical arena because of successful partnerships which were developed around a patient-first model.

There are five terms that the authors submit are necessary to understand for delivering ethical clinical care in the face of industry collaboration: transparency, disclosure, hypocrisy, recusal, and conflict. Transparency is important to maintain ethical boundaries between physicians' clinical practice and their responsibility to their working relationship with industry [10]. Transparency dictates that the physician divulges all industry relationships which has the potential toward clinician bias. Disclosure is the active release of this information [11]. The failure to disclose conflicts with industry is an example of hypocrisy [12]. "Recusal" is a term reserved for practitioners to abstain from making professional decisions based on a perceived or real complex of interest with a working partner [13]. Furthermore, conflict in this context is often a dollar sum which is considered by most to have the potential to cause clinician bias; most academic institutions standardize this amount to $10,000.

Corporate entities often approach physicians who have a skill set that is valuable to the vendor and knowledge base which advances their product(s). The fair market value leading to a financial offer is proportional to the curriculum vitae of the practitioner, experience, demographics, as well as the consultant's ability to engage either an audience within the corporation or to improve other practitioners' use of the product and improve the safety and efficacy.

Basic medical consulting often involves a clinical practitioner speaking on behalf of a company in order to increase either the use of the device or improve the safety and efficacy of the use of the technique. Public on-label discussions are important to mitigate legal repercussions on the clinician and corporation. The authors here do suggest that clinicians interested in working for industry select companies that have a track record of honest and moral clinical and public relations. It is important for the clinicians not to use industry-sponsored events as a local reach for patients, nor should it be used for local practice referrals.

There are several ways that clinicians can become involved with medical corporations in addition to consulting. An example of a role is as a member of a medical advisory board. The desirability of the physician for this type of project increases if the physician has a special skill set, such as creation of a randomized controlled trial (RCT) or other research designs for the company. There should be a valid need for the physician's expertise and unique skill set that can contribute to the team. Furthermore, industry may ask for clinicians to help in product development/improvement or develop a unique idea/patent.

Clinician practitioners may also become investors of medical device/pharmaceutical companies. Small start-up companies may remunerate physicians by payment in stock options if they do not have fluid cash on hand. Companies invest in the clinician based upon the fair market value that is commensurate with the strength of the receiving. It is strongly advised that clinician investors, or family members of clinicians, with a 5% or greater stake in a company disclose this information to maintain conflict of interest standards [14]. In addition, in order to work in an equity-based option model, there must be fair market value for the work done to equal the stock grant; furthermore, this should be carefully documented on time-based documents. In addition, if a spouse or close relative invests in a company, disclosure to any professional or clinical entity who may be influenced by the physician-industry relationship is still needed. Furthermore, since the Sunshine Act, a United States legal requirement for company disclosure, does not exist in other countries, we encourage international physicians to be transparent when consulting [15].

Irrespective of the relationship a clinician has with industry, the transparency of work relationships and financial investments are important to determining long-term success with medical corporate entities and mitigating conflicts which may lend itself to legal reprisal.

It is the opinion of the authors here that clinicians interested in corporate relationships invest in a compliance attorney, as guidelines and recommendations for clinical relationships, investment, and disclosures may have geographic and individual variability on a case-by-case basis.

Rules of Consulting

Physician skills and knowledge should be applicable for the work needed such as teaching or research.

The amount of reimbursement for consulting work should be based on fair market value, a term which is derived from the physicians' achievements, research, and publications.

The use of a product or service should not be directly related to the consulting work done for a company. The payment for use of a device or service is non-compliant and should not be tied to any work done.

The physician should be transparent with any conflicts of interest.

The physician should disclose conflicts of interest when relevant.

The physician should only agree to work with an entity when patient efficacy and safety is the main goal or concern of the interested parties.

Research Integration in Clinical Practice

Integrating research into clinical practice can expand the scope of one's clinical expertise, act as a source of new engagement with the academic community, and improve patient care. Possessing an extensive research background is not necessary to begin academic work. However, knowledge of fundamental research principles, including ethical standards in research and study design, is essential for success. Moreover, setting up a research center in a practice requires investment in research infrastructure, budgeting, and developing an institutional review board (IRB) relationship.

Ethical principles in pain research evolved significantly during the twentieth century following a larger referendum on paternalistic and abusive research practices common during that time period [16]. Early pain research was conducted by psychologists using painful stimuli to study learning and behavior [17]. As attitudes toward human subject research changed, the American Psychological Association published an ethics code detailing requirements for research involving deception and physical pain [17, 18]. Additionally, the Declaration of Helsinki and other pain management societies, such as International Association for the Study of Pain, have further developed guidelines for ethical practices specific to pain research [19].

One of the fundamental principles in research ethics holds that the pursuit of knowledge cannot infringe upon the safety and rights of human subjects [20]. Furthermore, research should be guided by the principles of beneficence, justice, and respect, first conceived of in the Belmont Report [21]. Comprehensive informed consent processes should be central to subject recruitment, and there should be provisions in place for vulnerable population protection and IRB oversight [20]. Pain trials should be designed to maximize benefit to participants so that they may reap the benefits of the study at its conclusion [22].

The application of these principles to RCTs has drawn scrutiny. Some ethicists hold that the routine use of placebo in RCTs is deceptive and offers little benefit to participants [23, 24]. Subjects risk untreated pain for the duration of the trial and lack of access to potentially beneficial therapies. Crossover RCT design may address this issue since subjects are exposed to both treatment and control study arms [22]. Other ethical issues in pain RCTs include studies that offer only incremental improvement in pain symptoms. Although the magnitude of treatment effect is often unknown prior to an RCT, studies anticipating only minor improvement in pain endpoints offer diminished benefit to participants [22].

Pain research utilizing laboratory animals poses unique challenges to the pain investigator. Since informed consent is immaterial in animal research, the burden of designing a scientifically sound study falls on the research investigator. The ethical debate of pain research in animals is predicated on the notion that since pain is a known negative and unpleasant force, it should be minimized in animal subjects. Vocalization, avoidance, and nursing behaviors are witnessed across animal species [17]. However, the pain experienced in non-sentient beings may not accurately represent the conscious interpretation of pain in humans [25, 26]. The ability to sense pain may be universal, but the capacity for suffering may be unique to humans. Pain research in animals is likely most suited for gathering basic science data and understanding the physiology of pain pathways. Animal studies relying on nursing and withdrawal behaviors are of less value when generalizing to humans [17, 27].

Investigators must also provide adequate justification for exposing animals to pain [28]. Exposure should be maintained at the minimum level needed to achieve the study goals [29]. This requires that the design of the study is clearly thought through, with the goal of bridging the gap between animal and human pain experiences. Practically speaking, researchers must be familiar with normal behavior in the animals they are studying and be able to recognize pain behavior [29]. Additionally, there should be protocols in place to provide animals with analgesia, if consistent with the study design, and for animal removal from the study if the pain becomes debilitating [30]. Finally, the pain researcher must adhere to all governmental guidelines regulating laboratory animal research.

Chronic pain research frequently utilizes a variety of study designs. RCTs are considered the gold standard for studying interventional and pharmacologic exposures. However, they can be resource intensive and carry ethical implications as previously mentioned [31]. Observational studies can be designed to overcome some of the practical limitations of RCTs but are prone to selection and measurement biases. Choosing a study design depends on the goals of the study and the resources at the disposal of the investigator. Designing any clinical research study begins with formulating a question that addresses the "who" and "what" of the project [32]. The research question determines the exposure of interest, designates the patient population, and defines the scope of the study. If pursuing an RCT, the next steps in study design involve determining recruitment, outcomes, and controlling systematic biases.

Recruitment for chronic pain trials should be limited to patients suffering from moderate to severe chronic pain. Registering participants without significant pain symptoms at baseline will underestimate the effects of the intervention [32]. The study should be designed to maximize benefits to the participants, and the outcome measures should reflect this goal. Other quality-of-life metrics (i.e., sleep quality, mobility, and employment capacity) and changes in medication utilization should be measured when possible [32, 33].

RCTs in general produce higher level evidence than observational studies because they more reliably link causation between exposures and outcomes due to the advantage of randomization and blinding. Yet, they are also susceptible to biases. For instance, chronic pain patients typically experience the greatest magnitude of the treatment effect early on after a study intervention, with diminishing benefits at longer intervals. Thus, short-duration studies can overestimate the effect of the therapy due to duration bias [32, 34]. Attrition and imputation bias reflect patients who withdraw or who are lost to follow-up; RCTs that have high attrition rates or carry forward data from withdrawn participants will overestimate treatment effect size. Finally, studies lacking sufficient sample sizes will also tend to overestimate effect size [32]. Therefore, investigators should carefully consider these factors to improve the fidelity of their studies.

Developing a research center requires research infrastructure, including personnel that can vary in composition but often includes nurses, research assistants, data managers, and administrative support staff. A research coordinator who is experienced with practice operations is important for managing the research team, overseeing individual projects, and delegating tasks [35]. These tasks include, but are not limited to, patient screening, gathering informed consent, submissions to the IRB, coordinating patient visits, data collection, budgeting, site audits, and safety reporting. Personnel training and the assignment of clear roles are critical for ensuring proper execution of study protocols. Receiving IRB approval is also often a hurdle for study investigators that can take months and delay study initiation. Clinicians affiliated with a hospital or university may use their institutional IRB, while community providers without such access can consider an external commercial or central IRB. Central IRBs are preferred for multicenter trials where a single protocol can be approved and used for multiple sites.

Financial support is essential for all research centers. Insight is needed on start-up fees and recurring costs to sustain a research practice. If institutional or federal support cannot be obtained, alternative sources such as grants from professional societies, academic groups, or industry can be considered. Researchers should also be aware that per-patient reimbursements may not be received until after enrollment and may not cover all operational costs. Furthermore, standardizing formats for clinical study contracts and processes for reimbursements help to expedite contract agreements between potential sponsors and leave any major negotiations to project-specific issues.

Ethical principles in research continue to change as investigators negotiate the process of scientific inquiry with the need for research subject protection. Therefore, it is incumbent upon the pain investigator to be knowledgeable of current research ethical standards and to be proficient in research study design. Although instituting a research practice requires an initial intellectual and capital investment, future research endeavors will benefit from a comprehensive approach toward practice development.

Innovation and Patents

Physicians can change the scope of medical care through innovation. Being directly engaged in patient care, they are best suited to recognize the shortcomings and inefficiencies within the system. Most physicians identify these problems, and many have ideas for solutions. However, the execution of transitioning these ideas to reality can be intimidating.

Prescription drugs are some of the most important interventions in medicine. They fundamentally changed the prognosis of once fatal cardiopulmonary and infectious diseases into curable or manageable conditions. However, on account of major side effects and public health crises that followed the widespread use of prescription drugs, major regulations were imposed on drug testing and advertising with more focus on drug safety than drug efficacy. These regulations gave rise to prolonged, expensive approval process.

Following the birth defects associated with thalidomide, the Kefauver-Harris Drug Act was passed in 1962 including the main elements for testing of a new drug before approval by the FDA [36].

There are four elements required by the FDA before approving a drug to be sold in the US market [37]:

First, there is the drug discovery that includes the identification of the compound that acts on a clinical pathway through pivotal basic science. This is followed by translational studies and testing on animals. Depending on the risk profile, testing on multiple animal species may be advised.

Afterward, the drug sponsor will submit an investigational new drug application (IND) to the FDA which includes the drug's acting ingredients, excipients, the manufacturing process, and the indication that will be studied in the clinical trials. A committee in the FDA will review the application and will determine if the animal studies are sufficient to start testing on humans.

Subsequently, clinical trials in three phases are established. Phase 1 clinical trials emphasize safety and including healthy volunteers. Phase 2 clinical trials emphasize drug effectiveness and include hundreds of patients followed by Phase 3 clinical trials, ideally randomized, controlled, and blinded that stress both safety and effectiveness of the drug in different populations and different doses.

During the application review, the FDA may require changes to drug labeling and may inspect the drug manufacturing facilities before final drug approval.

Furthermore, the FDA may require Phase 4 trials to test for safety in the population.

After the clinical trial, the drug sponsor will file the new drug application (NDA). Once the NDA is received, the FDA has 6 months for review if the NDA is granted priority review and 10 months for standard review. Determination is based on benefit-risk profile and no minimum threshold for effectiveness is required.

The De Novo development process entails on average 8 years from the time of the IND submission to approval of the NDA. Total drug development is longer since the time of preclinical development must be added to these 8 years.

In contrast, drug repurposing may cost less as it skips the initial phases of drug discovery, screening, and Phase 1 clinical trials.

In addition, in conditions where the FDA determines that the drug needs urgent review, approval may occur after Phase 2 trials.

Medical Device

While pharmaceutical innovation and medical device innovation share broad similarities in the pathway from inception to market, medical device innovation has unique factors that must be considered [38].

Medical devices are typically cheaper to bring to market as compared to pharmaceuticals. This is largely due to a reduction in costs associated with obtaining regulatory permission to bring products to market. Therefore, proof of concept becomes vital with regard to valuation of the product, which is usually embodied in prototyping. Additionally, the pathway for medical device regulatory permission is different compared to that of pharmaceuticals.

Prototyping

Once the viability and necessity of a product in the market has been clarified, the next step is patenting and prototyping. Prototyping is an iterative process. At its infancy, it is used to demonstrate proof of concept. As it continues to mature, it begins to resemble the end user product. Therefore, the following prototyping process will be described broadly as "proof-of-concept" phase and "refining" stages.

In the "proof-of-concept" phase, the first step is to define the product's goals. These goals are multifaceted, such as the goal of the product itself, the requirements of the product as it pertains to the end user, the regulatory requirements that the product is intended to obtain, and the quality assurance requirements for the product for manufacturing and distribution.

As the clinician, it is imperative that product goals and end-user requirements are outlined by the physician. While it is not necessary to employ regulatory and quality assurance requirements in preliminary prototyping, it can avoid redundancy or setbacks in future stages of prototyping. Advice on regulatory and quality assurance requirements of the products can be obtained through engineering and legal partners.

Once a "proof-of-concept" prototype has been demonstrated, the "refining" phase begins. In this phase, the product is transitioned from prototype to an end-user product. This includes the abovementioned regulatory board approval and quality assurance costs, such as analysis of product liability insurance and warranty, as well as creating cost-efficient product manufacturing and distribution. As the clinician, it is important to take an active role in end-user testing of the prototype to improve the product, as most times the clinician is best suited to evaluate end-user outcomes. Engaging with engineering partners is important to trial different materials and processes to reduce costs while maintaining standards of end-user outcomes. It is common at this stage to approach manufacturers to determine the current cost of goods and quality assurance measures that will be needed for efficient mass production and distribution. Once the prototype approaches the end-user ready product, it can be submitted for regulatory approval.

Regulation

There is high variance in medical device regulation from a worldwide perspective. In the United States, medical devices are regulated by the Food and Drug Administration. All medical devices are categorized into three classes, based largely on risk and safety of the device [38]. Class 1 and 2 devices are considered the lowest and moderate risk potential for harm, respectively. Class 3 devices are considered the highest risk for potential harm, such as devices that sustain or support life, are implanted, or present potential unreasonable risk of illness or injury. All medical devices require general controls, such as labeling and device listing. Some Class 2 devices may require special controls, such as special labeling, design characteristics, performance standards, or premarket data requirements. Class 3 devices require premarket approval (PMA), which encompasses most stringent control. There are exemptions that exist for a few Class 1 and some Class 2 medical devices, such as premarket notification (510 k), which can bypass regulatory testing if a device fulfills the criteria of a pre-approved device on the market.

The costs of obtaining regulatory approval are dramatically increased as a device is categorized in higher classes, particularly for non-exempt Class 2 and Class 3 devices. Therefore, it is imperative to research the potential classification for your medical device, prior to patenting and prototyping, to estimate the value of the product in the market.

Patenting

In the United States, an invention must meet three criteria to be patentable: novel, nonobvious, and useful [38, 39]. Therefore, when considering patenting an idea, it is important to assess the existing patents in the field or industry, commonly referred to as prior art. It is important to note that all issued patents are available for public review and can be researched through patent databases. However, leaning on legal partners at this early stage can be useful, especially in navigating prior art claims that may impede the invention's patentability.

Once an inventor determines that an invention can be patented, there are two routes to patenting: nonprovisional patent application or provisional patent followed by nonprovisional patent application. Patents are examined and issued from nonprovisional patent applications. Filing provisional patent applications allows inventors 12 months from provisional application date to file a nonprovisional patent application.

Benefits of provisional patent application include ability to safely disclose invention information prior to patent issuance and cost-spreading of legal fees, while risks include longer time period until patent issuance. Benefits of nonprovisional patent applications include quicker patent issuance, but higher upfront costs.

Conclusion

Clinical practice is the mainstay of most physicians' professional careers. With the uniqueness as well as the evolution and development of the specialty, pain medicine also provides numerous opportunities for clinicians to expand beyond the traditional patient care practice. These opportunities, from medical consulting to involvement in research to business endeavors, highlight non-traditional pathways beyond the typical clinical setting. Medical legal consulting, from expert witness to IME, enables the clinician to expand on and utilize their clinical expertise. Involvement and integration of research into and beyond the traditional clinical practice is another common opportunity. With the development of pharmaceuticals and biotechnology, industry-centered consulting has further enabled physicians to expand and participate in various roles: consultants, advisors, researchers, and educators. Though less common, innovation from pharmaceuticals to medical devices patents further allow the entrepreneurial clinicians to translate their expertise and skillsets. For all these potential avenues, clinical practice serves as the foundation for ever-evolving prospects for diverse, challenging, and stimulating careers. All these opportunities need thoughtful preparation and understanding but can be exciting and fulling while providing significant satisfaction and reward to those who participate.

References

1. Snyder L. Guidelines for the physician expert witness. American College of Physicians. Ann Intern Med. 1990;113(10):789.
2. Cohn B, Berger J. Guidelines for expert witness testimony in medical liability cases (S93-3). Pediatrics. 1994;94(5):755–6.
3. Murphy JL. When clinicians are summoned to testify in court: orientation to the process and suggestions on preparation. SAGE Open Nurs. 2018;4:2377960818757097.
4. Henson N. A taste of their own medicine: examining the admissibility of experts' prior malpractice under the Federal Rules of evidence. Vand L Rev. 2018;71:995.
5. Sullivan JD. The medico-legal expertise: solid medicine, sufficient legal and a measure of common sense. McGill J Med MJM. 2006;9(2):147.
6. Bal BS. The expert witness in medical malpractice litigation. Clin Orthop Relat Res. 2009;467(2):383–91.
7. Ky P, Hameed H, Christo PJ. Independent medical examinations: facts and fallacies. Pain Physician. 2009;12(5):811–8.

8. Greatbatch W, Holmes CF. History of implantable devices. IEEE Eng Med Biol Mag. 1991;10(3):38–41.
9. Penn RD, Savoy SM, Corcos D, Latash M, Gottlieb G, Parke B, et al. Intrathecal baclofen for severe spinal spasticity. N Engl J Med. 1989;320(23):1517–21.
10. Levay C, Waks C. Professions and the pursuit of transparency in healthcare: two cases of soft autonomy. Organ Stud. 2009;30(5):509–27.
11. Campbell EG, Rao SR, DesRoches CM, Iezzoni LI, Vogeli C, Bolcic-Jankovic D, et al. Physician professionalism and changes in physician-industry relationships from 2004 to 2009. Arch Intern Med. 2010;170(20):1820–6.
12. Wallace RJ. Hypocrisy, moral address, and the equal standing of persons. Philos Public Aff. 2010;38(4):307–41.
13. Barrocas A, Geppert C, Durfee SM, Maillet JOS, Monturo C, Mueller C, et al. ASPEN ethics position paper. Nutr Clin Pract. 2010;25(6):672.
14. Resnik DB. Conflict of interest in medical research, education, and practice. National Institute of Environmental Health Sciences; 2010.
15. Grande D. Limiting the influence of pharmaceutical industry gifts on physicians: self-regulation or government intervention? J Gen Intern Med. 2010;25:79–83.
16. Schwenzer KJ. Best practice & research in anaesthesiology issue on new approaches in clinical research ethics in clinical research. Best Pract Res Clin Anaesthesiol. 2011;25(4):569–82.
17. Schatman ME. Ethical issues in chronic pain management. 1st ed. Baton Rouge: CRC Press; 2006.
18. Ethical principles of psychologists and code of conduct. Am Psychol. 2002;57(12):1060–73.
19. Charlton E. Ethical guidelines for pain research in humans. Committee on Ethical Issues of the International Association for the Study of Pain. Pain. 1995;63(3):277–8.
20. World Medical Association Declaration of Helsinki. Ethical principles for medical research involving human subjects. JAMA. 2013;310(20):2191–4.
21. Knudson PL. Ethical principles in human subject research. Arch Med Res. 2001;32(5):473–4.
22. Casarett DJ, Karlawish J. Beyond informed consent: the ethical design of pain research. Pain Med. 2001;2(2):138–46.
23. Waisel DB. Ethics of research for patients in pain. Curr Opin Anaesthesiol. 2017;30(2):205–10.
24. Kaptchuk TJ, Hemond CC, Miller FG. Placebos in chronic pain: evidence, theory, ethics, and use in clinical practice. BMJ. 2020;370:m1668.
25. Tannenbaum J, Rowan AN. Rethinking the morality of animal research. Hast Cent Rep. 1985;15(5):32–43.
26. Knopp KL, Stenfors C, Baastrup C, Bannon AW, Calvo M, Caspani O, et al. Experimental design and reporting standards for improving the internal validity of pre-clinical studies in the field of pain: consensus of the IMI-Europain consortium. Scand J Pain. 2015;7(1):58–70.
27. Mogil JS. Animal models of pain: progress and challenges. Nat Rev Neurosci. 2009;10(4):283–94.
28. National Research Council Committee on R, Alleviation of Pain in Laboratory A. The National Academies Collection: Reports funded by National Institutes of Health. Recognition and Alleviation of Pain in Laboratory Animals. Washington, DC: National Academies Press (US) Copyright © 2009, National Academy of Sciences; 2009.
29. Tannenbaum J. Ethics and pain research in animals. ILAR J. 1999;40(3):97–110.
30. Zimmermann M. Ethical guidelines for investigations of experimental pain in conscious animals. Pain. 1983;16(2):109–10.
31. Noordzij M, Dekker FW, Zoccali C, Jager KJ. Study designs in clinical research. Nephron Clin Pract. 2009;113(3):c218–21.
32. Moore RA, Derry S, Wiffen PJ. Challenges in design and interpretation of chronic pain trials. Br J Anaesth. 2013;111(1):38–45.
33. Van Zundert J. Clinical research in interventional pain management techniques: the clinician's point of view. Pain Pract. 2007;7(3):221–9.

34. Gewandter JS, Dworkin RH, Turk DC, McDermott MP, Baron R, Gastonguay MR, et al. Research designs for proof-of-concept chronic pain clinical trials: IMMPACT recommendations. Pain. 2014;155(9):1683–95.

35. Scoglio D, Fichera A. Establishing a successful clinical research program. Clin Colon Rectal Surg. 2014;27(2):65–70.

36. Novack GD. The accelerated drug approval. Ocul Surf. 2010;8(4):205–7.

37. Darrow JJ, Avorn J, Kesselheim AS. FDA approval and regulation of pharmaceuticals, 1983–2018. JAMA. 2020;323(2):164–76.

38. Sastry A. Overview of the US FDA medical device approval process. Curr Cardiol Rep. 2014;16:1–5.

39. Nadeem M, Weiss A-PC. Medical product development. Part 2: Patent and FDA issues. J Hand Surg Am. 2021;46(10):918–23.

Index